AF744013

Detection and Assessment of Dental Caries

Andrea Ferreira Zandona
Christopher Longbottom
Editors

Detection and Assessment of Dental Caries

A Clinical Guide

Springer

Editors
Andrea Ferreira Zandona
Department of Comprehensive Care
Tufts University School of Dental Medicine
Boston, MA
USA

Christopher Longbottom
King's College London Dental Institute
London, UK

ISBN 978-3-030-16965-7 ISBN 978-3-030-16967-1 (eBook)
https://doi.org/10.1007/978-3-030-16967-1

© Springer Nature Switzerland AG 2019, corrected publication 2019
This work is subject to copyright. All rights are reserved by the Publisher, whether the whole or part of the material is concerned, specifically the rights of translation, reprinting, reuse of illustrations, recitation, broadcasting, reproduction on microfilms or in any other physical way, and transmission or information storage and retrieval, electronic adaptation, computer software, or by similar or dissimilar methodology now known or hereafter developed.
The use of general descriptive names, registered names, trademarks, service marks, etc. in this publication does not imply, even in the absence of a specific statement, that such names are exempt from the relevant protective laws and regulations and therefore free for general use.
The publisher, the authors, and the editors are safe to assume that the advice and information in this book are believed to be true and accurate at the date of publication. Neither the publisher nor the authors or the editors give a warranty, expressed or implied, with respect to the material contained herein or for any errors or omissions that may have been made. The publisher remains neutral with regard to jurisdictional claims in published maps and institutional affiliations.

This Springer imprint is published by the registered company Springer Nature Switzerland AG
The registered company address is: Gewerbestrasse 11, 6330 Cham, Switzerland

Foreword I

A Clinical Guide to Dental Caries Detection and Assessment has been constructed carefully by two authors who are deeply skilled in the art and science of caries detection and assessment and who have worked for years to build the often-fragile link bridging *best evidence* to *best clinical practice*. Together, they have assembled a formidable array of international talent to provide a much needed, comprehensive, accessible, well-illustrated, and authoritative guide for clinicians.

The Guide's structure provides a logical flow from the essential background required to understand the preparation for, conduct of, and limitations associated with clinical visual assessment of caries. This is followed by descriptions of a range of available visual detection criteria which are distinguished by some important differences. Intriguingly, many criteria systems also share very substantial commonalities. Detection during caries excavation is also addressed.

There follows a comprehensive series of chapters addressing additional detection methods as aid to caries lesion diagnosis. These range through radiographic film based and digital methods in both 2D and 3D, the use of white and near-infrared light, followed by fluorescence, bioluminescence, and photothermal radiometry. After considerations of what's in the pipeline (which often remains a frustratingly long one), important chapters cover making treatment decisions after caries detection and an essential appendix on the thorny but important topic of definitions.

The authors and contributors are to be congratulated on producing a focused and very useful Clinical Guide. I share the hope of the Editors that "this book will give the reader additional confidence to manage dental caries in the early stages with non-surgical approaches by using more precise and objective methods of assessment" and trust that this will help clinicians provide better care for their patients.

London, UK Nigel Pitts

Foreword II

Following the characterization of the initial phases of the dental caries process and the repeated demonstration that subsurface demineralization could be reversed by remineralization, many dental scientists focused their research on the identification and development of strategies and technologies for the very early detection of the caries process. For the past 40 years, numerous international dental scientists have meticulously and successfully investigated a wide variety of clinical methodologies and instrumental technologies for early caries detection resulting in a remarkable number of scientific publications in the dental literature.

A Clinical Guide to Dental Caries Detection and Assessment has been developed by two of these scientists who have been intimately involved in this research for more than 20 years and they have enlisted additional renowned scientists with similar experiences. The knowledge and experiences of this team of investigators has resulted in the compilation of this unique state-of-the-art review of research in this area. In developing this *Guide*, the authors have carefully included both clinical and instrumental technologies noting both the technical abilities of the strategies and their limitations. This material will be quite useful for the clinical control and management of dental caries by dental practitioners using non-surgical procedures.

In addition, the information presented in the *Guide* will be useful for the future development of even more effective procedures for the prevention of dental caries. Due to time and cost considerations, the development and clinical validation of more effective caries-preventive methods has become virtually impossible using historical procedures for clinical caries trials accepted by governmental agencies. However, these newer technologies will permit the assessment of significant caries-preventive benefits in much shorter time periods in much smaller cohorts of panelists. Without doubt this material will serve as a reference text for current as well as future cariologists and the authors are collectively acknowledged for their efforts.

Indianapolis, IN, USA George K. Stookey

Contents

Introduction

1

Andrea Ferreira Zandona and Christopher Longbottom

Dental caries detection is the cornerstone of every general dental practice. However, limited time is spent in the dental schools' curriculum; teaching dental caries detection and calibration of faculty is regarded as a great challenge [1–5]. Extensive lesions are usually easy to detect due to obvious clinical or radiological signs. Lesions in the early stages, however, are challenging. The visual signs can be subtle, and there can be many confounding effects. These lesions in the early stages, with no cavitation and no radiographic sign of demineralization, are considered questionable caries. A recent study with 82 practitioners and 6910 patients indicated that up to 34% of patients had questionable occlusal caries [6]. Clinical experience does not seem to reduce the number of surfaces deemed with questionable caries [6–8].

Dental caries remains a prevalent disease affecting millions of people worldwide [9]. Given the widespread use of fluoride, the burden of disease has decreased [10] but more than 90% of all United States dentate adults and more than two thirds of all children still experience dental caries [11]. With more adults retaining teeth later in life, we can expect an increase in surfaces with questionable caries. Many of these questionable caries surfaces will not progress toward cavitation [12]; therefore, it is paramount to both determine if there is a lesion and to assess caries activity. A paradigm shift pushing the management of dental caries from an operative/surgical approach to a nonsurgical approach in the last decades has led to a rise in interest on more detailed and objective caries detection methods [13].

A. Ferreira Zandona (✉)
Department of Comprehensive Care, Tufts University School of Dental Medicine, Boston, MA, USA
e-mail: Andrea.Zandona@tufts.edu

C. Longbottom
King's College London Dental Institute, London, UK
e-mail: Christopher.longbottom@kcl.ac.uk

© Springer Nature Switzerland AG 2019

A. Ferreira Zandona, C. Longbottom (eds.), *Detection and Assessment of Dental Caries*, https://doi.org/10.1007/978-3-030-16967-1_1

Dental explorers and air drying are the methods most commonly used for detection of caries (91%) with magnification and radiographs used on only half the lesions [6]. Several criteria have been developed based on visual examination, aiming to decrease subjectivity and improve the ability to monitor lesions (see Chaps. 3, 5–8). However, there is a myriad of detection aids available which can help dentists to more confidently monitor early initial lesions (see Chaps. 11–21). Once a lesion is detected and surgical intervention is proposed, distinguishing the different layers of carious dentin once a tooth is excavated prior to a restorative procedure (see Chaps. 9 and 10) is another challenging area for dentists who aim to preserve tooth structure.

For the practicing clinician, it is difficult to keep up with all the new methods and devices available, determine when and where to use them, and compare across all methods. This book aims to assist students and dentists on a better understanding of the several methods and devices available for caries detection. They are grouped based on the modality used (visual, x-rays, transillumination, fluorescence, and others). The chapters follow a standard template which should facilitate comparison among the methods. The chapters' authors are experts in their fields and have provided the latest evidence-based information for each of the methods. This book is not an all-encompassing review of all devices available. We do not discuss caries risk assessment, beyond discussing the role of caries detection in caries risk assessment: identifying the presence of caries lesions and assessing caries lesions activity are key procedures for an accurate diagnosis and prognosis. We also do not discuss caries management strategies beyond discussing treatment decision-making (see Chap. 22). We do discuss extensively the characteristics of tooth surfaces when they are affected by dental caries and changes in enamel and dentin properties as surfaces demineralize and remineralize. Many of the methods described rely on these changes to distinguish between sound surfaces and surfaces affected by dental caries. Some redundancy related to enamel/dentin properties and characteristics was allowed across the chapters to facilitate the understanding of the method in discussion without requiring the reader to go back to previous chapters.

Although there are clear distinctions among the methods discussed, there are also some clear messages across all chapters: teeth must be free of plaque prior to being examined to provide optimal conditions for the method being used; early caries detection methods can support clinical decision-making and allow for monitoring outcomes on nonsurgical interventions; methods should support visual examination and not be used in place of visual examination; users should be familiar with the limitations of each method and use sound judgment, especially when considering surgical intervention. Since many of the methods discussed in this book aim to improve detection of early lesions, we cannot overemphasize that this improvement in sensitivity is valuable for monitoring lesion behavior, and it is not a license to increase surgical intervention.

We hope this book will give the reader additional confidence to manage dental caries in the early stages with nonsurgical approaches by using more precise and objective methods of assessment.

References

1. Fontana M, Guzmán-Armstrong S, Schenkel AB, Allen KL, Featherstone J, Goolsby S, Kanjirath P, Kolker J, Martignon S, Pitts N, Schulte A, Slayton RL, Young D, Wolff M. Development of a core curriculum framework in cariology for U.S. dental schools. J Dent Educ. 2016;80(6):705–20.
2. Martignon S, Gomez J, Tellez M, Ruiz JA, Marin LM, Rangel MC. Current cariology education in dental schools in Spanish-speaking Latin American countries. J Dent Educ. 2013;77(10):1330–7.
3. Raphael SL, Foster Page LA, Hopcraft MS, Dennison PJ, Widmer RP, Wendell Evans R. A survey of cariology teaching in Australia and New Zealand. BMC Med Educ. 2018;18:75. https://doi.org/10.1186/s12909-018-1176-4.
4. Schulte AG, Buchalla W, Huysmans MC, Amaechi BT, Sampaio F, Vougiouklakis G, Pitts NB. A survey on education in cariology for undergraduate dental students in Europe. Eur J Dent Educ. 2011;15(Suppl 1):3–8.
5. Tikhonova S, Girard F, Fontana M. Cariology education in Canadian dental schools: where are we? Where do we need to go? J Dent Educ. 2018;82(1):39–46. https://doi.org/10.21815/JDE.018.006.
6. Makhija SK, Gilbert GH, Funkhouser E, et al. Characteristics, detection methods, and treatment of questionable occlusal carious lesions: findings from the National Dental Practice-Based Research Network. Caries Res. 2014;48(3):200–7. https://doi.org/10.1159/000354841.
7. Ferreira Zandona AG, Al-Shiha S, Eggertsson H. Student versus faculty performance using new visual criteria for the detection of caries on occlusal surfaces: an in vitro examination with histological validation. J Oper Dent. 2009;34(5):598–604. PMID: 19830976.
8. Lara JS, Braga MM, Shitsuka C, Wen CL, Haddad AE. Dental students' and lecturers' perception of the degree of difficulty of caries detection associated learning topics in Brazil. J Educ Eval Health Prof. 2015;12:56. https://doi.org/10.3352/jeehp.2015.12.56. Published 2015 Dec 25.
9. Frencken JE, Sharma P, Stenhouse L, Green D, Laverty D, Dietrich T. Global epidemiology of dental caries and severe periodontitis—a comprehensive review. J Clin Periodontol. 2017;44(Suppl 18):S94–S105. https://doi.org/10.1111/jcpe.12677.
10. Pitts NB. Are we ready to move from operative to non-operative/preventive treatment of dental caries in clinical practice? Caries Res. 2004;38:294–304.
11. Dye BA, Mitnik GL, Iafolla TJ, Vargas CM. Trends in dental caries in children and adolescents according to poverty status in the United States from 1999 through 2004 and from 2011 through 2014. J Am Dent Assoc. 2017;148(8):550–65, e557.
12. Ferreira Zandona AG, Santiago E, Eckert GJ, Katz BP, Pereira de Oliveira S, Capin OR, Mau M, Zero DT. The natural history of dental caries lesions—a 4 year observational study. J Dent Res. 2012;91(9):841–6. PMID: 22821238. PMCID: PMC3420396.
13. Ferreira Zandona A, Epure E. Evolution of caries diagnosis. J Multidisc Care Decisions Dent. 2018;4(2):43–6.

Part I

Background

Preparing Teeth for a Clinical Examination

2

Christopher Longbottom and Andrea Ferreira Zandona

2.1 Introduction

In this chapter examination condition, including the need for prophylaxis, air syringe, magnification and tooth separation are discussed. Additionally, susceptibility of different teeth and surfaces to caries are presented. Caries lesions can occur in the crowns (enamel), the roots (dentin) of teeth and adjacent to restorations in either/both of these tissues. The initial pathology of enamel or dentin is defined as primary caries, the latter being traditionally labelled 'secondary caries', although in reality this 'secondary' attack is generally the primary caries process adjacent to a restoration or sealant, hence the new, more appropriate, term CARS (Caries Adjacent to a Restoration or Sealant). In addition, the term 'residual caries' applies to aspects of caries lesions remaining after operative interventions. The focus initially in this text will be on the clinical examination in relation to primary caries lesions, with additional discussion of CARS and 'residual' caries.

2.2 Examination Conditions

Before examining teeth for visual signs of caries lesions, they should be: clean, dry (dried), and well-illuminated.

C. Longbottom (✉)
King's College London Dental Institute, London, UK
e-mail: Christopher.longbottom@kcl.ac.uk

A. Ferreira Zandona
Department of Comprehensive Care, Tufts University School of Dental Medicine, Boston, MA, USA
e-mail: Andrea.Zandona@tufts.edu

© Springer Nature Switzerland AG 2019

A. Ferreira Zandona, C. Longbottom (eds.), *Detection and Assessment of Dental Caries*, https://doi.org/10.1007/978-3-030-16967-1_2

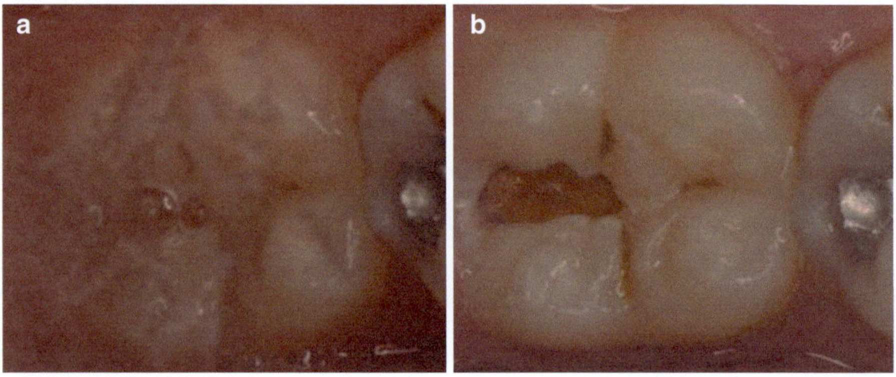

Fig. 2.1 Cavitated caries lesion before (**a**) and after (**b**) plaque removal

2.2.1 Clean

The earliest optical changes of carious changes in enamel (and dentin) are very subtle and are best visualized if the surface integuments—pellicle and plaque—as well as any food debris, have been removed from that surface. Caries lesions always occur under plaque, which is not transparent—a clinician cannot see through plaque—hence it must be removed prior to the visual examination of the actual surface of the tooth (Fig. 2.1a, b). This prophylaxis is best carried out using a rotating brush with a paste (or an air-polisher).

Failing this, the use of a toothbrush by the patient will remove the bulk of the plaque and the clinician can supplement this by the careful use of a probe—using the long edge of the probe to remove buccal and lingual surface plaque and a delicate 'dredging' technique with the probe tine to remove plaque from pits and fissures. The latter should be used with no pressure, but with 'the weight of the wing of a butterfly', i.e. simply 'resting' or 'balancing' the probe on the tooth surface and 'pulling' it gently along the fissure pattern with no pressure in the direction of the pulp. Flossing to remove interproximal plaque is essential prior to the examination of the approximal surfaces.

2.2.2 Dry/Dried

Isolating the teeth in a sextant, using cotton rolls and a saliva ejector, as well as retraction of the cheeks and tongue, prior to detailed examination of each tooth surface will aid clarity of the field by helping to reduce the risk of contamination by saliva (Figs. 2.2 and 2.3).

Air-drying of a tooth site will fully enhance the effect of the difference between the refractive index of enamel (1.6) and that of air (1.0). Normally the enamel pores are filled with water (refractive index 1.3), hence there is a smaller difference in refractive index prior to air-drying and the subtle optical changes due to demineralization are less readily distinguished by the clinician's eye.

However, it is important to try to assess the extent of any mineral changes present—a lesion which can only be visualized AFTER air-drying has generally produced less

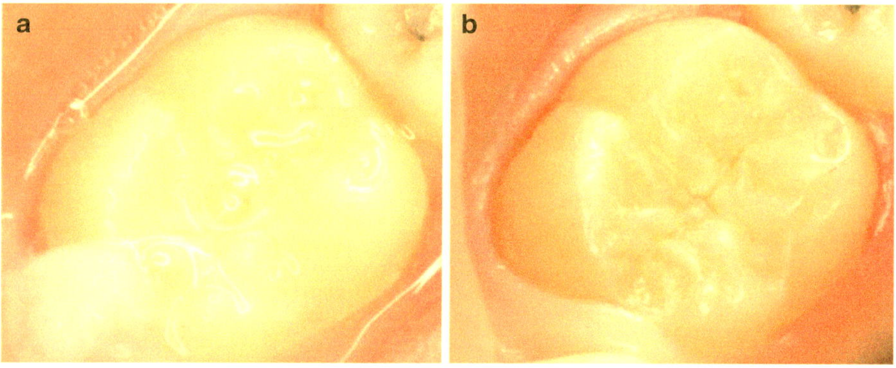

Fig. 2.2 Sound occlusal surface before (**a**) and after (**b**) drying

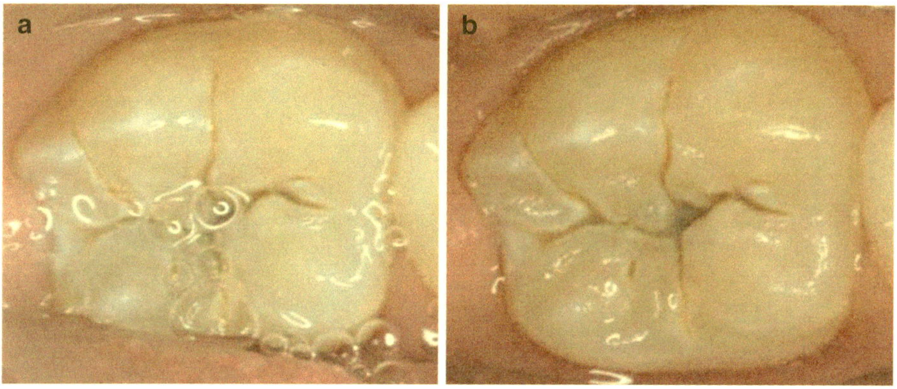

Fig. 2.3 (**a**, **b**) Occlusal surface with a caries lesion before and after drying

demineralization than one which is visible PRIOR to air-drying (since the amount of back-scattered light must be much greater to overcome the diminished refractive index difference brought about by the ingress of water into the enamel pores) (Fig. 2.4). In addition, for some lesions where dentin caries is present, the grey shadowing which results from such changes is often best visualized when the teeth are wet.

Hence in order to help assess the stage of progress (in terms of depth) of any lesion present, it is useful to visualize the tooth surface:

- **prior** to air-drying (i.e. a moistened tooth, not one covered in a thick layer of saliva)
- and
- then again after air-drying. Studies have indicated that 5 s of air-drying per surface will highlight the optical changes described above. This technique is used when using the visual ICDAS method—see below for details.

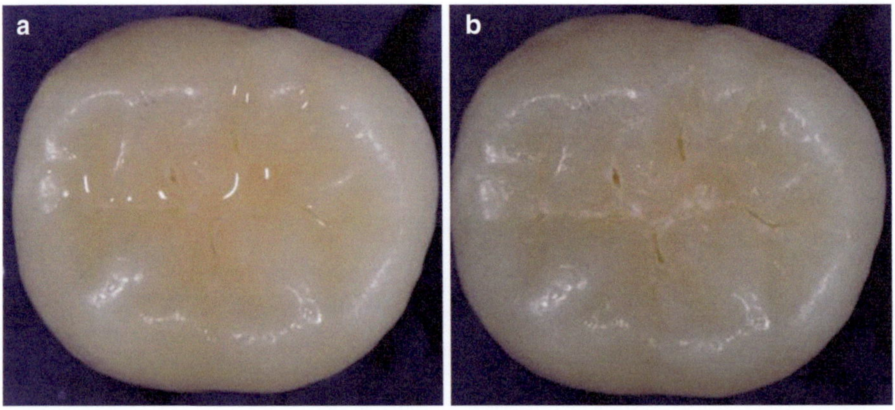

Fig. 2.4 (**a**, **b**) Occlusal surface with a caries lesion before and after drying. Note the white lesion only visible after drying

2.2.3 Well-Illuminated

The dental operating light can be used optimally by moving/tilting it and/or the patient's head to maximally illuminate the teeth in different regions of the mouth and in the two separate arches. The dental mirror should also be used to best effect by moving it in the three orthogonal planes, thereby reflecting the operating light on to the different surfaces of the tooth being examined in order to enhance any optical changes which have been produced by the caries process. Observing whether shadows within a tooth move or are stationary when a bright light is shone through a tooth from different angles can inform the operator about the likely source of these shadows—this is the fundamental process behind the use of transillumination, which enhances optical effects within a tooth—see below and in the Chap. 14. Viewing the teeth both directly and in the dental mirror will maximize the visual information gathered. If the operator also moves his/her head in the three planes, this will help provide 3D information about specific aspects of tooth morphology, particularly in relation to fissures, and aid lesion detection. The judicious use of a mirror when examining adjacent approximal surfaces will allow the operator to visually access the embrasure region and facilitate identification of caries lesions around and under approximal contact area/points.

2.3 Where to Look for Caries Lesions

2.3.1 Likely Teeth

During the last 70 years or so, a large amount of epidemiological data on permanent teeth has been collected worldwide. Analysis of this data has revealed patterns of susceptibility of teeth and specific surfaces of teeth.

The pattern of susceptibility in teeth and their surfaces occurs in groups, but by individual teeth is as follows, in order, decreasing from the highest to the lowest susceptibility to caries, as a child grows from the age of 5–6 years onwards:

- Lower first molar
- Lower second molar
- Upper first molar
- Upper second molar
- Upper and lower second premolars
- Upper first premolar
- Upper lateral and central incisors
- Lower first premolars
- Upper canine
- Lower incisors
- Lower canine

The overall epidemiological picture is nowadays confounded by the widespread use of pit and fissure sealants and topical fluorides, which help to prevent caries lesions, thus modulating the sites at which caries lesions occur. However, this fundamental underlying 'core' order of susceptibility of the teeth/sites appears to remain the same, probably due to the general eruption sequence of teeth, as well as their morphology and position/arrangement in the mouth.

There appears to be a considerable left-right symmetry of occurrence of caries lesions—hence, if a lesion appears in the occlusal fissure of the lower right first permanent molar of a patient, there is a high probability that the same site in the contra-lateral tooth, i.e. the lower left first permanent molar, will succumb or be highly susceptible to the development of a caries lesion.

From the above information, it is possible to derive general clinical implications in relation to examinations for caries lesions and the assessment of a patient's caries risk. By way of example, if a patient over the age of 15 years has no signs of caries lesions or restorations in any of the pits and fissures of the molar teeth, it is highly unlikely that there will be signs of caries lesions in the teeth below these molars on the above list. An exception to this would be where a patient has had successful pit and fissure sealants placed earlier in life which have prevented the development of lesions at these sites—if sealants have not also been placed on the premolars and incisor palatal pits of these patients, these sites should be very carefully monitored for the initial signs of disease, since the sealants have effectively skewed the caries-risk pattern in this patient.

By contrast, if a child patient aged 9 years has caries lesions present in the upper incisors the probability of caries lesions developing in the occlusal pits and fissures of ALL the as yet unerupted molars and premolars, after they erupt, is extremely high. It is virtually certain that by the age of 9 this child will have had caries lesions in the pits and fissures of the first permanent molars, although, as above, this may have been prevented by the timely and efficient placement and maintenance of pit and fissure sealants on these teeth. However, if the second primary molar is still present, the mesial (approximal) sites on these first permanent molar teeth will be highly susceptible to caries lesion development and should be examined extremely carefully for signs of disease.

Generally speaking, most individuals will lie somewhere between the two extremes of the above examples, but the same ‘rough indications’ apply—for example, if there are no signs of caries lesions in the fissures of any of the second premolars, in the absence of fissure sealants on these teeth, the probability is that the fissures of the first premolars and the upper lateral incisor pits will not be susceptible to caries lesion development.

These ‘rough indications’ are exactly that—approximate guides to what will occur—and the clinician must use his/her experience and knowledge of the disease process generally and in that patient in particular (especially with respect to the level of caries risk) to decide which teeth and sites are likely to be susceptible to caries lesion development. There are always exceptions to rules and the clinician should be ever-conscious of the potentially unexpected.

2.3.2 Likely Sites

As a general guideline, pits and fissures are more susceptible initially to caries lesion development than approximal sites, which in turn are more susceptible than free smooth (buccal and lingual/palatal) sites. This stems from tooth morphology and the relative difficulty (in that sequence order) for the patient in efficiently removing plaque from each of these sites.

The detailed morphology of occlusal fissure patterns varies enormously but the frequency of the different types of fissure morphology has been reported by several authors. In summary, there are effectively four different fissure types, each with their own prevalence and caries susceptibility. The name (letter) given to each type of morphology is based on its physical shape, e.g. the I-type is a narrow deep fissure.

The prevalence figures relate to how often each fissure type occurs when large numbers of teeth are sectioned and examined under a microscope—the prevalence does NOT relate to individual teeth but to the frequency across ALL fissure sites, e.g. teeth surfaces can have all these different fissure types within a single occlusal surface.

The least caries-susceptible fissure type is the U-type (14%) which is readily cleansable, thus plaque can be brushed off before it instigates the caries process. The V-type pattern (39%) is narrower than the U-type at its base so it presents a slightly more challenging fissure pattern to clean and is therefore more susceptible to caries. The I-type pattern (46%) is even narrower and because of its length and narrowness the base of it is virtually impossible to clean with a toothbrush, so is at considerable risk of developing caries lesions. Finally, the least prevalent (1%) bottle-type fissure, whose base is wider than its walls at the fissure entrance, is the most susceptible to caries since its base is inaccessible to toothbrush bristles.

One or more of these fissure types can occur on the same fissure pattern, so it is vital that the clinician uses the knowledge about these different types and their different susceptibilities when examining a tooth for signs of caries lesions. The different visual signs corresponding approximately to the stages of the progress of a caries lesion at a tooth site are incorporated in the visual ICDAS codes listed below.

The more difficult a fissure pattern is to clean the more likely it is to be an I-type or bottle-type fissure and is therefore more susceptible to caries lesion development. The plaque will sit on the enamel at the entrance to the fissure, hence this is where the first stage of the disease appears in the enamel. The clinician should therefore concentrate his visual attention initially on the enamel at the entrances to the fissures. Demineralization in enamel eventually produces an increase in the back-scattering of incident light to produce a white spot lesion—this will generally, but not always, appear at the fissure entrance, not in the depths of a fissure.

The more complex and convoluted the fissure pattern, the more difficult it will be to keep clean and the higher its susceptibility to caries lesion development. Thus, narrow steep-walled deep fissures (I-type), intersections (of different parts) of the fissure patterns and narrow pits will all present difficulties for the patient in keeping them free from plaque. These will be generally more susceptible sites than broader flatter fissure patterns (U-type). Examination and assessment of each patient's detailed pit and fissure morphology will highlight which specific sites within a fissure pattern are likely to be more vulnerable than others.

The use of an explorer/probe to 'catch' a fissure pattern to detect primary caries lesions has been shown to be of no diagnostic value, i.e. it adds no valid extra information on caries lesion presence or extent to what can be gleaned by a careful detailed visual assessment. This has been reported by several different authors over the last 60 years. It has also been shown that for non-cavitated lesions probing can irreversibly damage the tooth surface, effectively creating a micro-cavity within a lesion where none previously existed, making the lesion more prone to disease progression.

On older patients exposed root surfaces are at higher risk for developing caries lesions. Crown margins, especially those ending in dentin will be particularly at risk as well (see below).

2.4 Temporary Elective Tooth Separation

A number of authors have reported the use of elastomeric separating modules (commonly used in orthodontic treatment) to create, temporarily, a small space between contacting teeth which allows direct visual access of the two adjacent approximal surfaces. This process involves the placement of a small elastomeric band between these teeth (around the contact areas/points) and leaving it in place for 2–7 days. Hence a second visit, to remove the band and visually identify the presence or absence of any approximal lesions and assess their surface integrity for signs of micro- or macro-cavitation. This latter assessment can be aided by the use of FOTI, as well as by the taking of a small impression of the expanded embrasure area, to identify any breaks in the enamel surface morphology (Fig. 2.5).

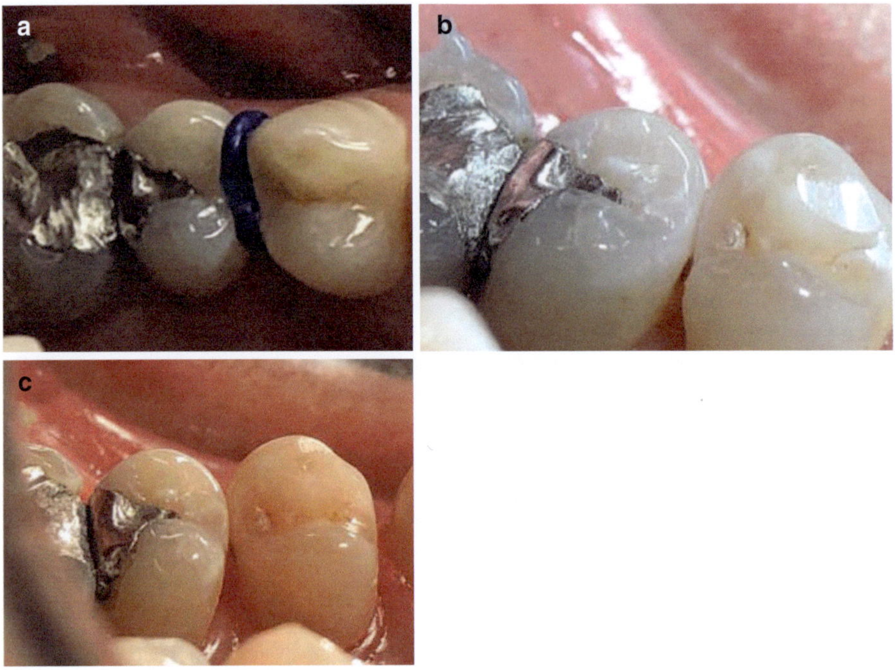

Fig. 2.5 (**a**–**c**) A lesion was observed on the distal surface of the first premolar and the mesial surface of the second premolar. An ortho separator was left in place for 48 h. Both lesions were non-cavitated

2.5 Magnification

The wearing of magnification aids can help clinicians to identify changes in the surface characteristics of enamel. The extent of the literature on the effectiveness of using magnification aids in caries lesion detection and diagnosis is surprisingly limited and has produced some mixed results.

The latter may be the result of limitations in research methods, since the very process of magnification of an image increases the level of detail available compared to the naked eye view. This should facilitate and enhance the identification of the various visual changes which occur during the caries process.

2.6 Caries Lesions in Primary Teeth

The morphology of primary molars and permanent posterior teeth is significantly different—primary molars have broader contact areas than permanent posterior teeth, which makes it more difficult to visualize into the embrasures to assess the enamel beneath the contact points and also leads to a greater potential for plaque retention.

The shapes of the fissures on the occlusal surfaces of primary molars are generally less pronounced than for permanent teeth, hence they tend to be less caries-susceptible than in their permanent tooth equivalents.

Separators can be used in children, from as young as 4 or 5 years upwards to adulthood, to aid visual caries lesion detection—they are well tolerated as their use by orthodontists for over 5 decades attests.

2.7 Root Caries Lesions

See the ICDAS criteria (Chap. 6)—although visual indicators such as colour (darkening) and glossiness seem to be helpful in differentiating between active and inactive root caries lesions, essentially the texture (softness) of a lesion using a ball-ended probe appears to be the best detection aid for the presence of an active root caries lesion and the increased hardness of a lesion over time is a good indicator that the lesion is arresting.

2.8 CARS

See the ICDAS criteria (Chap. 6). CARS lesions are primary caries lesions adjacent to restorations or sealants, hence the same visual signs for primary caries lesions are appropriate for CARS lesions. The specific 'added' factor to be taken into account is the potential presence of a 'plaque-trap' caused by the presence of a restoration or sealant, e.g. a ledge (restoration), or a breakdown of the marginal integrity of the restoration or sealant (fracture and/or loss of seal between the enamel and the restoration/sealant). The routine use of floss can aid the identification of ledges on approximal restorations.

2.9 Concluding Remarks

The detection of dental caries lesions is not a simple task and requires careful and systematic visual techniques to identify the subtle changes in the various characteristics of tooth tissues brought about by the pathological processes involved. Each tooth site being examined should be clean, dry (dried), and well-illuminated for optimum visual assessment. Even then, meticulous visual examination is not sufficient to detect totally accurately all lesions and assess the stage of each lesion at the different sites at which they occur. There are well-recognized patterns of susceptibility of tooth sites to caries attack in both the permanent and primary dentitions. Knowledge of these site-risk patterns will aid the clinician in the optimization of the visual assessment method of caries lesion detection.

Caries lesion detection is the first step in a three-stage process, which then involves lesion characterization and subsequent assimilation of the lesion information, together with patient data, to lead the clinician to a diagnosis relating to the activity (or otherwise) of any detected lesion(s) and his/her subsequent treatment-decision with regard to each lesion.

References

1. Selwitz RH, Ismail AI, Pitts NB. Dental caries. Lancet. 2007;369:51–9.
2. Longbottom C, Huysmans M-C, Pitts NB, Fontana M. Glossary of key terms. In: Pitts NB, editor. Detection, assessment, diagnosis and monitoring of caries, Monographs in oral science, vol. 21. Basel: Karger; 2009. p. 207–15.
3. Pitts NB, Stamm J. International Consensus Workshop on Caries Clinical Trials (ICW-CCT)—final consensus statements: agreeing where the evidence leads. J Dent Res. 2004;83(spec iss C):125–8.
4. Neuhaus KW, Ellwood R, Lussi A, Pitts NB. Traditional lesion detection aids. In: Pitts NB, editor. Detection, assessment, diagnosis and monitoring of caries. Basel: Karger; 2009. p. 42–3.
5. Bader JD, Shugars DA, Bonito AJ. Systematic reviews of selected dental caries diagnostic and management methods. J Dent Educ. 2001;65(10):960–8.
6. Bader JD, Shugars DA. A systematic review of the performance of a laser fluorescence device for detecting caries. J Am Dent Assoc. 2004;135(10):1413–26. Review.
7. Batchelor PA, Sheiham A. Grouping of tooth surfaces by susceptibility to caries: a study in 5–16 year-old children. BMC Oral Health. 2004;4:2.
8. Pitts NB, Longbottom C. Preventive care advised (PCA)/operative care advised (OCA)—categorizing caries by the management option. Community Dent Oral Epidemiol. 1995;23:55–9.

The Visual Presentation of Dental Caries

3

Andrea Cortés, Stefania Martignon, and Gail Douglas

3.1 Introduction

A caries lesion is the result of diverse local metabolic events that lead to pH fluctuations at the interface between the biofilm and the tooth structure [1]. The production of organic acids resulting from bacterial metabolism generates H^+ and a decrease in the pH. The H^+ react with the PO_4^{-3} and $-OH^-$ ions from the enamel to form phosphates (HPO_4^{-2} and $H_2PO_4^{-1}$), phosphoric acid, and water, thus generating a subsaturation environment that favors mineral loss [2]. The study of the histopathology of dental caries has contributed to the understanding of the behavior of the enamel, the dentin, and the cementum in the demineralization process [3–5] and has provided an essential understanding of its visual appearance [6]. When the ion loss in the surface is higher than the ion gain, over a period of time [1], a visible caries lesion may be detected during the clinical examination. If the metabolic events in the biofilm continue without being disturbed over a long period of time, the caries lesion progresses, manifesting different visual characteristics as severity worsens.

Current understanding of the tooth structure recognizes the enamel structure as a nanocomposite bioceramic which helps to protect the tooth from the assaults which is constantly exposed to in the oral environment. The enamel is formed by thickly packed

A. Cortés (✉)
UNICA Caries Research Unit, Research Vice-Rectory, Universidad El Bosque, Bogotá, Colombia
e-mail: cortesandrea@unbosque.edu.co

S. Martignon
UNICA Caries Research Unit, Research Vice-Rectory, Universidad El Bosque, Bogotá, Colombia

King's College London Dental Institute, Dental Innovation and Translation Centre, Guy's Hospital, London, UK

G. Douglas
School of Dentistry, University of Leeds, Leeds, UK

© Springer Nature Switzerland AG 2019

A. Ferreira Zandona, C. Longbottom (eds.), *Detection and Assessment of Dental Caries*, https://doi.org/10.1007/978-3-030-16967-1_3

crystals made up of calcium, phosphate, hydroxyl groups ($Ca_{10}[PO_4]_6[OH]_2$), and other ions such as fluoride, magnesium, sodium, chlorine, potassium, and carbonate [2].

Careful visual and tactile examination to search for enamel changes related to caries lesions, after careful cleaning of the teeth (see Chap. 2), can be combined with other diagnostic methods to make the evaluation more accurate [7, 8] (see Part III, Chaps. 11–18).

A good visual-tactile detection and assessment system for caries should include a clinical assessment which: (1) is useable for both the primary and permanent dentition; (2) records the status of all surfaces; and (3) includes the assessment of caries from the early stages. These are important characteristics to assist clinicians in proposing patient care focused upon preventing new caries lesions, arresting any active caries lesions and to support the patient achievement of good oral health. Additionally, caries detection and assessment systems should be compatible for use by clinicians, researchers, educators, and epidemiologists to facilitate communication about caries between these fields.

Based upon this understanding of the dental caries process, different classifications systems such as Nyvad [9] (see Chap. 5), ICDAS [10] (see Chap. 6), ADA CCS [11] (see Chap. 7), and CAST [12] (see Chap. 8) have been devised to detect caries lesion at all stages, especially in early caries phases when the lesions are difficult to be detected by traditional systems.

The appearance of normal enamel and early caries to the naked eye is influenced by how light interacts with the tooth surface. Sound enamel is translucent and has a refractive index of 1.6.

3.2 Initial Caries Lesions (A)

As net mineral loss occurs during the caries process, the first mineral which is lost is from dissolution of the crystals located at the prismatic surface and from the interprismatic space. This results in an increase in enamel pore-volume. These gaps between the crystals in the very initial stage of caries however do not change the visual appearance of the enamel as the small gaps between crystals are filled with fluid with a similar refractive index to the enamel itself (1.33) and light passes through the lesion in a similar way to the surrounding normal enamel. These lesions can be visualized by driving off the moisture from the enamel by prolonged air drying for around 5 s with the three-in-one air syringe. If the caries lesion continues to progress, and the loss of mineral from the lesion causes the gaps between the prisms to become large enough to be air filled (refractive index = 1.0), then the lesion becomes visible clinically as a whitish area. Light hitting the surface of the porous caries lesion is refracted differently from that hitting sound enamel [3]. If the lesion's progression is arrested or significantly slowed down, then lesions may take up color from the oral environment and become more brownish [13].

3.3 Moderate Caries Lesions (B)

If demineralization continues, the caries progresses further until the gaps between the crystals become so large and the structure becomes fragile and vulnerable to mechanical forces. The enamel surface starts to break down causing microcavitation at first then visually detectable breakdown of the enamel surface itself [13, 14]. As the lesion extends to involve the dentin, it becomes darker in color which creates a shadow that can be seen through the surface enamel [15].

3.4 Extensive Caries Lesions (C)

At some point, when the depth and width of carious dentin undermines the top layer of fragile enamel, the surface caves in creating a cavity which exposes the dentin [16] (Table 3.1).

Table 3.1 Some expels of clinical and histological caries stages

Caries severity	Clinically	Histology
Sound	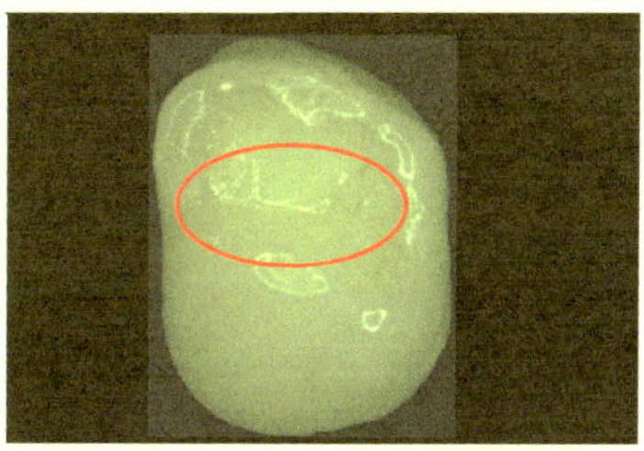	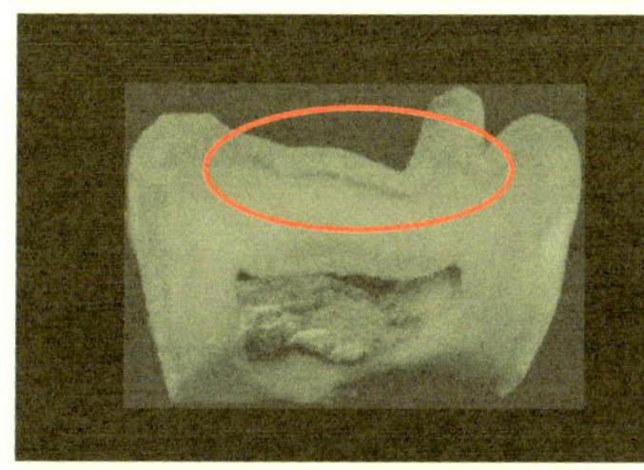
Coronal caries [9–12, 14]	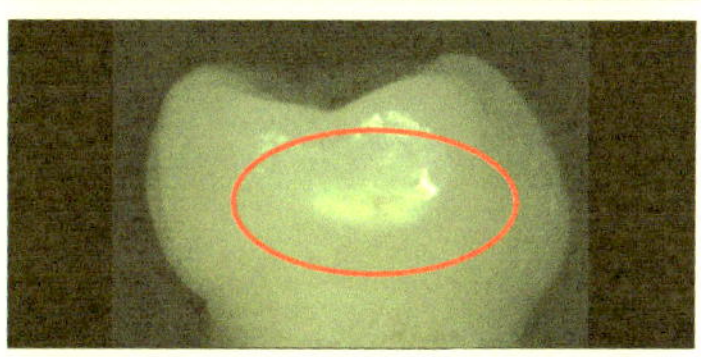	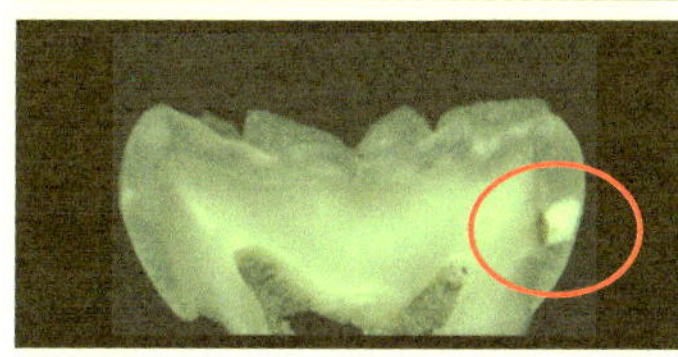
	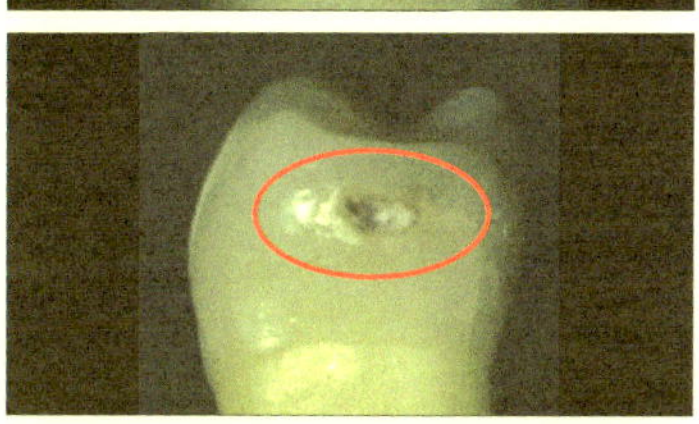	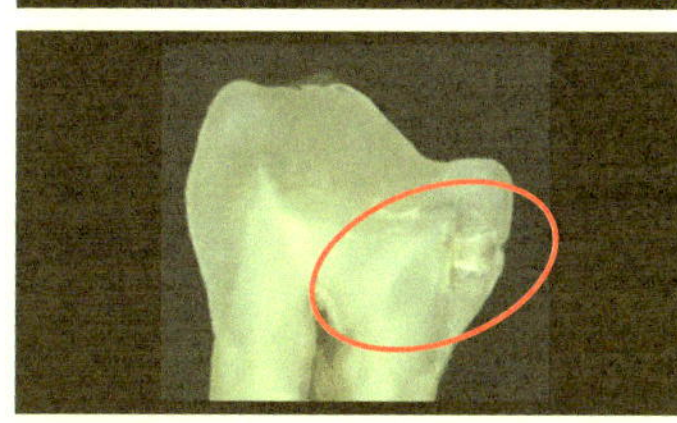
	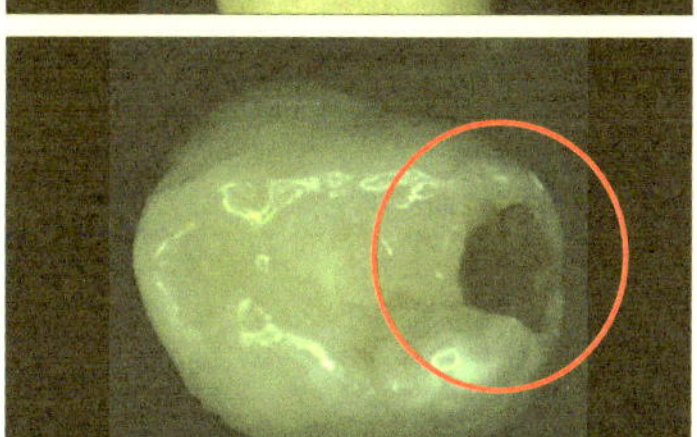	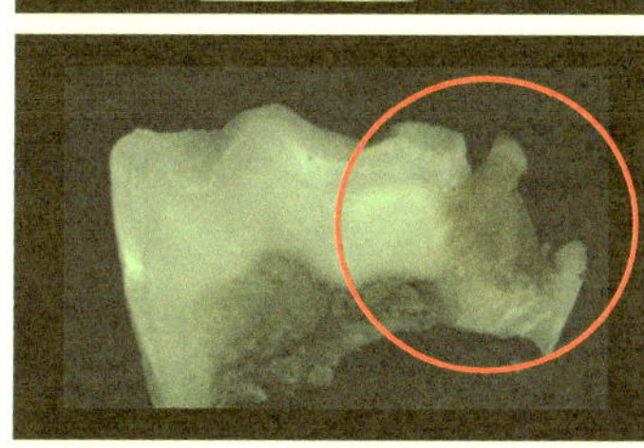
Caries adjacent to restorations [17, 18]	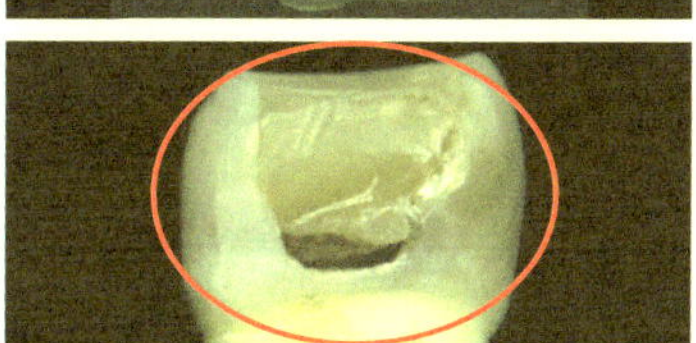	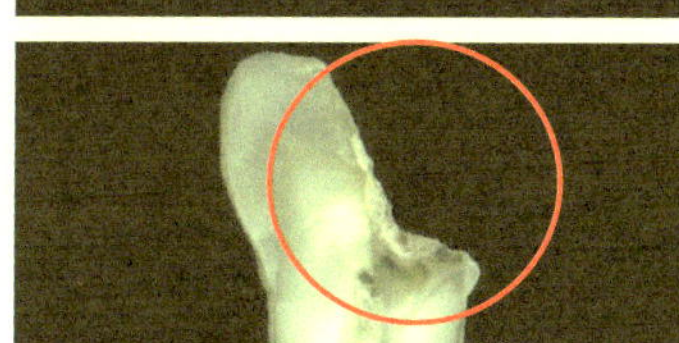

(continued)

Table 3.1 (continued)

Caries severity	Clinically	Histology
Root caries [19]	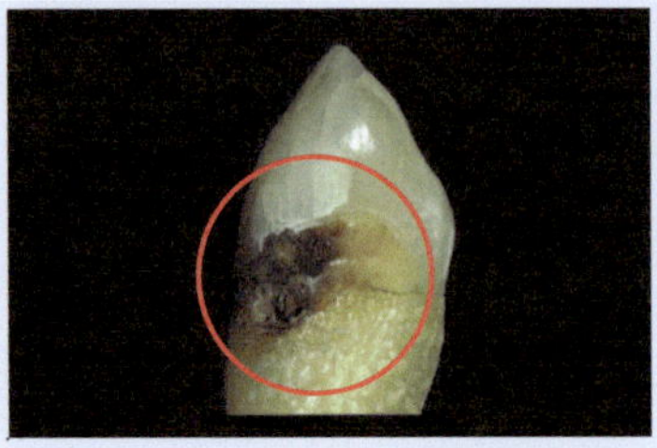	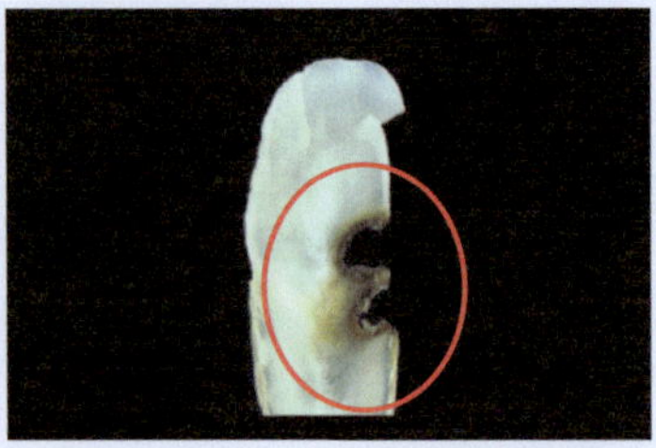

3.5 Clinical Technique

Visual-tactile assessment begins with detecting whether there is presence of a caries lesion or not (caries lesion detection). If a caries lesion is present, the severity (initial (A), moderate (B), or extensive (C) caries lesion) of the lesion should be determined [20] and an assessment made of whether the lesion is active or inactive.

Dental caries is located in areas where plaque tends to be retained for longer periods (see Chap. 2). Caries prone areas include natural areas in the mouth that are harder to clean as well as man-made zones where plaque may be trapped, e.g., by fixed and removable devices such as orthodontic appliances, crowns, bridges, and dentures. Plaque stagnation areas vary depending on the tooth surface [21]:

Coronal Caries [9–12]:

– Pit and fissures in occlusal and buccal/lingual surfaces

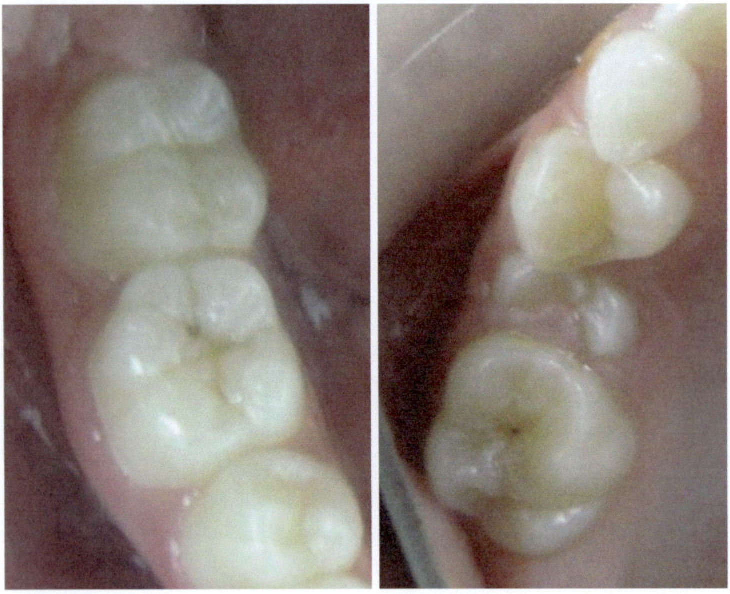

– Smooth surfaces at the gingival margin of the buccal surfaces

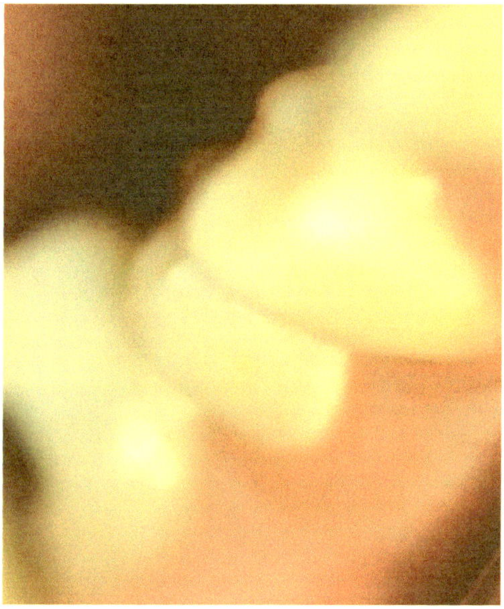

– Proximal surfaces from the contact point/area to the gingival margin and around the contact point/area

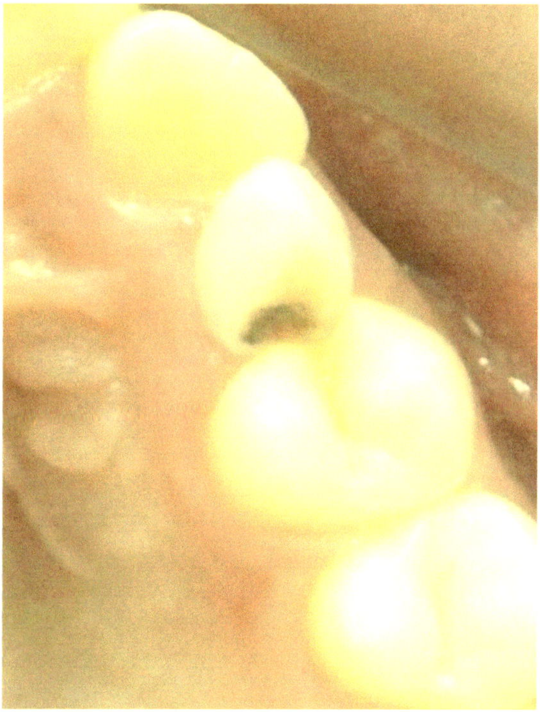

Secondary Caries [17, 18]:

- Adjacent to restorations, particularly those with gaps and rough edges

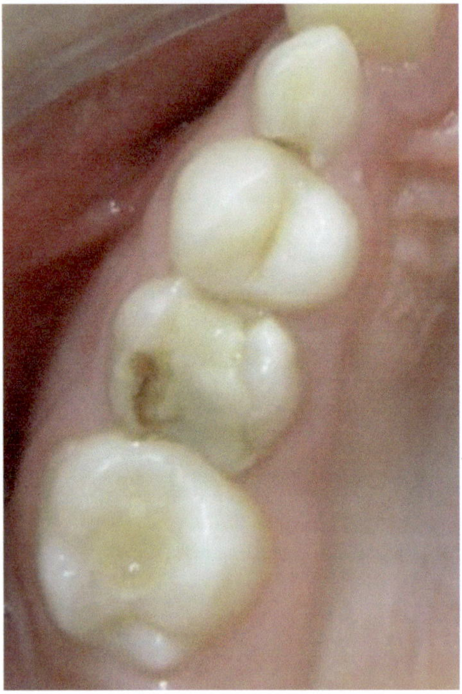

Root Caries [19]:

- Exposed root surfaces

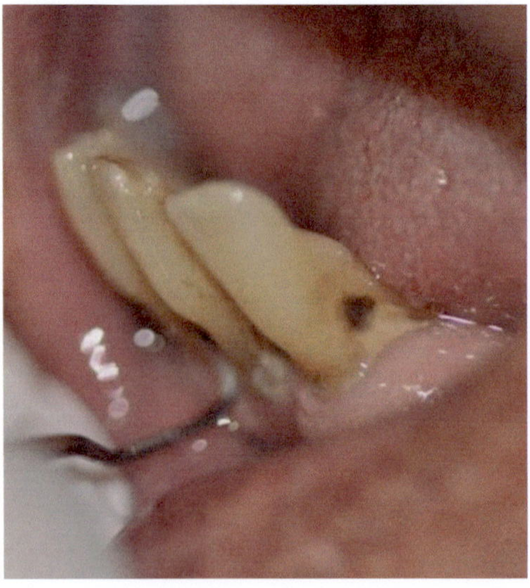

Visual caries diagnosis of the proximal surfaces is very difficult when there is an adjacent tooth. However, it is possible to visualize and feel these surfaces using temporary separation. Placing an elastic band between teeth for 2 days can facilitate access to the surface which is particularly useful to help determine if the enamel is broken or not. This procedure can create a space of around 0.7 mm between teeth [22] (Fig. 3.1) (see Chap. 2).

As caries forms beneath stagnant plaque, it is essential to clean the teeth adequately before undertaking a clinical examination (Fig. 3.2).

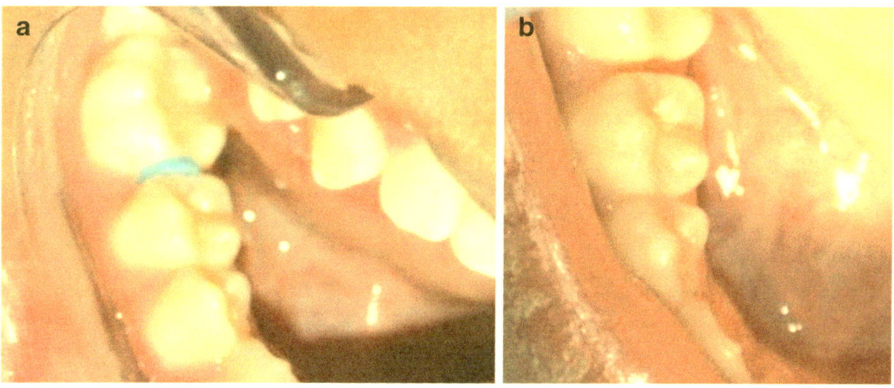

Fig. 3.1 Elective temporary separation. (**a**) An elastic band was inserted between second premolar first permanent molar; (**b**) The elastic band was removed after 2 days and gave access to the proximal surface

Fig. 3.2 The visual diagnosis procedure. (**a**) No plaque removal; (**b**) Cleaning the surfaces; (**c**) Isolation with cotton rolls and remove excess saliva before examining the surfaces

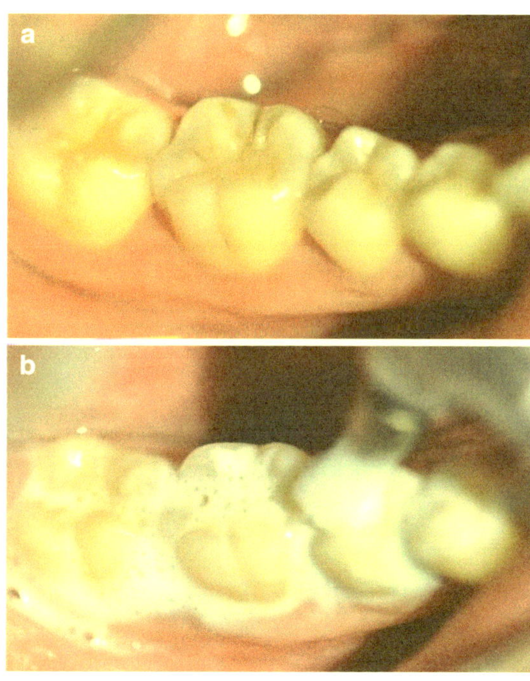

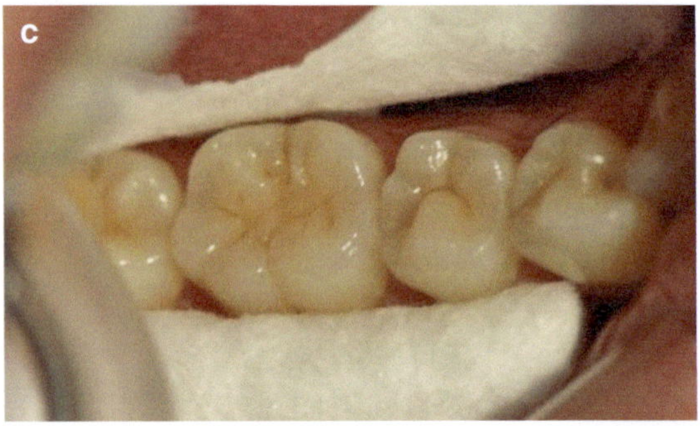

Fig. 3.2 (continued)

3.6 Concluding Remarks

The visual-tactile detection and assessment of caries is a qualitative method that requires an understanding of the caries process and training to be of use. It must always be bear in mind that the caries process makes lesions vulnerable to mechanical force and the use of a probe therefore can cause further damage. An optimal visual-tactile diagnostic system should provide all the necessary information for an appropriate management plan which takes into account both the patient-level factors which influence risk of progression as well as tooth surface status in order to determine personalized treatment plans including preventive measures [23].

Summary table

Bitewing radiography	Visual-tactile			
Which surfaces/ sites is it useful for	Occlusal (pits and fissures)	Proximal/ (approximal)	Smooth surface (buccal and lingual)	Root caries and which of the four surfaces?
	Y	**Y**	**Y**	**Y, all the four surfaces**
What type of lesion is it valuable for	Primary coronal	Secondary coronal	Primary root caries	Secondary root caries
	Y	**Y**	**Y**	**Y**
What type of dentition	Primary		Permanent	
	Y		**Y**	
Lesion severity	Enamel lesions		Dentinal lesions	
	Y		**Y**	
Sensitivity	Literature reported range of 42% for occlusal surfaces and 12–50% for cavitated caries lesions in proximal surfaces			
Specificity	Literature reported range of 94% in occlusal surfaces and 90–97% for cavitated caries lesions in proximal surfaces			
Perceived Ease Of Use (PEOU)[a]	1. "Visual-tactile examination" is easy to use 2. It is easy to become skillful at using "visual-tactile examination" 3. Learning to operate "visual-tactile examination" is easy 4. "Visual-tactile examination" is flexible to interact with 5. My interaction with "visual-tactile examination" is clear and understandable 6. It is easy to interact with "visual-tactile examination"			

Advantages/ disadvantages	*Advantages* 1. No expensive tools required to undertake examination 2. No exposure to ionizing radiation required 3. Clinical setting ideal but not vital for examination 4. Acceptable to patients of all ages *Disadvantages* 1. Proximal surfaces difficult to visualize 2. Lesions beneath restorations not detectable 3. Teeth need to be cleaned before examination
Time	Approximate time per patient 3 min in primary dentition and 4 min in permanent dentition Around 10 s for each tooth
Cost	Minimal

[a]Davis (1989) [24]

References

1. Fejerskov O. Changing paradigms in concepts on dental caries: consequences for oral health care. Caries Res. 2004;38:182–91.
2. Castellanos JE, Marín LM, Úsuga MV, Castiblanco GA, Martignon S. La remineralización del esmalte bajo el entendimiento actual de la caries dental. Univ Odontol. 2013;32:49–59.
3. Silverstone LM. Structure of carious enamel, including the early lesion. Oral Sci Rev. 1973;3:100–60.
4. Thylstrup A, Bruun C, Holmen L. In vivo caries models—mechanisms for caries initiation and arrestment. Adv Dent Res. 1994;8:144–57.
5. Ekstrand KR, Luna LE, Promisiero L, Cortes A, Cuevas S, Reyes JF, Torres CE, Martignon S. The reliability and accuracy of two methods for proximal caries detection and depth on directly visible proximal surfaces: an in vitro study. Caries Res. 2011;45:93–9.
6. Kidd EA, Fejerskov O. What constitutes dental caries? Histopathology of carious enamel and dentin related to the action of cariogenic biofilms. J Dent Res. 2004;83 Spec No C:C35–8.
7. Pitts NB, Renson CE. Image analysis of bitewing radiographs: a histologically validated comparison with visual assessments of radiolucency depth in enamel. Br Dent J. 1986;160:205–9.
8. Pretty IA, Ekstrand KR. Detection and monitoring of early caries lesions: a review. Eur Arch Paediatr Dent. 2016;17:13–25.
9. Nyvad B, Machiulskiene V, Baelum V. Reliability of a new caries diagnostic system differentiating between active and inactive caries lesions. Caries Res. 1999;33:252–60.
10. Ekstrand KR, Gimenez T, Ferreira FR, Mendes FM, Braga MM. The International Caries Detection and Assessment System—ICDAS: a systematic review. Caries Res. 2018;52:406–19.
11. Young DA, Nový BB, Zeller GG, Hale R, Hart TC, Truelove EL, American Dental Association Council on Scientific Affairs, American Dental Association Council on Scientific Affairs. The American Dental Association Caries Classification System for clinical practice: a report of the American Dental Association Council on Scientific Affairs. J Am Dent Assoc. 2015;146:79–86.
12. Leal SC, Ribeiro APD, Frencken JE. Caries Assessment Spectrum and Treatment (CAST): a novel epidemiological instrument. Caries Res. 2017;51:500–6.
13. Pitts NB, Ekstrand KR, ICDAS Foundation. International Caries Detection and Assessment System (ICDAS) and its International Caries Classification and Management System (ICCMS)—methods for staging of the caries process and enabling dentists to manage caries. Community Dent Oral Epidemiol. 2013;41:e41–52.
14. Ekstrand KR, Ricketts DN, Kidd EA. Occlusal caries: pathology, diagnosis and logical management. Dent Update. 2001;28:380–7.

15. Ekstrand KR, Kuzmina I, Bjorndal L, Thylstrup A. Relationship between external and histologic features of progressive stages of caries in the occlusal fossa. Caries Res. 1995;29:243–50.
16. Fejerskov O, Nyvad B, Larsen MJ. Human experimental caries models: intra-oral environmental variability. Adv Dent Res. 1994;8:134–43.
17. Özer L, Thylstrup A. What is known about caries in relation to restorations as a reason for replacement? A review. Adv Dent Res. 1995;9:394–402.
18. Kidd EA. Diagnosis of secondary caries. J Dent Educ. 2001;65:997–1000.
19. Carrilho MRO. Monographs in oral science—root caries: from prevalence to therapy. Basel: Karger; 2017.
20. Pitts NB, Stamm JW. International Consensus Workshop on Caries Clinical Trials (ICW-CCT)—final consensus statements: agreeing where the evidence leads. J Dent Res. 2004;83 Spec No C:C125–8.
21. Pitts N. Monographs in oral science—detection, assessment, diagnosis and monitoring of caries. Basel: Karger; 2009.
22. Cortes A, Martignon S, Qvist V, Ekstrand KR. Approximal morphology as predictor of approximal caries in primary molar teeth. Clin Oral Investig. 2018;22:951–9.
23. ICCMS™ 2018. International Caries Classification and Management system (ICCMS™) Web site. https://www.iccms-web.com/.
24. Davis FD. Percieved usefulness, percieved ease of use, and user acceptance of information technology. MIS Quarterly. 1989;319–40.

The Concept of Hidden Caries

4

Christopher Deery

4.1 Introduction and Historical Perspective

During the period of decline in caries prevalence starting in the late 1960s or early 1970s, there were reports that the diagnosis of occlusal caries has become more difficult [1]. This phenomenon was labelled "hidden" or "occult" caries, defined as dentin caries which was not evident clinically but only detected radiographically (Fig. 4.1).

The initially accepted explanation for this was the exposure of the dentition to fluoride, particularly in toothpaste, over the same period. The hypothesis suggested to account for this is that fluoride results in delayed cavitation because the surface layer of the carious lesion continues to remineralise and therefore cavitates at a later

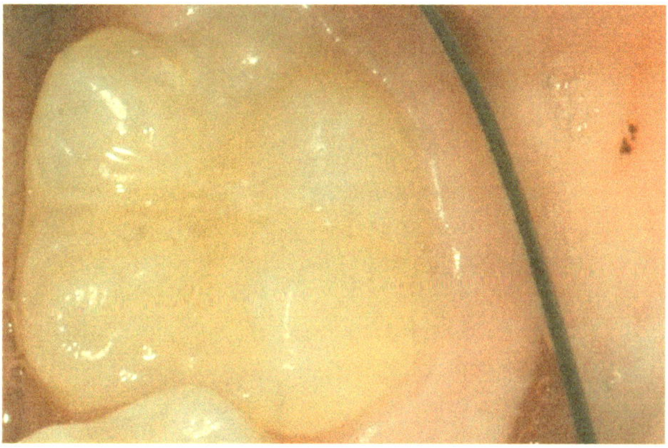

Fig. 4.1 A clinically sound occlusal surface with no evidence of enamel or dentinal caries. For there to be true hidden dentinal caries, a radiograph would have to reveal dentinal caries to be present

C. Deery (✉)
School of Clinical Dentistry, University of Sheffield, Sheffield, South Yorkshire, UK
e-mail: C.deery@sheffield.ac.uk

© Springer Nature Switzerland AG 2019

A. Ferreira Zandona, C. Longbottom (eds.), *Detection and Assessment of Dental Caries*, https://doi.org/10.1007/978-3-030-16967-1_4

stage than it would have in the absence of fluoride. This later point of cavitation results in a more difficult diagnosis of the presence of caries.

This explanation was quickly questioned as a possible aetiological link between hidden caries and the use of fluoride using data collected in the 1960s, by Backer Dirks, Houwink and Kwant (1961) [2] from 15-year-old inhabitants of two Dutch towns (Tiel and Culemborg), participating in a trial of artificially fluoridated water [3]. This study reported hidden caries to be evident in both the non-fluoridated control town and the fluoridated study town, thus demonstrating that hidden caries is not a new phenomenon. In fact, the fluoridated town had less occurrence of hidden caries than the control town, which implies that the fluoride ion is not responsible for hidden caries, at least when delivered in water. The authors suggest that the decline in caries prevalence associated with the beneficial action of fluoride has resulted in more clinically sound occlusal surfaces being evaluated, thus focusing the attention of clinicians on lesions which have not been detected clinically. The hypothesis that fluoride has not altered the appearance of caries is also supported by an Irish study, which found no difference between the prevalence of clinically cavitated and non-cavitated dentin lesions between fluoridated and non-fluoridated communities [4] and a more recent Brazilian study which again found more hidden caries in the non-fluoridated water area [5]. These latter studies have the advantage of reporting populations where fluoride was available from both water and toothpaste, indicating that the unlikely possibility that fluoride acts differently in water than toothpaste is not the case.

Prior to the "fluoride era", it is not clear how simple was the diagnosis of occlusal caries. Konig (1963) stated that "…caries lesions of pits and fissures may be diagnosed and the nature and extent of destruction estimated fairly accurately by visual inspection alone…" [6]. This view is similar to that of Sognnaes (1940) [7], although others have reported the diagnosis of caries in pits and fissures to be problematic [8]. It is highly likely that in the absence of radiographs many lesions were being missed.

Following some discussion in the dental press, Sawle and Andlaw (1988) [1] investigated whether occlusal caries in molar teeth had become more difficult to diagnose by visual-tactile examination (caries into dentin threshold). For this study, radiographs of 14–16-year-old children who had participated in fluoride toothpaste trials in 1974 and 1982 were used as the validating criterion. A total of 10.3% of dentin lesions were not diagnosed clinically in the 1974 sample, compared to 32.2% not diagnosed clinically in the 1982 sample ($p < 0.001$). Their conclusion was that occlusal caries had become more difficult to diagnose clinically.

A number of other studies have examined this phenomenon, which has variously been described as "hidden", "occult" or "clinically undetected caries" [9, 10]. These studies have likewise used radiographs as the validating criterion. Although not the ideal validating criterion, which would be histological validation, radiographs are acceptable in these studies as they are the only available technique. It must be remembered that radiographic diagnosis of occlusal dentin caries has been reported to have a low false-positive rate [11].

Creanor et al. (1990), like Sawle and Andlaw (1988), used visual and tactile clinical diagnostic methods. They examined a large sample of adolescents ($n = 2623$) in Lanarkshire, Scotland, and reported the prevalence of undetected dentinal caries

[1, 10]. This study confirmed the presence of clinically undetected occlusal dentinal caries as a problem. Further they found this to be a greater problem in the lower than the upper arch: 12.1% of lower molars and 3.1% of upper molars showed evidence of dentinal caries in the absence of a "firm clinical" diagnosis of dentin caries.

Likewise, a study of 15-year olds in the Isle of Wight, UK in 1987, reported a significantly greater prevalence of undetected dentinal caries in the lower than the upper arch, 12.9% and 6.3%, respectively, a higher prevalence than that reported in the Scottish study [12]. However, no difference in the presence of undetected lesions in upper and lower jaws was found by the two Dutch studies, although both studies agreed hidden dentinal caries was a problem [9, 13]. One of these Dutch studies with a sample of 359 children attending a dental hospital was examined in a dental surgery, rather than under the less than optimal conditions of the other studies [9].

Direct comparison of the results of these studies must be undertaken with caution due to variation in the training of examiners, criteria used to define caries and methods of diagnosis used both clinically and radiographically. For example, the teeth in the Lanarkshire study were not dried with compressed air, whereas the teeth in the Isle of Wight study were dried [10, 12]. It is also not clear how well trained and calibrated the examiners were in some of the studies. Similarly, the samples vary in their size, age group and how representative they are, for example the Dutch dental hospital sample may have a bias in terms of caries risk compared to a sample drawn from the general population [9].

4.2 Prevalence

The prevalence of undetected dentinal caries appears to be of the order 2–25% in adolescents, depending on the diagnostic criteria employed (Table 4.1). A prevalence of 13–15% of completely sound teeth (apparently clinically free of enamel and dentin caries) were found to have radiographically detectable dentinal caries in these projects [9, 10]. The study of Weerheijm et al. (1992) reported a higher prevalence of such lesions, 26% in a sample of 14-year olds, similar to the 32% reported by Sawle and Andlaw for their 1982 sample of 14–16-year olds and 25% reported by Kidd, Naylor and Wilson (1992) [1, 12, 13]. The latter three studies only included clinically diagnosed dentin lesions in their criteria for a positive diagnosis of caries. These more restricted criteria may explain the different prevalence from the studies which included enamel lesions.

One study has reported a higher prevalence of hidden caries in an older age group, 20-year olds [13]. This study found a prevalence of 50% for molar teeth,

Table 4.1 Estimated prevalence of radiographically diagnosed dentinal occlusal caries not diagnosed using various diagnostic thresholds

Method	Prevalence (%)
Traditional dentin caries threshold [12]	25
Enamel caries threshold [9, 10]	13–15
Meticulous caries diagnostic system [19]	2

which is higher than that reported for younger subjects. However, this study did include sealed surfaces, which may have masked caries that may otherwise have been diagnosed clinically [14]. One study explicitly excluded sealed surfaces from the analysis, whilst the other studies referred to did not explicitly deal with this issue [10]. In this sample of 14-year-old subjects, 32% of "sound" sealed teeth ($n = 174$) had a radiolucency in dentin. These radiolucencies may be due to either caries or the presence of radiolucent materials used in sealant restorations. This situation is now further complicated by changes in our understanding of caries and its management, which mean we would now routinely seal non-cavitated occlusal dentin lesions [15].

Only one study has reported the prevalence of clinically undetected dentinal caries at a subject, rather than tooth level, in which it was reported that 7.5% of 12-year-old children in a dental hospital sample had clinically undetected dentinal caries [9].

Despite variation in design, all of the studies discussed here suggest that clinically undetected dentinal caries is a problem for both clinicians and epidemiologists alike.

The presence of hidden caries has in part lead to the development of tools to aid with caries diagnosis such as laser fluorescence devices. However, no clinical study has reported the ability of fibre optic transillumination, fluorescence, laser fluorescence devices or electrical impedance devices to specifically identify hidden caries.

One further complication is that pre-eruptive intra-coronal resorption has been reported with a prevalence of up to 2%, it is unclear if this accounts for some of the hidden caries identified [16].

Although some of the studies reporting hidden caries have worked at the enamel carious lesion level of diagnosis, few have used a modern validated meticulous caries diagnostic systems (such as those described in Chaps. 5, 6, 7 and 8); using such a system the prevalence of "hidden" caries is lower at 2% [17, 18]. Unfortunately,

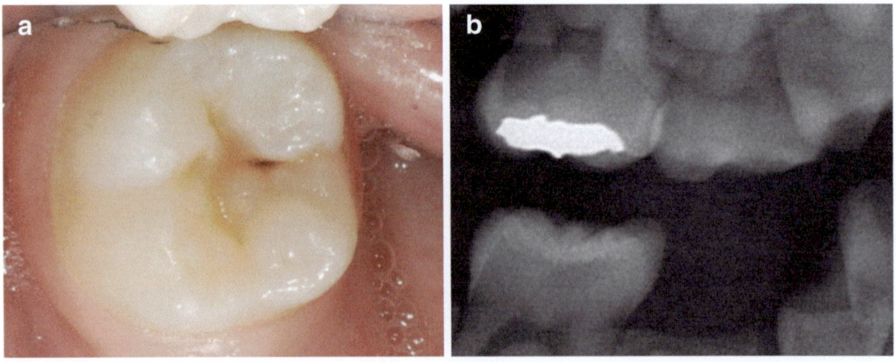

Fig. 4.2 (**a**, **b**) What appears to be enamel caries lesion (ICDAS code 2) revealing a lesion halfway into dentin, dentin in some studies this would be considered "hidden" caries but of course it is not hidden, even if more advanced than clinically apparent

no study has reported the prevalence of hidden occlusal dentinal caries in unsealed or restored teeth, with radiographic validation using one of these systems.

Overall using diagnostic systems that include enamel caries, the prevalence of hidden caries is much lower than initially reported. However, radiographs are required to ensure lesions are not missed and to confirm the depth of the lesion (Fig. 4.2a, b).

4.3 Concluding Remarks

In summary, studies suggest that hidden caries is a problem for clinicians and epidemiologists. The use of diagnostics aids as those described in Part II of this book can significantly reduce the prevalence of hidden caries. The available evidence does not support the concept that fluoride either in water or toothpaste has altered the clinical presentation of caries.

References

1. Sawle RF, Andlaw RJ. Has occlusal caries become more difficult to diagnose? A study comparing clinically undetected lesions in molar teeth of 14–16-year old children in 1974 and 1982. Br Dent J. 1988;164:209–11.
2. Backer Dirks O, Houwink B, Kwant GW. The results of 6.5 years of artificial fluoridation of drinking water in the Netherlands: the Tiel-Culemborg experiment. Arch Oral Biol. 1961;5:284–300.
3. Weerheijm KL, Kidd EAM, Groen HJ. The effect of fluoridation on the occurrence of hidden caries in clinically sound occlusal surfaces. Caries Res. 1997;31:30–4.
4. Whelton H, O'Mullane DO, McLoughlin J. Caries levels in Ireland according to varying diagnostic criteria. J Dent Res. 1996;75:85.
5. Hashizume LN, Mathias TC, Cibils DM, Maltz M. Effect of the widespread use of fluorides on the occurrence of hidden caries in children. Int J Paediatr Dent. 2013;23:72–6.
6. Konig KG. Dental morphology in relation to caries resistance with special reference to fissures as susceptible areas. J Dent Res. 1963;42:461–76.
7. Sognnaes RF. The importance of a detailed clinical examination of carious lesions. J Dent Res. 1940;19:11–5.
8. Slack GL, Jackson D, James PMC, Lawton FE. A clinical investigation into the variability of dental caries diagnosis. Br Dent J. 1958;104:399–404.
9. Weerheijm KL, Gruythuysen RJM, van Amerongen WE. Prevalence of hidden caries. J Dent Child. 1992;59:408–12.
10. Creanor SL, Russell JI, Strang DM, Stephen KW, Burchell CK. The prevalence of clinically undetected occlusal dentine caries in Scottish adolescents. Br Dent J. 1990;169:126–9.
11. Wenzel A, Fejerskov O, Kidd E, Joyston-Bechal S, Groeneveld A. Depth of occlusal caries assessed clinically, by conventional film radiographs, and by digitized, processed radiographs. Caries Res. 1990;24:327–33.
12. Kidd EAM, Naylor NM, Wilson F. Prevalence of clinically undetected and untreated molar occlusal dentine caries in adolescents on the Isle of Wight. Caries Res. 1992;26:397–401.
13. Weerheijm K, Groen HJ, Bast AJJ, Kieft JA, Eijkman MAJ, van Amerongen WE. Clinically undetected occlusal dentine caries: a radiographic comparison. Caries Res. 1992;26:305–9.
14. Deery C, Fyffe HE, Nugent Z, Nuttall NM, Pitts NB. The effect of placing a clear pit and fissure sealant on the validity and reproducibility of occlusal caries diagnosis. Caries Res. 1995;29:377–81.

15. Deery C. Caries detection and diagnosis, sealants and management of the possibly carious fissure. Br Dent J. 2013;214:551–7.
16. Spierer WA, Fuks AB. Pre-eruptive intra-coronal resorption: controversies and treatment options. J Clin Pediatr Dent. 2014;38(4):326–8.
17. Pitts NB, Ekstrand KR, ICDAS Foundation. International Caries Detection and Assessment System (ICDAS) and its International Caries Classification and Management System (ICCMS)—methods for staging of the caries process and enabling dentists to manage caries. Community Dent Oral Epidemiol. 2013;41:e41–52.
18. Nyvad B, Machiulskiene V, Baelum V. Construct and predictive validity of clinical caries diagnostic criteria assessing lesion activity. J Dent Res. 2003;82:117–22.
19. Machiulskiene V, Nyvad B, Baelum V. A comparison of clinical and radiographic caries diagnoses in posterior teeth of 12-year-old Lithuanian children. Caries Res. 1999;33:340–8.

Part II

Visual Detection Criteria

5 Nyvad Criteria for Assessment of Caries Lesion Activity and Severity

Vita Machiulskiene

5.1 Introduction

Dental caries lesions develop as a result of continuous interactions between the microbial biofilm and the tooth surface. Depending on the pH fluctuations in the biofilm, there are periods of dominating mineral loss and alternatively, mineral gain. As long as these episodes are in balance, no caries progression occurs. However, shifting the reactions towards mineral dissolution would eventually produce demineralized areas called caries lesions.

This chapter describes the clinical alterations that are visible due to the changes that occur in enamel and dentin during the demineralization and remineralization process. It also delineates how to conduct the clinical examination.

5.2 Background

The first clinically visible alterations of the "sound" dental enamel appear as changes in luster, color, or texture. These changes occur due to increased porosity of the subsurface enamel layer, and the subsequent change of light transmission in the demineralized area. It was shown years ago by Thylstrup and coworkers that the surface characteristics of caries lesions reflect the underlying mechanisms of de- and re-mineralization and that actively progressing enamel lesions exhibit matt/chalky and rough surfaces [1, 2]. However, in situations of predominating mineral uptake from the oral environment, the surface texture becomes shiny and smooth. Such lesions are usually characterized by a pronounced surface abrasion and by an increased mineralization of the surface layer [3, 4]. Clinical status of the caries

V. Machiulskiene (✉)
Clinical Department of Dental and Oral Pathology, Faculty of Odontology, Medical Academy, Lithuanian University of Health Sciences, Kaunas, Lithuania
e-mail: vita.maciulskiene@lsmuni.lt

© Springer Nature Switzerland AG 2019

A. Ferreira Zandona, C. Longbottom (eds.), *Detection and Assessment of Dental Caries*, https://doi.org/10.1007/978-3-030-16967-1_5

lesions can change depending on the oral environment. As suggested by the Dutch researcher Otto Backer Dirks back in 1966 [5], the transition of active, progressing lesions into arrested or even regressing lesions is a result of the altered environmental conditions due to masticatory cleansing effect and mechanical removal of bacterial accumulations from the surfaces of teeth. A number of clinical and experimental studies, later on, have confirmed that this process can be successfully controlled by means of regular biofilm removal and fluoride presence in the oral environment.

From the clinical point of view, it is important to determine whether the caries lesions detected on the tooth surfaces show signs of progression and therefore need to be taken care of, or appear inactive and do not require any external intervention (see Chap. 22). Clinical differentiation of the detected lesions according to their stage of activity *(active/progressing or inactive/arrested)* helps the dental professionals to choose the appropriate management strategy and to control the progression of the detected lesions. Demineralization and remineralization reactions do occur in enamel, and in dentin [6]. Therefore, progression of the caries process can be controlled not only in the lesions confined to enamel but also in the cavities extending through the enamel into dentin, provided that the surface is accessible to mechanical cleaning and to exchange of minerals with the surrounding environment.

Following the above-described investigations, a set of visual-tactile caries diagnostic criteria for caries lesion activity assessment was developed in the last decade of the twentieth century by Nyvad and coworkers and, later on, tested in the clinical trials for their reliability and validity. The scoring system has been shown to have good reliability and also construct and predictive validity for the assessment of caries lesion activity [7, 8].

The criteria are designed for use in clinical practice as well as for public health needs. They can be used for scoring caries lesions in primary as well as in permanent teeth. Most importantly from the patient's perspective, there are clear prognostic benefits in assessing caries lesion activity. As confirmed in the longitudinal clinical trials, the active non-cavitated lesions run a significantly greater risk of progressing to a cavity than do the inactive (arrested) non-cavitated lesions [8]. The risk is lower in the subjects regularly brushing their teeth with fluoride toothpaste. Caries lesion activity assessments may be used to estimate the treatment needs and linked with subsequent treatment decisions for the individual patients [9] as well as to monitor the clinical course of the detected caries lesions [10–12].

In summary, determination of the lesion activity reflects the present status of the lesion and is therefore linked with the subsequent treatment strategy. The rationale of differentiating caries lesions according to their stage of activity is based on the argument that active, progressing lesions need active care, whereas inactive or arrested caries lesions do not. The surfaces of arrested lesions are usually free of the dental biofilm, and therefore, the underlying de-mineralization and re-mineralization processes are in balance. Thus, such lesions do not need any treatment. The determined stage of the lesion activity can change any time, depending on the oral environment, thus requiring revision of the treatment strategy.

5.3 Clinical Procedure

As described above, the Nyvad criteria are based on the patho-anatomical surface characteristics of the caries lesions, rather than on the depth of lesion penetration. Nevertheless, the scoring system incorporates two levels of severity: non-cavitated and cavitated. The non-cavitated level of caries detection is used to define lesions located in enamel without visible surface breakdown, while the localized enamel discontinuities as well as overt cavities fall into the category of "cavitated lesions." The reason for including the severity aspect in the clinical classification of the lesion is that the surface characteristics of enamel and dentine lesions differ, so do the management options. Although the non-operative treatment approach is generally preferable, in cases of non-cleansable cavities in dentin, surgical intervention cannot be avoided.

The teeth need to be free from dental plaque prior to the dental examination. The patients are usually asked to clean their teeth with toothbrush and toothpaste. Performance of professional cleaning with rotor-aided cups is not advised since it may abrade the superficial layer of the lesion, and consequently, certain characteristics pertaining to lesion activity assessment (e.g., plaque stickiness to the surface of an active lesion, or surfaces roughness) may be lost.

When assessing the activity status of caries lesions, a combination of several visual-tactile surface characteristics needs to be considered: texture, translucency/opacity, lesion location, and partially, surface color. It is important to note that all of these characteristics can be evaluated clinically when an examination is performed in a standard dental surgery setting, using routine tools for dental inspection, i.e., dental mirror and explorer. The examination conditions do require proper lighting as well as compressed air to be available. Each dental surface under examination should be carefully dried with a blast of air for 10–15 s, in order to prevent saliva entering the examination field. Extensive overdrying is not recommended as desiccated enamel surface appears whitish and can mask signs of demineralization. The clinical experience with the Nyvad criteria has shown that sharp dental explorer is a more helpful supplementary tool for the evaluation of the surface morphology than a ball-ended probe. By means of the explorer, dental plaque remnants can be carefully removed from the lesion, and integrity as well as roughness of the surface layer can be sensed through vibrations of the instrument. Although use of sharp explorers in the caries detection process has been criticized for their potential to damage demineralized areas of the enamel [13], no evidence exists about the clinical relevance of this phenomenon, particularly with regard to caries lesion progression. Of course, caution should be taken when examining the dental surface, in order to minimize harmful effects of probing for the enamel. Thus, the tip of the probe should be moved gently across the surface at an angle of 20–30°, with no vigorous poking into the surface.

Most of the surface features, such as *translucency/opacity*, *location*, and *color*, can be evaluated visually.

Active enamel caries lesions are characterized by matt/chalky, whitish, or yellowish appearance. They feel rough when explorer is gently moved across the surface. Such lesions are typically located in pits and fissures of the occlusal surfaces or close to gingival margin on the smooth surfaces. Very often the active lesions may be covered with a thin, sticky plaque layer remaining on the tooth surface even after toothbrushing. Therefore, careful removal of such remnants by means of the explorer is indicated to check for the absence or presence of lesion beneath the plaque.

Active lesions in dentin present similar surface characteristics. However, since dentin has a higher organic component, active lesions will fell softer rather than rougher. In cases of the transitional stage from active to inactive, it may feel leathery and somewhat resistant to probing. The color is not a decisive factor. However, light/yellowish color in combination with soft texture mostly represents active progression while brownish discoloration of the rubbery texture is more typical for transitional or slowly progressing lesions.

In contrast, inactive caries lesions are glossy and smooth on probing. The color of such lesions in enamel may vary from whitish to brownish or black. In fact, the lesion color is only a secondary diagnostic feature as in cases of relatively early and shallow arrested lesions; due to lack of acquired pigmentation, it can be as white as an active lesion. Inactive enamel lesions can be detected in pits and fissures of the occlusal surfaces; on the smooth surfaces, they are located at a distance from gingival margin. Inactive lesions are usually free from dental plaque.

Inactive/arrested lesions in dentin feel smooth and hard on gentle probing, with varying degree of discoloration. It is important to note that for a dentin lesion to be defined as inactive, no enamel margins overhanging the cavity floor should be present. Presence of the enamel overhangs may mask active parts of the lesion that are not accessible to mechanical cleaning.

Of course, in practice, there are situations when clinical appearance of a caries lesion does not match the typical description of the activity stage. Due to the dynamic nature of dental caries, the same lesion may contain active and inactive parts of progression. In case of a "mixed" set of characteristics, the lesion is considered active and needs to be controlled to prevent further progression.

The Nyvad classification includes scores for secondary caries that are based on the same criteria as for primary caries lesions. In other words, when a caries lesion is detected next to a filling, it should be evaluated for its severity (non-cavitated or cavitated) and for the activity stage (active or inactive). From the treatment perspective, many fillings surrounded with discolored margins or micro-gaps without signs of activity can be saved from repeated restoration procedures. Likewise, the fillings accompanied by active non-cavitated lesions can still be monitored non-operatively, based on the same principles as for primary non-cavitated active lesions.

Root caries lesions are scored following the same principle as coronal dentin lesions (Fig. 5.1 and Tables 5.1 and 5.2).

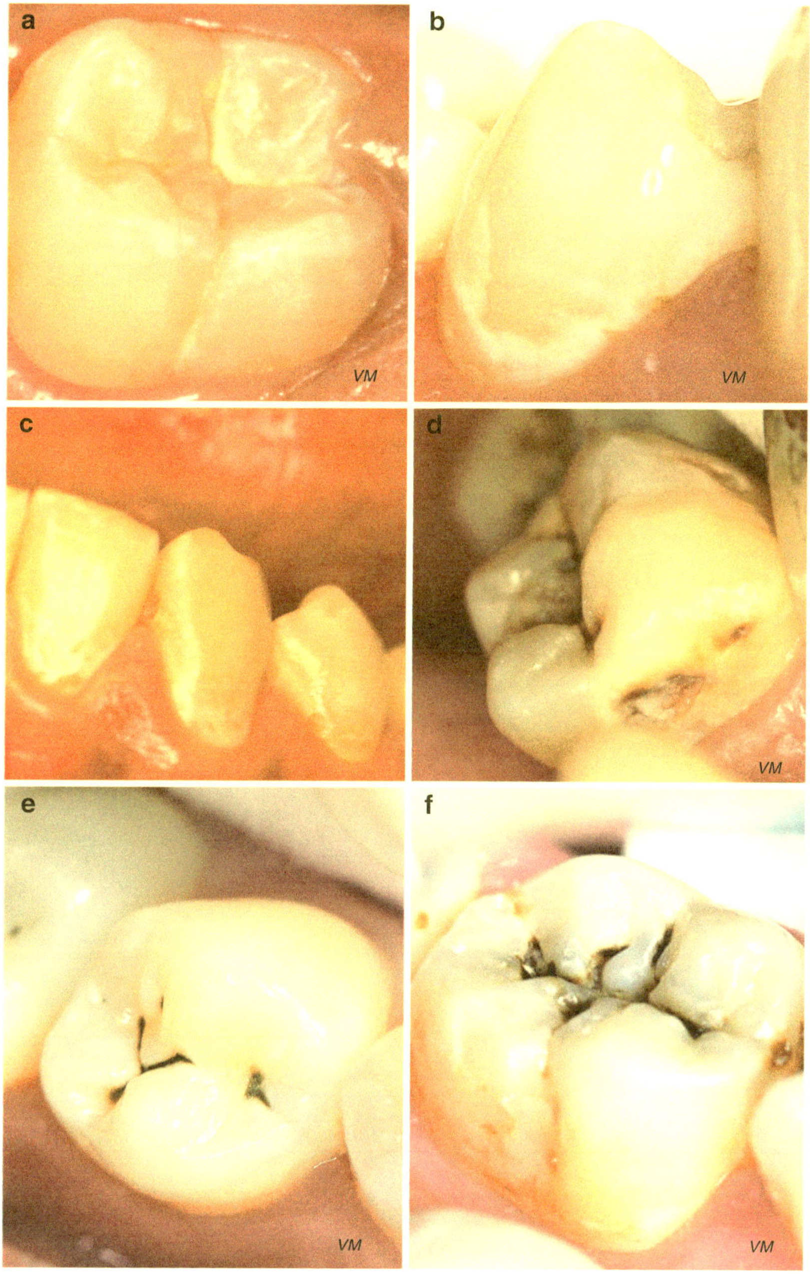

Fig. 5.1 Examples of Nyvad clinical criteria for caries lesion activity assessment. (**a**) Active, non-cavitated lesion; score 1, occlusal surface. (**b**) Active, non-cavitated lesion, score 1, smooth surface. (**c**) Active microcavity, score 2, approximal and smooth surface. (**d**) Active cavitated lesion, score 3, approximal surface. (**e**) Inactive non-cavitated lesion, score 4, occlusal surface. (**f**) Inactive microcavity, score 5, occlusal surface. (**g**) Inactive microcavity, score 5, smooth surface. (**h**) Filling + active caries, score 7, occlusal surface. Inactive non-cavitated, score 4, smooth surface. (**i**) Filling + inactive caries, score 8, smooth and occlusal surfaces

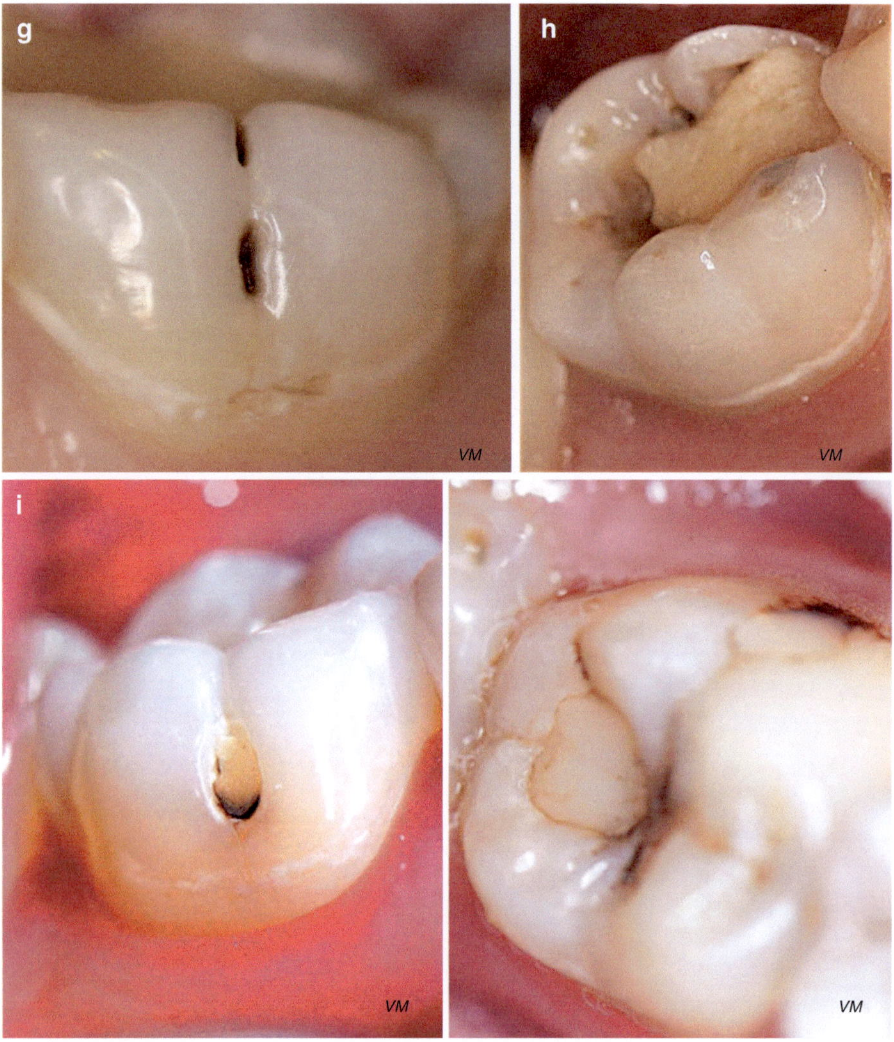

Fig. 5.1 (continued)

Table 5.1 Description of codes for scoring activity and severity of enamel, coronal, and root dentin caries lesions [7]

Score	Category	Criteria
0	**Sound**	Normal enamel translucency and texture (slight staining allowed in the fissure)
1	**Active, non-cavitated**	Whitish/yellowish opaque with loss of luster; feels rough when the tip of the explorer is moved across the surface; usually covered with plaque. No clinically detectable loss of substance Smooth surface: lesion typically located close to the gingival margin Pit/fissure: intact fissure morphology, lesion extending along the walls
	Active, cavitated	
2	Surface discontinuity	Same as score 1. Localized surface defect (micro-cavity) in enamel only
3	Cavity	Enamel/dentin cavity visible with the naked eye; surface feels soft or leathery on gentle probing. There may or may not be pulpal involvement
4	**Inactive, non-cavitated**	Whitish-brownish, or black. The surface is shiny, feels hard, and smooth when the tip of the explorer is moved across the surface. No clinically detectable loss of substance Smooth surface: lesion typically located at a distance from gingival margin Pit/fissure: intact fissure morphology, lesion extending along the walls
	Inactive cavitated	
5	Surface discontinuity	Same as score 4. Localized surface defect (microcavity) in enamel only
6	Cavity	Enamel/dentin cavity visible with the naked eye; the surface may be shiny, feels hard on gentle probing. No pulpal involvement
7	**Filling**	
8	**Filling + active caries**	Active (criteria as above) lesion next to filling may be non-cavitated or cavitated
9	**Filling + inactive caries**	Inactive (criteria as above) lesion next to filling may be non-cavitated or cavitated

Table 5.2 Summary

Nyvad criteria for clinical assessment of caries lesion activity				
Which surfaces/ sites is it useful for	Occlusal (pits and fissures)	Proximal/ (approximal)	Smooth surface (buccal and lingual)	Root caries (all surfaces)
	Y	**Y**	**Y**	**Y**

(continued)

Table 5.2 (continued)

Nyvad criteria for clinical assessment of caries lesion activity				
What type of lesions is valuable for	Primary coronal	Secondary coronal	Primary root caries	Secondary root caries
	Y	**Y**	**Y**	**Y**
What type of dentition	Primary		Permanent	
	Y		**Y**	
Lesion severity	Enamel lesions		Dentinal lesions	
	Y		**Y**	
Sensitivity[a]	0.78–0.90%[b]			
Specificity[a]	0.74–0.81%[b]			
Perceived ease of use (PEOU)	It is easy to become skillful at using "Nyvad criteria"			
Advantages of Nyvad criteria	1. Are linked to various treatment options 2. Have a prognostic value 3. Can be used for the estimation of treatment outcomes 4. Can be applied for research purposes, in clinical studies of caries management 5. Easily applicable in standard clinical settings			
Restrictions	Are not advised to be used without a proper understanding of the biological background of the criteria, in non-standardized examination conditions			
Time	30–50 s for each tooth surface; might take a couple of minutes for drying the surface and adjusting the light prior to inspection			

[a]It is not appropriate to validate the criteria for caries lesion activity histologically as they are based on the surface characteristics rather than on the lesion depth. Reliability of the Nyvad criteria was evaluated in the clinical settings by several research groups and showed very good or excellent reproducibility of the scores, both in permanent and in primary dentition [7, 14]. The criteria were shown to have predictive and construct validity as they reflected the well-known caries inhibiting effect of fluoride [8, 15]

[b]There is only one study [16] that attempted to estimate the accuracy of the Nyvad criteria, in relation to lesion depth, but not to the activity status

5.4 Concluding Remarks

The Nyvad visual caries classification criteria reflect the visual-tactile surface characteristics of the caries lesions such as integrity, texture, translucency/opacity, lesion location and surface color. The criteria incorporates scores for active/progressing and inactive/arrested lesions at two levels of severity, non-cavitated and cavitated. Clinical differentiation of the detected lesions according to their stage of activity allows dental professionals to identify lesions that are in need of treatment, to choose the appropriate management strategy, and to monitor the course of the disease.

References

1. Holmen L, Thylstrup A, Ogaard B, Kragh F. A polarized light microscopic study of progressive stages of enamel caries in vivo. Caries Res. 1985;19:348–54.
2. Holmen L, Thylstrup A, Ogaard B, Kragh F. A scanning electron microscopic of progressive stages of enamel caries in vivo. Caries Res. 1985;19:355–67.
3. Silvestrone LM. Remineralization phenomena. Caries Res. 1977;11:59–84.
4. Thylstrup A, Bruun C, Holmen L. In vivo caries models—mechanisms for caries initiation and arrestment. Adv Dent Res. 1994;8:44–57.
5. Backer Dirks O. Post eruptive changes in dental enamel. J Dent Res. 1966;45:503–11.
6. Kidd EA, Fejerskov O. What constitutes dental caries? Histopathology of carious enamel and dentin related to the action of cariogenic biofilms. J Dent Res. 2004;83 Spec No C:C35–8.
7. Nyvad B, Machiulskiene V, Baelum V. Reliability of a new caries diagnostic system differentiating between active and inactive caries lesions. Caries Res. 1999;33:252–60.
8. Nyvad B, Machiulskiene V, Baelum V. Construct and predictive validity of clinical caries diagnostic criteria assessing lesion activity. J Dent Res. 2003;82:117–22.
9. Nyvad B, Fejerskov O. Assessing the stage of caries lesion activity on the basis of clinical and microbiological examination. Community Dent Oral Epidemiol. 1997;25:69–75.
10. Carvalho JC, Thylstrup A, Ekstrand KR. Results after 3 years of non-operative occlusal caries treatment of erupting first permanent molars. Community Dent Oral Epidemiol. 1992;20:187–92.
11. Machiulskiene V, Richards A, Nyvad B, Baelum V. Prospective study of the effect of post-brushing rinsing behaviour on dental caries. Caries Res. 2002;36:301–7.
12. Maltz M, et al. Result after two years of non-operative treatment of occlusal surfaces in children with high caries prevalence. Braz Dent J. 2003;14:48–54.
13. Stookey G. Should a dental explorer be used to probe suspected carious lesions?. No—use of an explorer can lead to misdiagnosis and disrupt remineralization. J Am Dent Assoc. 2005;136:1527.
14. Sellos MS, Soviero M. Reliability of the Nyvad criteria for caries assessment in primary teeth. Eur J Oral Sci. 2011;119:225–31.
15. Nyvad B, Baelum V. Nyvad criteria for caries lesion activity and severity assessment: a validated approach for clinical management and research. Caries Res. 2018;52:397–405.
16. Braga MM, Mendes FM, Martignon S, Ricketts DN, Ekstrand KR. In vitro comparison of Nyvad's system and ICDAS-II with lesion activity assessment for evaluation of severity and activity of occlusal caries lesions in primary teeth. Caries Res. 2009;43:405–12.

Visual Detection Criteria Using the International Caries Detection and Assessment System (ICDAS)

6

Kim R. Ekstrand and Mariana M. M. B. Braga

6.1 Introduction and Historical Perspective

The international Caries Detection and Assessment system (ICDAS) was devised to allow for a means to more reliable communicate regarding caries classification. This chapter describes the ICDAS criteria, provides guidelines for its' use and clinical considerations for the management of dental caries relating to the different ICDAS scores. At the beginning of this millennium, it was the general feeling that reliabilities and accuracies of the available caries detection/diagnostic systems (at that time) were not strong [1, 2]. A conference was held in Dundee, Scotland, in 2002 with the aim of devising a caries scoring system which was reliable with regard to coronal caries, root caries, and caries adjacent to restorations. Concerning coronal caries, it was suggested to use the Ekstrand, Kidd, Ricketts system (ERK-system) as a base, because that system had used histology as validation [3–6]. Activity assessment of the lesions had also been done [4]. It was decided to expand the 5-score ERK-system to a 7-score-system. The scoring system devised for caries adjacent to restorations eventually got the same 7 scores, while for classifying root caries the scores were restricted to 3. The participants at the congress named the new scoring system "The International Caries Detection and Assessment System," in short ICDAS [7–9].

At follow-up meetings in 2005 and 2007, criteria for activity assessment of the lesion and a radiographical scoring system were both devised [9–11], completing the addressed needs for caries lesion assessment in clinical practice.

K. R. Ekstrand (✉)
Department of Odontology, University of Copenhagen, Copenhagen, Denmark
e-mail: kek@sund.ku.dk

M. M. M. B. Braga (✉)
Pediatric Dentistry, University of São Paulo, São Paulo, SP, Brazil
e-mail: mmbraga@usp.br

© Springer Nature Switzerland AG 2019

A. Ferreira Zandona, C. Longbottom (eds.), *Detection and Assessment of Dental Caries*, https://doi.org/10.1007/978-3-030-16967-1_6

6.2 The Detection Part of the Scoring System

The ICDAS stages the severity of the lesion and assesses lesion activity on primary caries lesions and caries lesions adjacent to restorations on both coronal surfaces and the roots [7–11]. The surface is used as a unit. Detection wise, it is a two-digit scoring system (Fig. 6.1a, b). The first digit is used to describe the status of the surface, for example, if the surface is restored with amalgam (score 4). The second digit is used to describe the caries severity (ICDAS score 0–7) at the surface.

The ICDAS for coronal caries detection is histologic-based [9, 12, 13]. The study by Ekstrand et al. [12] showed that, if a surface is scored ICDAS 0 (sound), 95% of them are actually histological without demineralization. If the lesion is scored ICDAS 1, 95% shows no demineralization or the demineralization is restricted to the outer half of the enamel. A total of 83% of ICDAS 2 lesions are characterized to be histologically wise in the inner half of the enamel or, if in dentin, restricted to the outer 1/3 of the dentin. ICDAS lesions scored as 3 or 4 are characterized by the overall majority (67%) having demineralization reaching the middle 1/3 of the dentin. Finally, the overall majority of ICDAS score 5 and 6 lesions (84%) shows histologically demineralization in the inner 1/3 of the dentin, thus close to or already in the pulp. The substantial relation between the ICDAS scores and histology relates to both primary teeth and permanent teeth [12, 14].

In **clinical settings** it may be easier to state the diagnoses as "Initial" (ICDAS scores 1 and 2), "Moderate" (ICDAS scores 3 and 4), and "Extensive" (ICDAS scores 5 and 6), rather than using the full 7 scores [15]. The 7 scores may be more relevant for some epidemiological investigations or clinical follow-up of patients in investigations.

The ICDAS root caries lesions are less well related to histology; however, one study showed that score 2 was significantly deeper than score 1 [10].

Figure 6.2a–i shows an example of how to score a particular surface with the ICDAS scores (two digits) presented in Fig. 6.1a, b.

6.2.1 The Activity Assessment of the Scoring System

To decide if a lesion is active or arrested at the time of the examination is sometimes difficult. Lesions scored as ICDAS score 3, 4, 5, and 6 concerning coronal caries and score 2 concerning root caries have a high probability for being active. Cavitated lesions harbor plaque, which is difficult to remove. The shadowed lesions (score 4) are related to demineralization reaching the middle 1/3 of the dentin, and studies have shown that there are microorganisms at the enamel–dentin junction, which is not the case in ICDAS score 1 and 2 [6]. It is more difficult to decide if lesions scored as ICDAS 1 or 2 are active or arrested.

Lesion location, visual appearance, tactile feeling, and gingival bleedings (Fig. 6.3) are variables, which have shown evidence for being able to indicate if a lesion is active or arrested, when related to ICDAS [12–19]. Each variable can then be dichotomized or divided into three scripts concerning the lesion or the gingiva next to the lesion. Whether gingiva bleeds or not is only useful to assess

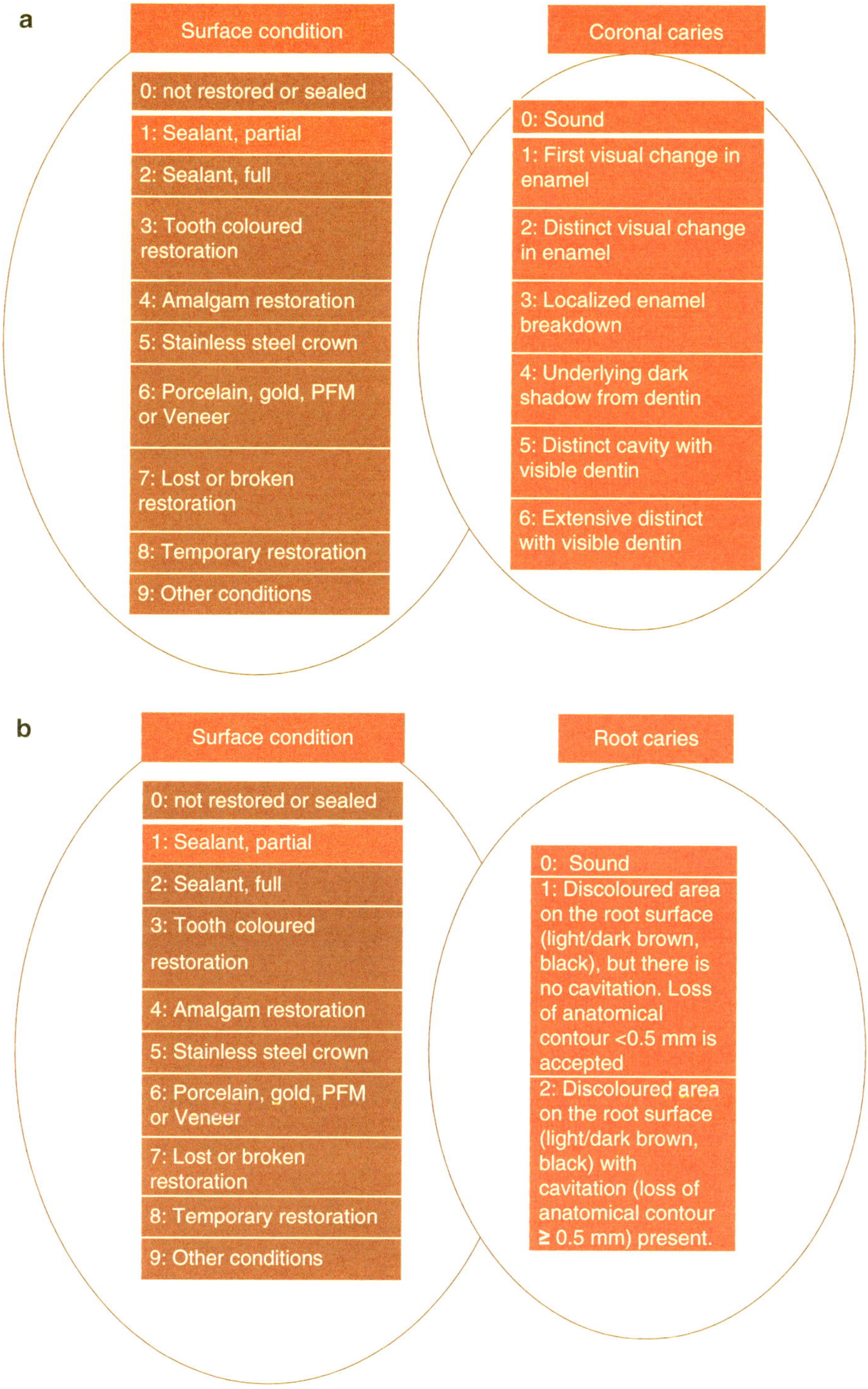

Fig. 6.1 (**a**) ICDAS scores devised for tooth status (1. digit) and coronal caries (2. digit). (**b**) ICDAS scores devised for tooth status (1. digit) and root caries (2. digit)

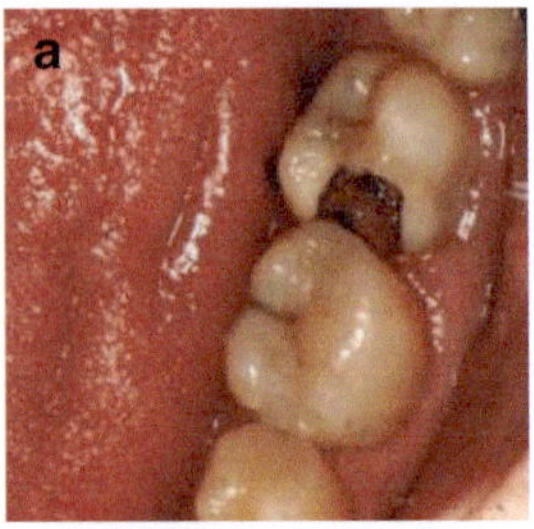

2nd molar Occlusally 3, 5
2nd molar Mesially 0, 6

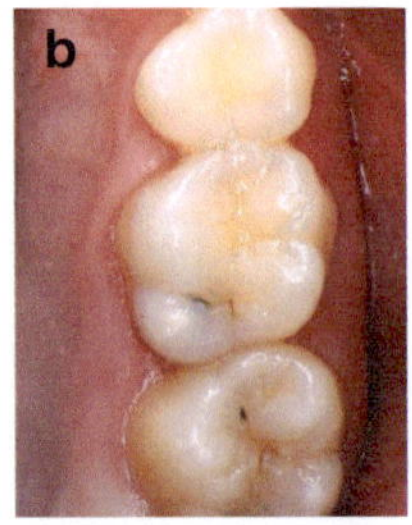

2nd premolar Occlusally 0, 0
1st molar Occlusally 0, 4
2nd molar Occlusally 0, 3

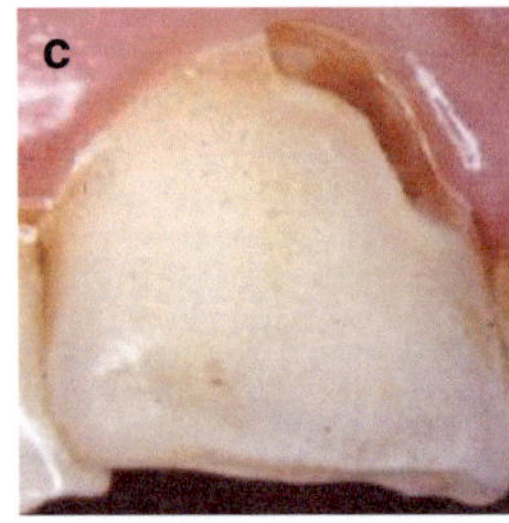

Central incisor Buccally 0, 5

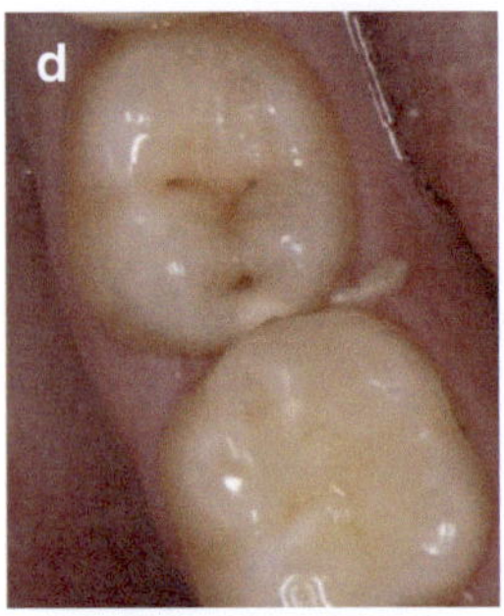

2nd molar Mesially 0, 4;
1st molar Occlusally 5, 0

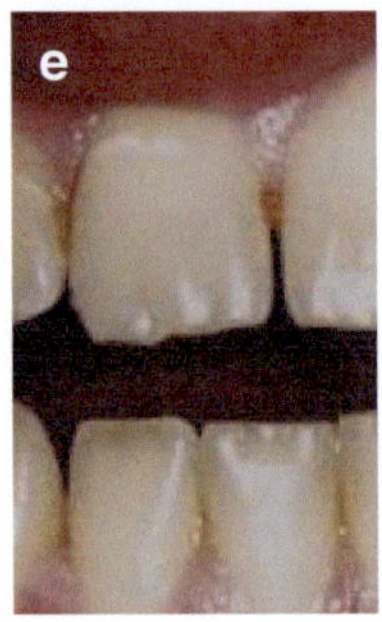

Central incisor Buccally 0, 2

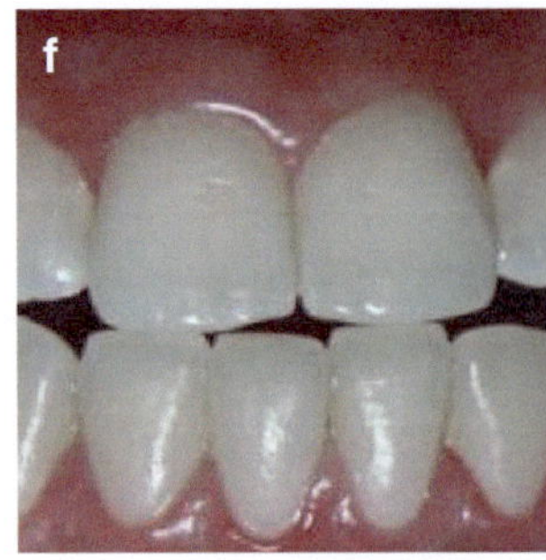

Left lateral Mesially 0, 2
Right lateral Mesially 0, 2

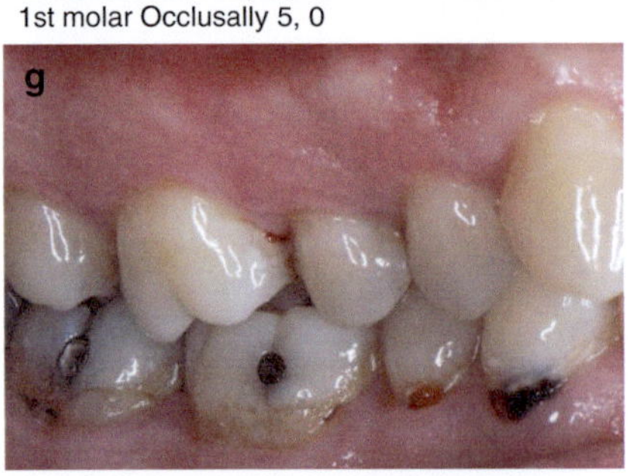

2nd mandibular premolar buccally 0, 2 root caries
1st mandibular premolar buccaly 0, 2 root caries

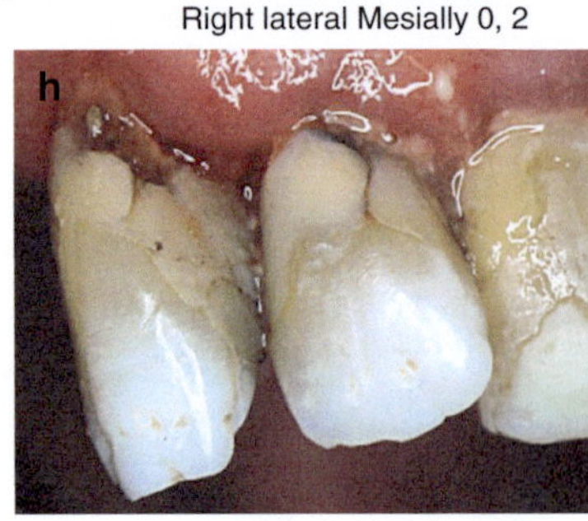

Cuspid buccally 3, 2 root caries

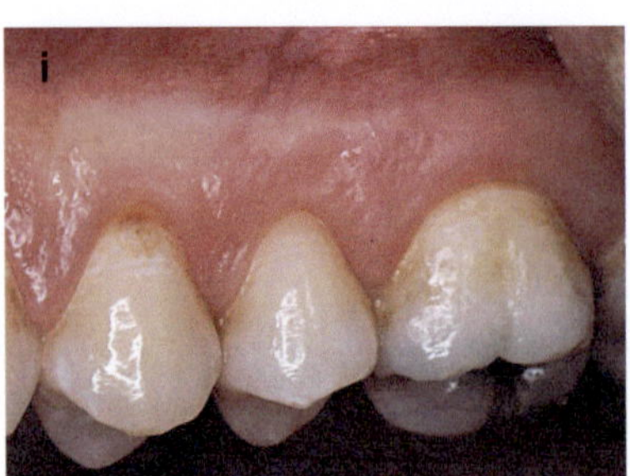

1st premolar buccally, 0, 1 root caries
2nd premolar buccally, 0, 0

Fig. 6.2 (**a**–**i**) Images of tooth surfaces and the related ICDAS scores. (1) Digit the status of the surfaces, (2) digit the caries stages

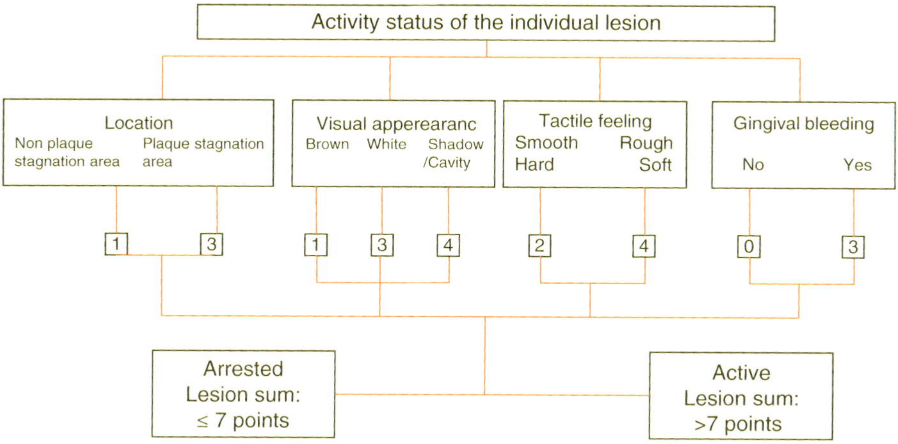

Fig. 6.3 Variables and scripts used to assess activity status of coronal lesions. Each script's predictive power is expressed in points. If the total score adding up the points for each script is less than 7 points, the lesion is arrested. If 7 points or more, the lesion is active

when the lesion is located close to the gingiva, such as on approximal or smooth surfaces [19].

Some papers have used these scripts for activity assessment of the lesions judged over a couple of years [17, 18]. The final assessment if the lesion was active or arrested was then done based on the gut feeling combining those scripts, thus rather subjectively. Ekstrand et al. [12] suggested a more objective approach because a study showed that the predictive power of the different scripts was different (Fig. 6.3). These predictive values were calculated based on the validation of activity status of lesions using a pH-sensitive impression material [12]. The highest predictive power for lesion activity was when the lesion was cavitated, the enamel was rough, and the dentin soft. If the lesion was located in a plaque stagnation area (in the groove fossa system, approximately between molar teeth or along the gingiva), the predictive power was lower than those above. This was also the case if the lesion appeared whitish. Those scripts with lowest predicting power for a lesion is active if the lesion was smooth or hard to probing, the lesion was brown, and the lesion was not located in a plaque stagnation area (>1 mm away from the gingiva). Figure 6.3 shows the points allocated to each script related to their predictive power. The study [12] further revealed that if the points from the scripts were added up, then arrested lesions got at a maximum of 7 points, while active lesions achieved more than 7 points.

Concerning the first upper right molar occlusally (Fig. 6.2b) on an 18-year-old individual, the lesion is located in a plaque stagnation area and will achieve **3 points**; the lesion appeared shadowed (**4 points**); and the lesion was rough to probing (**3 points**) given a total of 10 points, therefore active. The lesion buccally on 11 in Fig. 6.2e on a 34-year-old individual achieved 6 points: (location **1 point**; visual appearance **3 points**, tactile feeling **2 points**, and gingiva bleeding **0 points**). The lesion is then considered arrested. Finally, the two mesial lesions on the laterals in Fig. 6.2f on a 25-year-old individual are both active (totally 13 points).

6.3 Diagnoses and Treatment

Active lesions demand management, while inactive lesions only need to receive intervention if there is a need to reestablish aesthetics or function (see Chap. 22). Considering different approaches to control caries lesions, we should consider that extensive and most moderate lesions will require a restorative intervention (operative treatment) or any kind of sealing/controlling to be arrested [15]. Initial caries lesions can be arrested by using non-operative approaches. For active lesions, Fig. 6.4 presents the relationship between the 7 ICDAS scores, when the scores are merged into initial (ICDAS score 1 and 2), moderate (ICDAS score 3 and 4), and extensive (ICDAS score 5 and 6) and the related management possibilities.

Based on the above, the diagnoses, for example, of the occlusal lesion on 16 (Fig. 6.2b) is an ICDAS score 4, active (10 points), and in need of operative intervention. The lesion on the buccal surface in Fig. 6.2e is a score 2, inactive (6 points), and does not need any intervention (surgical or non-surgical). The lesions on the laterals, in Fig. 6.2f, are ICDAS score 2 as well, but active (13 points), and they need non-operative management.

The histological stage of caries lesions evidenced by clinical conditions scored by ICDAS also reflects on the prognosis of caries lesions concerning progression. Initial lesions tended to progress 2–4 times more than sound surfaces while microcavited lesions or shadowed lesions were more than 10 times prone to progression than the same sound surfaces [17, 18]. The merged codes presented similar prognosis and consequently demand similar treatments, if they have similar activity status.

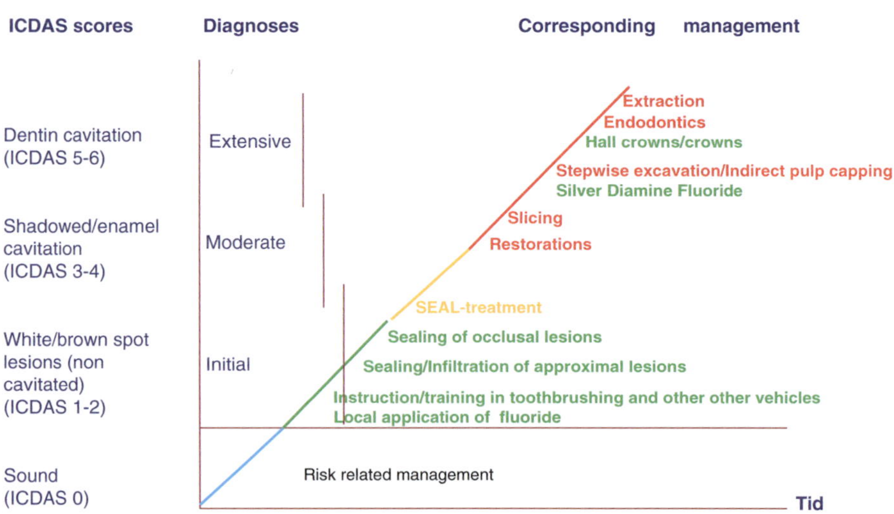

Fig. 6.4 The relation between individual ICDAS scores, merged scores, and management possibilities

6.4 Clinical Considerations

To score caries with the ICDAS requires teeth to be clean and dry [9]. Professional tooth cleaning either by means of rotating brushes or simply by manual tooth brushing would be adequate. Approximal surfaces are most easily cleaned by flossing. Cotton rolls are placed in the maxillary sulci to control saliva from the parotid glands. Each tooth is then examined following a logical, predetermined sequence to not miss any surface. For example, we could start in the maxilla in the right side of the mouth on the most posterior tooth, examining occlusal, lingual, buccal, and finally the mesial/distal interproximal surfaces. The examination proceeds in the anterior direction, completing first the upper and then the lower arch. A dental mirror is needed. Some prefer to use the three-in-one syringes to dry the consecutive teeth on the other hand and then pick up the probe when necessary. Others prefer to have a mirror on one hand and the ball-ended probe on the other hand. Please pay attention to not perform too hard probing in demineralized dental hard tissue as that can provoke defects [20, 21].

Figure 6.5 shows *one approach, among many possible*, on how to chart the observations in a patient file recording system, and the scores from Fig. 6.2a–f is placed related to tooth and surface. Red figures indicate that the lesion is active, and black indicates that the lesion is arrested. Blank cells mean that the tooth surfaces are healthy (Fig. 6.5a). In Fig. 6.5b, we present the scores after the treatment of the

a **Name** ______________________ **ID number** ______________

Teeth	18	17	16	15 55	14 54	13 53	12 52	11 51	21 61	22 62	23 63	24 64	25 65	26	27	28
Tooth Present			1	0	0	0	0	1	1	0	0	0	0	1		
Occ		0, 3	0, 4			Upper Jaw										
Mes							0, 2			0, 2						
Buc								0, 2	0, 5							
Dis																
Ora																
Tooth Present			1	0	0	0	1	1	1	1	0	0	0	1		
Occ			3.0			Lower Jaw									3, 5	
Mes		0, 4													0, 6	
Buc																
Dis																
Ora																
Teeth	48	47	46	85 45	84 44	83 43	82 42	81 41	71 31	72 32	73 33	74 34	75 35	36	37	38

Fig. 6.5 (**a**) Example of how to record the ICDAS scores using the images 6.2a–f. (1) digit tooth status, (2) digit caries. (**b**) The changes of the scores in (**a**) after management

b **Name** ______________________ **ID number** ________________

Teeth	18	17	16	15 55	14 54	13 53	12 52	11 51	21 61	22 62	23 63	24 64	25 65	26	27	28
Tooth Present			1	0	0	0	0	1	1	0	0	0	0	1		
Occ		3, 0	3, 0			Upper Jaw										
Mes							0, 2			0, 2						
Buc								0, 2	3, 0							
Dis																
Ora																
Tooth Present			1	0	0	0	1	1	1	1	0	0	0	1		
Occ			3.0			Lower Jaw									6, 0	
Mes		3.0													6, 0	
Buc															6, 0	
Dis															6, 0	
Ora															6, 0	
Teeth	48	47	46	85 45	84 44	83 43	82 42	81 41	71 31	72 32	73 33	74 34	75 35	36	37	38

Fig. 6.5 (continued)

individual lesions. We would for example suggest to crown 37 which if done would mean that the score for tooth 37 on all surfaces would be 6, 0.

In regular practice, the time spent for the examination ranges from 9 to 14 min, depending on clinical experience and method used to activity assessment [22]. This time does not include the time required to clean the teeth. In many practices, regular patients are examined after the hygiene appointment, which would fit well with this protocol. For new patients, a cursory examination of hard tissues can take place, followed by a detailed examination after x-rays are obtained and hygiene appointment is completed.

6.5 Scientific Background

Recently, a systematic review including a meta-analysis gave the following values for the ICDAS system when it concerned ICDAS related to coronal lesions [23]. The pooled intra- and inter-reproducibility in terms of kappa values were 0.67 or above, indicating a substantial reproducibility. The pooled correlation between ICDAS scores and depth was also 0.67 and above, indicating a substantial correlation between the ICDAS scores and depth of the lesion. The pooled specificity and sensitivity were both 0.7, and the area below the ROC curves was ≥0.75.

There have been no or very few studies concerning ICDAS and root caries and ICDAS adjacent to restorations. Therefore, there is little evidence for the reliability and accuracies of these sections of ICDAS.

Concerning activity assessment, the systematic review [23] stated that the ICDAS activity assessment system can classify if a lesion is arrested or active at a moderate confidence level. However, further studies should be conducted to enhance evidence in activity assessment.

To summarize, the ICDAS is a robust caries recording system, which works quite well under most conditions.

Summary table

Bitewing radiography	ICDAS			
Which surfaces/sites is it useful for	Occlusal (pits and fissures)	Proximal/ (approximal)	Smooth surface (buccal and lingual)	Root caries and which of the four surfaces?
	Y	**Y**	**Y**	**Y all surfaces**
What type of lesions is valuable for	Primary coronal	Secondary coronal	Primary root caries	Secondary root caries
	Y	**Y**	**Y**	**Y**
What type of dentition	Primary		Permanent	
	Y		**Y**	
Lesion severity	Enamel lesions		Dentinal lesions	
	N		**N**[a]	
Sensitivity (primary coronal caries)	Literature reported range in 50–80%			
Specificity (primary coronal caries)	Literature reported range in 60–80%			
Perceived ease of use (PEOU)[a]	1. ICDAS is easy-to-use 2. It is easy to become skillful at using ICDAS 3. Learning to operate ICDAS is easy 4. ICDAS is flexible to interact with 5. My interaction with ICDAS is clear and understandable 6. It is easy to interact with ICDAS			
Advantages/ disadvantages	*Advantages* 1. Easy to use 2. No especial equipment needed 3. Can monitor lesion changes over time 4. Low cost *Disadvantages* 1. Somewhat subjective 2. Need to clean surface before use 3. Calibration of examiners recommended			
Time	6 s per surface (on average)			
Cost	US$5.56 per patient			

[a]Davis (1989) [24]

6.6 Concluding Remarks

The ICDAS stages the severity of the lesion and assesses lesion activity on primary caries lesions and caries lesions adjacent to restorations on both coronal surfaces and on the roots. The criteria have 7 stages of caries severity which correlate to histological depth of the lesion and clinical prognosis.

References

1. Bader JD, Shugars DA, Bonito AJ. A systematic review of selected caries prevention and management methods. Community Dent Oral Epidemiol. 2001;29:399–411.
2. Pitts NB, Stamm JW. International consensus workshop on caries clinical trials (ICW-CCT)—final consensus statements: agreeing where the evidence leads. J Dent Res. 2004;83 Spec No C:C125–8.
3. Ekstrand KR, Ricketts DN, Kidd EA. Reproducibility and accuracy of three methods for assessment of demineralization depth of the occlusal surface: an in vitro examination. Caries Res. 1997;31(3):224–31.
4. Ekstrand KR, Ricketts DNJ, Kidd EAM, Qvist V, Schou S. Detection, diagnosing, monitoring and logical treatment of occlusal caries in relation to lesion activity and severity: an in vivo examination with histological validation. Caries Res. 1998;32: 247–54.
5. Côrtes DF, Ekstrand KR, Elias-Boneta AR, Ellwood RP. An in vitro comparison of the ability of fibre-optic transillumination, visual inspection and radiographs to detect occlusal caries and evaluate lesion depth. Caries Res. 2000;34:443–7.
6. Ricketts DN, Ekstrand KR, Kidd EA, Larsen T. Relating visual and radiographic ranked scoring systems for occlusal caries detection to histological and microbiological evidence. Oper Dent. 2002;27:231–7.
7. Pitts N. "ICDAS"—an international system for caries detection and assessment being developed to facilitate caries epidemiology, research and appropriate clinical management. Community Dent Health. 2004;21:193–8.
8. Ismail AI, Sohn W, Tellez M, et al. The International Caries Detection and Assessment System (ICDAS): an integrated system for measuring dental caries. Community Dent Oral Epidemiol. 2007;35:170–8.
9. Pitts N. Monographs in oral science—detection, assessment, diagnosis and monitoring of caries. Basel: Karger; 2009.
10. Facetti M, Elizabeth C. Association between visual characterization of root caries and histological severity in vitro. MS (Master of Science) thesis. University of Iowa; 2010. http://ir.uiowa.edu/etd/856.
11. ICDAS Foundation. International Caries Assessment and Detection System (ICDAS). http://www.icdas.org.
12. Ekstrand KR, Martignon S, Ricketts DJ, Qvist V. Detection and activity assessment of primary coronal caries lesions: a methodologic study. Oper Dent. 2007;32:225–35.
13. Ekstrand KR, Zero DT, Martignon S, Pitts NB. Lesion activity assessment. Monogr Oral Sci. 2009;21:63–90.
14. Braga MM, Mendes FM, Martignon S, Ricketts DN, Ekstrand KR. In vitro comparison of Nyvad's system and ICDAS-II with lesion activity assessment for evaluation of severity and activity of occlusal caries lesions in primary teeth. Caries Res. 2009;43: 405–12.
15. Ismail AI, Pitts NB, Tellez M, Authors of International Caries Classification and Management System (ICCMS), Banerjee A, Deery C, Douglas G, Eggertsson H, Ekstrand K, Ellwood R, Gomez J, Jablonski-Momeni A, Kolker J, Longbottom C, Manton D, Martignon S, McGrady M, Rechmann P, Ricketts D, Sohn W, Thompson V, Twetman S, Weyant R, Wolff M, Zandona A. The International Caries Classification and Management System (ICCMS™) an example of a caries management pathway. BMC Oral Health. 2015;15(Suppl 1):S9. https://doi.org/10.1186/1472-6831-15-S1-S9. Epub 2015 Sep 15.
16. Braga MM, Ekstrand KR, Martignon S, Imparato JC, Ricketts DN, Mendes FM. Clinical performance of two visual scoring systems in detecting and assessing activity status of occlusal caries in primary teeth. Caries Res. 2010;44:300–8.
17. Guedes RS, Piovesan C, Ardenghi TM, Emmanuelli B, Braga MM, Ekstrand KR, Mendes FM. Validation of visual caries activity assessment: a 2-yr cohort study. J Dent Res. 2014;93(Suppl):101S–7S.

18. Ferreira Zandoná A, Santiago E, Eckert GJ, Katz BP, Pereira de Oliveira S, Capin OR, Mau M, Zero DT. The natural history of dental caries lesions: a 4-year observational study. J Dent Res. 2012;91:841–6.
19. Ekstrand KR, Bruun G, Bruun M. Plaque and gingival status as indicators for caries progression on approximal surfaces. Caries Res. 1998;32:41–5.
20. Ekstrand KR, Qvist V, Thylstrup A. Light microscope study on the effect of probing in occlusal surfaces. Caries Res. 1987;21:368–74.
21. Mattos-Silveira J, Oliveira MM, Matos R, Moura-Netto C, Mendes FM, Braga MM. Do the ball-ended probe cause less damage than sharp explorers?—an ultrastructural analysis. BMC Oral Health. 2016;16:39.
22. Gimenez T, Bittar DG, Piovesan C, Guglielmi CAB, Fujimoto KY, Matos R, Novaes TF, Braga MM, Mendes FM. Influence of examiner experience on clinical performance of visual inspection in detecting and assessing the activity status of caries lesions. Oper Dent. 2013;38:583–90.
23. Ekstrand KR, Gimenez T, Ferreira FR, Mendes F, Braga MM. Aims, advantages and limitations of the International Caries Detection and Assessment System—ICDAS. Caries Res. 2018;52(5):406–19. https://doi.org/10.1159/000486429. Epub 2018 Mar 8.
24. Davis FD. Perceived usefulness, perceived ease of use, and user acceptance of information technology. MIS Q. 1989;13(3):319–40. https://doi.org/10.2307/249008.

7 The American Dental Association Caries Classification System (ADA CCS)

Gregory Zeller, Douglas A. Young, and Brian Novy

7.1 Introduction

The American Dental Association (ADA), under the auspices of the ADA Council on Scientific Affairs (CSA), developed the ADA Caries Classification System (CCS) for use in clinical practice. This consensus development process started in 2008 and culminated in the final release of the ADA CCS in 2015. The ADA CCS offers the clinician the capability to categorize all stages of caries lesion by the surfaces involved, site of origin (when identifiable), extent, and when possible, activity level in a standardized, consistent manner over time [1]. The ADA CCS facilitates risk assessment to aid decision-making regarding which clinical treatments and therapeutic interventions will best control and treat these caries lesions. In the ADA CCS, facial and lingual smooth, cervical, and root surfaces receive similar consideration because these surfaces exhibit many similar characteristics and they are accessible for visible and tactile clinical examination.

The ADA CSA designed the ADA CCS to incorporate the latest scientifically based terminology and techniques used in US clinical practice. The ADA CCS is easy to learn, easily translates to other languages, is useful in a variety of clinical practice settings, and may be mapped to other caries classification systems used for clinical caries management and research. In particular, the international community

G. Zeller (✉)
University of Kentucky College of Dentistry, Lexington, KY, USA
e-mail: greg.zeller@uky.edu

D. A. Young
Department of Diagnostic Sciences, Arthur A. Dugoni School of Dentistry, University of the Pacific, San Francisco, CA, USA
e-mail: dyoung@pacific.edu

B. Novy
Department of General Dentistry, Loma Linda University School of Dentistry, Loma Linda, CA, USA

© Springer Nature Switzerland AG 2019

A. Ferreira Zandona, C. Longbottom (eds.), *Detection and Assessment of Dental Caries*, https://doi.org/10.1007/978-3-030-16967-1_7

has created a classification tool, the International Caries Detection and Assessment System (ICDAS), developed to facilitate epidemiological caries research and appropriate clinical management [2] (see Chap. 6). ICDAS and the associated International Caries Classification and Management System (ICCMS) are available for implementation to enable dentists to classify and manage caries lesions [3]. These international systems were developed using a global consensus approach to caries classification and management that allows for specific "local" implementations tailored for use in various geographic regions. Some clinicians believe that ICDAS may be too cumbersome to apply to all tooth sites in private practice settings where other metrics are already prevalent, such as bitewing radiographs for assessment of the approximal surface. However, ICDAS may offer a helpful approach to the occlusal surface, where there is no current metric available to accurately classify caries lesions [4]. This context contributed to the development of the ADA CCS.

7.2 Caries Disease Management

Caries disease management is not just management of individual caries lesions. A discussion of caries management by risk assessment is pertinent with regard to the ADA CCS. For purposes of this chapter, caries management by risk assessment (CAMBRA) is a disease-based approach focused on treating or minimizing caries risk factors unique to each patient to prevent, arrest, and reverse disease. This approach includes, when necessary, restorative repair of cavitated caries lesions using minimally invasive techniques. The basic CAMBRA approach means (1) assessing the risk for future caries lesions, (2) reducing the pathological factors, (3) enhancing the protective factors, and (4) using minimally invasive restorative care as indicated, resulting in control of the disease [5]. The CAMBRA philosophy is built on the understanding that dental caries is a disease initiated by a complex biofilm that varies dynamically depending on the environment and chemistry of the local tooth site, pellicle, and saliva, rather than one pathogen [6–8]. This approach is in stark contrast to the traditional "drill and fill" model. Rather than focusing solely on restoring damage to teeth made manifest in the end stages of caries disease or even concentrating on the elimination of one pathogen, the CAMBRA approach is to determine which of many possible caries risk factors are causing the expression of disease, and then take corrective therapeutic action at the earliest possible stage [5].

7.3 Terminology

Using the term "caries" by itself can be confusing. The term is open to several interpretations, and worse, if used incorrectly, could lead to the wrong clinical decision. Consider adding a second descriptor to the term "caries," such as "caries disease" or "caries lesion," because these two are clearly different in meaning. The caries lesion is the end result of caries disease. A caries lesion is a manifestation of the disease at a location on the tooth; however, the term "caries lesion" lacks specificity as well because it says nothing about the extent, severity, or activity of the caries lesion.

The term "surgical" refers to the need to remove tooth structure and usually results in a restoration. It is assumed that the restoration of caries lesions is performed in a manner that is minimally invasive and conserves natural tooth structure [9] in conjunction with appropriate non-surgical chemotherapeutic and behavioral interventions based on the caries risk assessment in order to reduce the risk of further caries disease [5].

The term "non-surgical" refers to treatment of the lesion through strategies such as physical barriers using sealants, biofilm modification, remineralization using chemotherapeutics, and behavioral modification. As discussed below, the decision to treat surgically or non-surgically should be based on whether or not the tooth surface is fully cavitated through enamel [5, 9] (for additional nomenclature, see definitions in Chap. 24).

7.4 The Clinical Significance of Cavitation

The term "cavitation" is used to denote a loss of surface integrity, which, in the case of enamel, expresses some degree of surface microcavitation not to dentin or full cavitation completely through the enamel exposing dentin [10]. The ADA CCS includes terminology for sound, noncavitated, and cavitated caries lesions and describes these caries lesions using clinical presentation without reference to specific treatment approaches. However, a key metric in the ADA CCS is the ability to classify a caries lesion with regard to the likelihood of the presence of infected dentin, which is a methodology for predicting full cavitation through the enamel. Intact enamel prevents bacteria from entering the dentin because the fluid-filled enamel diffusion channels are much too small and will not allow bacteria to enter [11]. Once the lesion fully cavitates through enamel to dentin, if the disease is left untreated, cariogenic bacteria will enter the dentin and most likely require surgical restoration. Conversely, a caries lesion not fully cavitated through enamel treated chemically can remineralize and become acid resistant in the presence of topical fluoride [12]. Thus, the clinical decision to surgically restore a caries lesion should be based on the likelihood of full cavitation. The ADA CCS categories of sound, initial, moderate, and advanced provide information regarding the likelihood of the presence of infected dentin with full cavitation. The ADA CCS also integrates research correlating radiographic radiolucency depth to clinical cavitation for approximal surfaces [13], which provides a visual method to monitor caries lesion activity by progression or regression of the caries lesion image radiodensity over time.

7.5 ADA CCS Use

Clinical application of the ADA CCS relies upon examinations conducted on a clean tooth dried with compressed air, the use of adequate lighting, and a rounded explorer or ball-end probe. Note that forcing an explorer into any site to detect a caries lesion can cause cavitation and eliminate the chance to remineralize the previously intact surface [14]. A rounded (blunt or dull) explorer or a ball probe should be used to evaluate surface texture as rough versus smooth by dragging the instrument over the surface in question. Indicated radiographs also should be available for the examination.

The visual and tactile examination of each accessible surface should be completed to determine if each surface is sound, or, if a caries lesion is present, then the lesion site of origin, surfaces involved, extent, and when possible, activity should be noted. The ADA CCS scores each surface of the dentition (occlusal, approximal, and facial/lingual) based on the following: tooth surface(s) involved, presence or absence of a caries lesion, suspected anatomic site of origin, severity of the change (sound, initial, moderate, or advanced), and estimation of lesion activity. For each severity level (initial, moderate, and advanced), there are descriptors for clinical appearance and the corresponding presence of infected dentin/cavitation to classify caries lesions and help with clinical decisions regarding treatment.

Table 7.1 below presents an integrated view of the overall criteria used in the ADA CCS.

Note that Table 7.1 combines both the clinical appearance and, in the case of the approximal caries lesions, the radiographic presentation for an overall assessment of a caries lesion. In the ADA CCS, the combined clinical and radiographic presentation for tooth surfaces is classified as either sound, an initial caries lesion, a moderate

Table 7.1 American Dental Association Caries Classification System (With permission from JADA)

	AMERICAN DENTAL ASSOCIATION CARIESS CLASSIFICATION SYSTEM			
	Sound	**Initial**	**Moderate**	**Advanced**
Clinical Presentation	No clinically detectable lesion. Dental hard tissue appears normal in color, translucency, and gloss.	Earliest clinically detectable lesion compatible with mild demineralization. Lesion limited to enamel or to shallow demineralization of cementum/dentin. Mildest forms are detectable only after drying. When established and active, lesions may be white or brown and enamel has lost its normal gloss.	Visible signs of enamel breakdown or signs the dentin is moderately demineralized.	Enamel is fully cavitated and dentin is exposed. Dentin lesion is deeply/severely demineralized.
Other Labels	No surface change or adequately restored	Visually noncavitated	Established, early cavitated, shallow cavitation, microcavitation	Spread/disseminated, late cavitated, deep cavitation
Infected Dentin	None	Unlikely	Possible	Present
Appearance of Occlusal Surfaces (Pit and Fissure)*,†	ICDAS 0 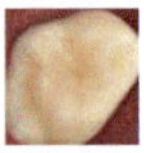	ICDAS 1 ICDAS 2 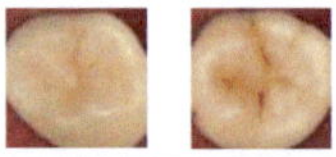	ICDAS 3 ICDAS 4 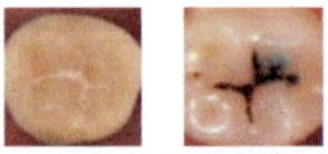	ICDAS 5 ICDAS 6 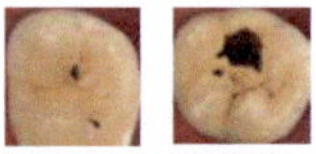
Accessible Smooth Surfaces, Including Cervical and Root‡	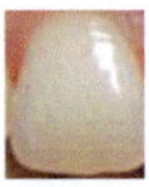	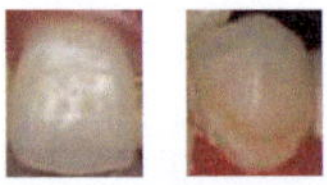	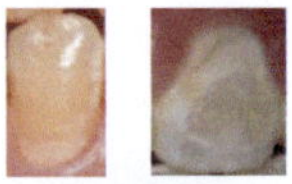	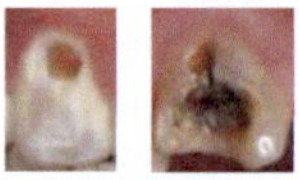
Radiographic Presentation of the Approximal Surface§	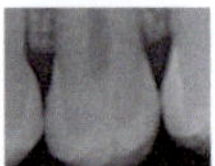 E0¶ or RO# No radiolucency	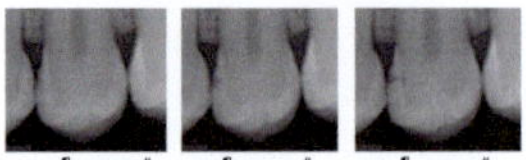 E1¶ or RA1# E2¶ or RA2# D1¶ or RA3# Radiolucency may extend to the dentinoenamel junction or outer one-third of the dentin. Note: radiographs are not reliable for mild occlusal lesions.	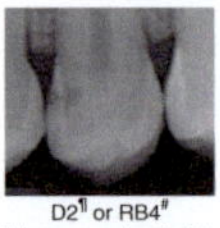 D2¶ or RB4# Radiolucency extends into the middle one-third of the dentin	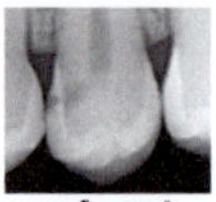 D3¶ or RC5# Radiolucency extends into the inner one-third of the dentin

* Photographs of extracted teeth illustrate examples of pit-and-fissure caries.
† The ICDAS notation system links the dintcal visual appearance of occlusal caries lesions with the hiscotogically determined degree of dentinal penetration using the evidence collated and published by the ICDAS foundation over the last decade; ICDAS also has a menu of options, including 3 levels of caries lesion classification, radiographic scoring and an integrated, risk-based caries management system ICCMS. (Pitts NB, Ekstrand KR. International Caries Detection and Assessment System [ICDAS] and its International Caries Classification and Management System [ICCMS]: Methods for staging of the caries process and enabling dentists to manage caries. *Community Dent Orol Epidemiol* 2013;41 [1]:e41-e52. Pitts NB, Ismail AI, Martignon S, Ekstrand K, Douglas GAV, Longbottom C. ICCMS Guide for Practitioners and Educators. Available at: https://WWW.fcdas.org/uploads/ICCMS-Guide_Full_Guide_US.pdf. Accessed April 13, 2015.)
‡ Includes any smooth surface lesion on or below the anotomical crown that is accessible through direct visual/tactile examination.
§ Simulated radiographic images.
¶ E0-E2, D1-D3 notation system.[15]
# RO, RA1-RA3, RB4, and RC5-RC6 ICCMS radiographic scoring system (RC6 = into pulp). Pitts NB, Ismail AI, Martignon S, Ekstrand K. Douglas GAV, Longbottom C. ICCMS Guide for Practitioners and Educators. Available at: https://www.icdas.org/uploads/ICCMS-Guide_Full_Guide_US.pdf. Accessed April 13, 2015.)

caries lesion, or an advanced caries lesion [1]. In addition to classifying the surfaces involved for a caries lesion, classifying the site of origin for a caries lesion, when identifiable, is useful for assessing the etiology of the lesion and for addressing the treatment options available for that caries lesion. Any caries lesion described in Table 7.1 may also be associated with an existing restoration or sealant.

Note also that Table 7.1 contains ADA CCS cross-mapping for the occlusal surfaces and visible smooth surfaces to specific criteria used in ICDAS. Additionally, Table 7.1 displays the cross-mapping for the ADA CCS categories E0, E2, E3, D1, D2, and D3 radiographic classifications [15] to specific criteria used for radiographic scoring in the ICCMS. The ADA CCS cross-mapping offers the flexibility, depending on the clinical practice, to use simpler, less complex terminology, such as sound, initial, moderate, and advanced, or to use more granular terminology, such as that present in the ICCMS. This flexibility makes the use of the ADA CCS attractive across a broad spectrum of clinical situations. More specific discussion of the clinical use of the ADA CCS follows.

7.6 The Occlusal Surface (Pits and Fissures)

The morphology of the pits and fissures may make determination of the degree of enamel cavitation problematic because direct visual and tactile examination of the enamel thickness over dentin is often not possible. In this case, histologic information may be the next best science for clinical decision-making. The ICDAS Coordinating Committee has published data correlating the clinical appearance of these occlusal pit-and-fissure lesions with the percent chance of histological penetration (not cavitation) of these caries lesions into the dentin on extracted teeth, manifested as demineralization (brown discoloration). Based on this published data [2, 4], ADA CCS initial pit-and-fissure caries lesions (ICDAS 1 and 2) could exhibit histologic dentin demineralization 9–50% of the time and ADA CCS moderate pit-and-fissure caries lesions (ICDAS 3 and 4) may demonstrate dentin demineralization histologically 50–88% of the time. ADA CCS advanced pit-and-fissure caries lesions (ICDAS 5 and 6), because they are fully cavitated through enamel, would be expected to demonstrate histologic demineralization of the dentin 100% of the time [1]. Even though expected histologic dentin penetration does not directly equate to enamel cavitation, the histologic data related to these probability ranges for dentin demineralization should be beneficial in any caries management system that includes treatment considerations based on the classification of the caries lesions.

7.7 The Approximal Surfaces

The approximal surfaces are examined using the visual and tactile method if possible. When direct access not available due to contact with an adjacent tooth, radiographs or elastomeric tooth separation may be used for examination. When sequential radiographs spanning an appropriate amount of time are available for an approximal caries lesion, Table 7.1 may be used to determine the radiographic progression or regression and can provide activity classification for the caries lesion over time.

In 1992, Pitts and Rimmer [13] correlated radiographic radiolucency depth for approximal caries to cavitation in posterior teeth. In this study, none of the teeth presenting a radiolucency in the outer one-half of the enamel were cavitated. If the radiolucency appeared radiographically in the inner one-half of the enamel, the percentage of cavitation was approximately 10.8% in permanent teeth and 2.9% in primary teeth. These percentages increased to 40.9% in permanent teeth and 28.4% in primary teeth if the lesion extended radiographically to the outer one-half of dentin and to 100% cavitation in permanent teeth and 48% in primary teeth if the lesion extended to the inner one-half of the dentin radiographically (see Chaps. 11–13 for additional information on radiographic detection of caries).

The ADA CCS, as shown in Table 7.1, uses nomenclature that divides the dentin into thirds instead of halves [15]. This ADA CCS nomenclature (E0, E1, E2, D1, D2, and D3) is simply a way to express the relative depth of a radiolucency as measured on a dental radiograph. Dividing the dentin into thirds instead of halves results in finer gradation and allows specific attention to the D1 area where, according to Pitts and Rimmer, cavitation is less likely [13]. Radiographic extent is only an estimate on the continuum of mineral loss described previously and may not always fit neatly into one lesion stage. For example, the middle of the D2 stage is exactly halfway from the dentinoenamel junction to the pulp, so there may be some early D2 radiolucencies that may not be clinically cavitated, whereas deeper D2 radiolucencies are more likely to be cavitated. Note again that the use of tooth separation for visualization can be helpful in confirming cavitation of a deep D1 or shallow D2 radiolucency. These correlations may be useful for making treatment decisions.

7.8 Facial and Lingual Smooth, Cervical, and Root Surfaces

Caries lesions on the facial and lingual smooth surfaces, regardless of involvement of the cervical or root surfaces, are usually easily accessible for direct visual and tactile examination. In other words, you can visually confirm if the surface is cavitated and you can more easily classify any caries lesion. In the ADA CCS, to classify these lesions, the clinician simply describes what is seen with regard to the caries lesion, such as white or brown coloration, partial or microcavitation, or fully cavitated to dentin. For each clinical caries lesion recorded in this manner, an estimate of lesion activity can also usually be determined as described below.

7.9 Caries Lesion Activity (or Inactivity)

The ADA CCS scores visible changes in tooth structures and, therefore, cannot score initial caries activity before visible structural changes occur. Longitudinal assessment of activity [16] is clinically valuable. When there are visible changes of

Table 7.2 Characteristics of active and inactive caries lesions* (With permission from JADA)

Activity assessment factor	Caries lesion activity assessment descriptors Likely to be inactive/arrested	Likely to be active
Location of the lesion	Lesion is not in a plaque stagnation area	Lesion is in a plaque stagnation area (pit/fissure, approximal, gingival)
Plaque over the lesion	Not thick or sticky	Thick and/or sticky
Surface appearance	Shiny; color: brown-black	Matte/opaque/loss of luster; color: white-yellow
Tactile feeling	Smooth, hard enamel/hard dentin	Rough enamel/soft dentin
Gingival status (if the lesion is located near the gingiva)	No inflammation, no bleeding on probing	Inflammation, bleeding on probing

*Source: Ekstrand KR, Zero DT, Martignon S, Pitts NB. Lesion activity assessment. Monogr Oral Sci 2009;21:63–90 (See Chaps. 4.1 and 4.3 for addional information on caries activity assessment)

caries lesions over time, it is often possible to determine whether the lesion is active or arrested. An inactive caries lesion may not need further treatment. Table 7.2 lists factors to consider when making a clinical determination of caries lesion activity or inactivity.

The lesion is classified as active when there are findings suggestive of continuing demineralization. This demineralization process can be monitored over time to judge the presence of disease activity, which may influence the decision regarding surgical or non-surgical therapeutic intervention. Detection of arrested lesions is an indication that the caries disease process is no longer active. "Affected dentin" is a term used to describe dentin that has been exposed to bacterial acids but may or may not be currently demineralizing. Depending on clinical assessment of caries lesion activity at the time of examination, affected dentin may be soft if demineralization is presently occurring (active) or may be tactilely hard if the lesion is "arrested" and already remineralized (inactive). Affected dentin is often stained or discolored, which is not a reason for surgical removal if the dentin has remineralized and is acid resistant [17].

Caries lesion activity assessment, despite any limitations, is a key factor for monitoring noncavitated lesion progression or regression over time and is a useful metric for gauging the effectiveness of chemotherapeutic treatment interventions. Lesion activity should be considered both clinically and radiographically. Evidence of lesion activity over time, based on changes (or lack thereof) in the radiolucency, can impact clinical treatment decisions. An arrested, remineralized, noncavitated lesion (white or brown) is acid resistant and does not indicate active caries disease. In fact, surgical removal of this protected layer is contraindicated.

7.10 Caries Risk Assessment (CRA) and Lesion Activity

The best predictor of caries risk is the presence of disease indicators such as current active caries lesions or evidence active of caries lesions in the recent past [18–21]. Thus, a careful clinical hard tissue examination must occur before the CRA process.

The identification and classification of new or progressing noncavitated or cavitated caries lesions or radiolucencies and recent restorations due to caries disease are considered heavily weighted statistically in the CRA process [21–23]. During the clinical dental examination, the surface(s), the site of origin (if identifiable), the extent, and, if possible, the activity of all caries lesions should be recorded in a reliable and valid way to classify current caries disease status as well as changes over time. Lesion activity should be considered when assigning caries risk status as part of a caries management system. In other words, an arrested caries lesion should not be considered a current disease indicator because it is neither a new nor a progressing caries lesion. The ADA CCS aids CRA through the application of an integrated system that uses both clinical and radiographic findings.

7.11 Hard Tissue Charting

If a caries lesion involves two (or more) tooth surfaces and the two (or more) surfaces are obviously joined together clinically, the surfaces involved are recorded together as a single caries lesion. However, only the suspected most likely site of origin would be recorded for that lesion. For example, a single advanced caries lesion involving the maxillary right first premolar consisting of the mesio-occlusal surfaces together for a single advanced caries lesion judged to be active and to have started on the approximal surface, would be recorded in the following manner: #4 mesio-occlusal surfaces, approximal origin, advanced extent, active.

Each current site of visible change can be scored as "inactive (I)" or "active (A)." Note that activity cannot be determined by radiographic manifestation alone except in those situations in which it is possible to compare sequential radiographic images of the same caries lesion exposed over an appropriate period of time. If the practitioner is unable to determine the activity of a caries lesion using the activity factors in Table 7.2 (Table 7.1 for sequential radiographs), the lesion activity should be recorded as "undetermined (UD)." If the practitioner decides not to assess activity level for a lesion, where such an assessment is possible using Table 7.2 (Table 7.1 for radiographs), it should be recorded as "not recorded (NR)."

The following are additional examples of caries lesion classification using the ADA CCS as detailed in Tables 7.1 and 7.2:

- #30 **occlusal** surface, **pit and fissure** origin, **advanced** (more specifically, **ICDAS 6**) extent, **active**
- #4 **facial** surface, **cervical**/smooth surface origin, **initial** (more specifically, **ICDAS 1** or **visually noncavitated white spot**) extent, **inactive**
- #2 **distal** surface, **approximal** origin, **moderate** (more specifically, **D2 radiographically**) extent, **active**
  - Explanation: Two bitewing radiographs taken 1 year apart support the clinical judgment of "active" based on progression of caries lesion (D1–D2) displayed on the bitewings and consistent with the "moderate extent" (D2) based on the Table 7.1 factors for this caries lesion.

Refer to the examples shown in Table 7.1 and to the criteria displayed in Table 7.2 to view additional specific details and examples that illustrate how the ADA CCS may be applied in clinical practice [1].

7.12 Concluding Remarks

Many practitioners currently use the G.V. Black system to classify caries lesions. Limiting the dental examination to cavitated lesions as classified in the G.V. Black system does not allow recognition of the earliest signs of caries lesions and also underestimates the prevalence and severity of disease. In addition, the G.V. Black approach describes only cavitated lesions, thus limiting the capacity to assess the effectiveness of preventive therapeutic interventions for the early stages of caries disease. The ADA CCS attempts to correct these limitations through an integrated use of clinical and radiographic examination findings that include reliable, reproducible criteria for detecting early lesions and for monitoring the clinical status of these early lesions over time.

To determine the effectiveness of caries management strategies aimed at improving patient care, a caries classification system must be reliable, valid, and usable in the local clinical setting in which it is implemented. The ADA CCS offers an integrated process that accommodates the use of all available useful criteria for capturing and classifying components of the caries disease process likely to be used in a US clinical practice. It can be tailored to fit any clinical practice by using simple categories such as sound, initial, moderate, or advanced, including, when possible, activity level, or, in contrast, it could be cross-mapped to more granular terminology often used in research, such as ICDAS [2, 4] and the E0, E1, E2, D1, D2, D3 nomenclature [15].

The ADA CCS will facilitate measuring the effectiveness of contemporary caries disease management strategies in clinical practice as the dental profession strives toward improving overall patient health through improved oral health. The ADA CCS is available now for the next implementation steps to test reliability and usability by practitioners in clinical and research settings [1].

Summary table

Bitewing radiography	ADA Caries Classification System			
Which surfaces/sites is it useful for	Occlusal (pits and fissures)	Proximal/ (approximal)	Smooth surface (buccal and lingual)	Root caries and which of the four surfaces?
	Y	**Y with visible inspection, where possible, and with bitewing radiographic comparisons over time**	**Y**	**Y (all surfaces)**

What type of lesions is valuable for	Primary coronal	Secondary coronal	Primary root caries	Secondary root caries
	Y	**Y**	**Y**	**Y**
What type of dentition	Primary		Permanent	
	Y		**Y**	
Lesion severity	Enamel lesions		Dentinal lesions	
	Y		**Y**	
Sensitivity	Literature reported range in 93.3% [24] Reported through extrapolation of other research			
Specificity	Literature reported range in 86.9% [24] Reported through extrapolation of other research			
Perceived Ease Of Use (PEOU)[a]	1. The ADA Caries Classification System is easy to use 2. It is easy to become skillful at using the ADA Caries Classification System 3. Learning to operate the ADA Caries Classification System is easy 4. The ADA Caries Classification System is integrated and flexible in order to interact with and map to other caries classification systems, e.g., ICDAS II and ICCMS 5. Interaction with the ADA Caries Classification System is clear and understandable 6. It is easy to interact with the ADA Caries Classification System, which maps to other caries classification systems, e.g., ICDAS II and ICCMS			
Advantages/ disadvantages	*Advantages*			
	1. Clinically oriented 2. No especial equipment needed 3. Visual exam			
	Disadvantages			
	1. Somewhat subjective 2. Validility extrapolated from other research			
Time	Approximate time for each tooth surface: Once the practitioner completes training on the ADA Caries Classification System, there is no increase in time or materials over current examination methods			
Cost	Approximate cost per unit and any disposables: Once the practitioner completes training on the ADA Caries Classification System, there is no increase in time or materials over current examination methods			

[a]Davis (1989) [25]

References

1. Young DA, Novy BB, Zeller GG, et al. The American Dental Association Caries Classification System for clinical practice: a report of the American Dental Association Council on Scientific Affairs. J Am Dent Assoc. 2015;146(2):79–86.
2. Pitts N. "ICDAS"—an International System for Caries Detection and Assessment being developed to facilitate caries epidemiology, research and appropriate clinical management. Community Dent Health. 2004;21(3):193–8.
3. Pitts N, Ekstrand KR. International Caries Detection and Assessment System (ICDAS) and its International Caries Classification and Management System (ICCMS)—methods for staging of the caries process and enabling dentists to manage caries. Community Dent Oral Epidemiol. 2013;41:e41–52.

4. Ismail AI, Sohn W, Tellez M, et al. The International Caries Detection and Assessment System (ICDAS): an integrated system for measuring dental caries. Community Dent Oral Epidemiol. 2007;35(3):170–78.
5. Young DA, Featherstone JD. Caries management by risk assessment. Community Dent Oral Epidemiol. 2013;41:e1–e12.
6. Takahashi N, Nyvad B. Caries ecology revisited: microbial dynamics and the caries process. Caries Res. 2008;42(6):409–18.
7. Takahashi N, Nyvad B. The role of bacteria in the caries process: ecological perspectives. J Dent Res. 2011;90(3):294–303.
8. Marsh PD, Percival RS. The oral microflora—friend or foe? Can we decide? Int Dent J. 2006;56(4 Suppl 1):233–9.
9. Ismail AI, Tellez M, Pitts NB, et al. Caries management pathways to preserve dental tissues and promote oral health. Community Dent Oral Epidemiol. 2013;41(1):e12–40.
10. Longbottom CL, Huysmans MC, Pitts NB, Fontana M. Glossary of key terms. Monogr Oral Sci. 2009;21:209–16.
11. Gonzalez-Cabezas C. The chemistry of caries: remineralization and demineralization events with direct clinical relevance. Dent Clin North Am. 2010;54(3):469–78.
12. Featherstone JD. The science and practice of caries prevention. J Am Dent Assoc. 2000;131(7):887–99.
13. Pitts NB, Rimmer PA. An in vivo comparison of radiographic and directly assessed clinical caries status of posterior approximal surfaces in primary and permanent teeth. Caries Res. 1992;26(2):146–52.
14. Stookey G. Should a dental explorer be used to probe suspected carious lesions? No—use of an explorer can lead to misdiagnosis and disrupt remineralization. J Am Dent Assoc. 2005;136(11):1527, 1529, 1531.
15. Anusavice KJ. Present and future approaches for the control of caries. J Dent Educ. 2005;69(5):538–54.
16. Ekstrand KR, Zero DT, Martignon S, Pitts NB. Lesion activity assessment. Monogr Oral Sci. 2009;21:63–90.
17. Kidd EA, Ricketts DN, Beighton D. Criteria for caries removal at the enamel-dentine junction: a clinical and microbiological study [see comments]. Br Dent J. 1996;180(8):287–91.
18. Fontana M, Zero DT. Assessing patients' caries risk. J Am Dent Assoc. 2006;137(9):1231–9.
19. Twetman S, Fontana M. Patient caries risk assessment. Monogr Oral Sci. 2009;21:91–101.
20. Twetman S, Fontana M, Featherstone J. Risk assessment—can we achieve consensus? Community Dent Oral Epidemiol. 2013;41:e64–70.
21. Domejean S, White JM, Featherstone JD. Validation of the CDA CAMBRA caries risk assessment—a six-year retrospective study. J Calif Dent Assoc. 2011;39(10):709–15.
22. Domejean S, Leger S, Rechmann P, White JM, Featherstone JD. How do dental students determine patients' caries risk level using the caries management by risk assessment (CAMBRA) system? J Dent Educ. 2015;79(3):278–85.
23. Domejean-Orliaguet S, Gansky SA, Featherstone JD. Caries risk assessment in an educational environment. J Dent Educ. 2006;70(12):1346–54.
24. Thompson V, Schenkel A, Penugonda B, et al. A pilot study of dentists' assessment of caries detection and staging systems applied to early caries: PEARL Network findings. Gen Dent. 2016;4(3):20–27.
25. Davis FD. Perceived Usefulness, Perceived Ease of Use, and User Acceptance of Information Technology. MIS Quarterly. 1989;13(3):319–340.

The Caries Assessment Spectrum and Treatment (CAST) Instrument

8

Soraya Leal, Ana Paula Dias Ribeiro, and Ana Luiza de Souza Hilgert

8.1 Introduction

The CAST instrument is a caries detection tool initially developed for application in epidemiological surveys. Its inclusion in this book aims to provide a tool that might be useful for those practicing in public health or community-based settings where an overall needs assessment is paramount. The rationale behind its development is that other current assessment systems do not cover the total spectrum of dental caries [1, 2], are not always easy to apply [3], and are difficult to report in a meaningful way [4]. These characteristics are of paramount importance in an epidemiological instrument for global use in order to allow the comparison of results from surveys carried out around the world. These conditions (ease and comparability) are, most probably, the reasons why the WHO criterion [5], which only assesses the presence of a dentin cavity and which expresses the findings in a dmf/DMF count [6], is still the major criterion used.

Considering that the prevalence of dental caries has decreased significantly in the last two decades, a cavitated dentin carious lesion is no longer frequently observed in many high-income countries [7]. Researchers, therefore, felt it necessary to develop caries detection systems that can also register the early stages of dental caries. Good examples of these systems are the ICDAS (see Chap. 6) [8] and the Nyvad criterion (see Chap. 5) [9].

S. Leal (✉)
Department of Dentistry, Faculty of Health Science, University of Brasília, Brasília, Brazil

A. P. D. Ribeiro
Department of Restorative Dental Sciences, College of Dentistry, University of Florida, Gainesville, FL, USA

A. L. de Souza Hilgert
Department of Dentistry, Pediatric Dentistry from the Military of Federal District, Brasília, Brazil

© Springer Nature Switzerland AG 2019

A. Ferreira Zandona, C. Longbottom (eds.), *Detection and Assessment of Dental Caries*, https://doi.org/10.1007/978-3-030-16967-1_8

The decline in the prevalence and severity of dental caries, however, has not been observed in all world communities, and, in many, caries prevalence still ranges from moderate to high [7, 10]. In Brazil, for example, for those aged 5 years who present a dmft score greater than 1, 80% of the index is represented by the d-component [11]. Nevertheless, the mean dmft score cannot identify the percentage of lesions that have already progressed to the severe stages (pulp exposure, fistula, and abscess). Such disease conditions are also not included in the caries detection systems mentioned above, even though identifying the severity of dental caries is extremely important for countries like Cambodia or the Philippines, where the consequences of carious lesions on soft tissues are many [2, 12].

The first index developed to assess the consequences of the severe stages of carious lesions was pufa/PUFA [2], which quantifies the prevalence and severity of oral conditions resulting from untreated dentin cavities. Therefore, pufa/PUFA is not a caries detection system, but merely a tool that complements caries detection systems such as ICDAS that cannot assess carious lesions reaching the pulp or abscesses/fistulas. This can be considered a limitation of the instrument, as the severity of the disease will only be recorded in cases where a decision is made to use pufa/PUFA.

In summary, none of the carious lesion assessment systems/indices/criteria in current use cover the total spectrum of carious lesion detection. In contrast, CAST was developed as an epidemiological instrument that includes the total spectrum of dental caries from a sound surface/tooth, to enamel carious lesions, to different levels of severity of dentin carious lesions to tooth loss due to dental caries and also includes the presence of dental treatments (sealants and restorations).

The aim of this chapter is to present the CAST instrument and highlight its applicability in epidemiological surveys. Moreover, different ways of presenting the CAST results will be discussed.

8.2 The CAST Instrument

The CAST instrument was first described in 2011 and was built on the strengths of both the ICDAS system and the pufa/PUFA index in addition to the provision of a link to the DMFT index [13]. CAST codes are organized in hierarchal order to facilitate the understanding of the severity of the disease, meaning that the higher the CAST code, the worse the situation (Table 8.1).

The CAST instrument has been validated and tested for reliability in various age groups [14, 15] and applied in several studies around the world, as shown in Table 8.2.

Table 8.1 CAST codes and descriptions

Characteristic	Code	Description
Sound	0	No visible evidence of a distinct carious lesion is present
Sealant	1	Pits and/or fissures are at least partially covered with a sealant material
Restoration	2	A cavity is restored with a (in)direct restorative material
Enamel	3	Distinct visual change in enamel only. A clear caries-related discoloration is visible, with or without localized enamel breakdown
Dentin	4	Internal caries-related discoloration in dentin. The discolored dentin is visible through the enamel, which may or may not exhibit a visible localized breakdown of enamel
	5	Distinct cavitation into dentin. The pulp chamber is intact
Pulp	6	Involvement of the pulp chamber. Distinct cavitation reaching the pulp chamber or only root fragments are present
Abscess/ fistula	7	A pus-containing swelling or a pus-releasing sinus tract related to a tooth with pulpal involvement
Lost	8	The tooth has been removed because of dental caries
Other	9	Does not correspond to any of the other descriptions

Table 8.2 Year, country, sample, age group, setting, and main findings from published studies using the CAST instrument

Year and country	Sample (*n*)	Age group	Setting	Main findings for CAST
2014, Poland [16]	542	6–8 years	School	– Reliable and promising tool – Categorizes teeth with restorations as functional: logical approach – Easy evaluation of the full caries spectrum – More information on disease prevalence, experience, and severity compared with DMF index is needed – Needs further in vitro and in vivo validation of its reliability
2014, Poland [17]	284	7–8 years	School	– Simple hierarchical structure – Caries process is categorized according to progression – Modern approach to filled teeth because of their inclusion in the category of sound teeth – Good intra-examiner reliability in both dentitions – Useful in epidemiological surveys
2014, Pakistan [18]	100	31 ± 17 years	Dental clinic	– A new paradigm to assess dental caries – Does not present overestimated caries prevalence – Scores the whole spectrum of dental caries

(continued)

Table 8.2 (continued)

Year and country	Sample (*n*)	Age group	Setting	Main findings for CAST
2014, Brazil [15]	1971	2–6 years 6–9 years 19–30 years	School and dental clinic	– A reliable tool – Reproducibility reached a substantial to a high level – Further testing on various age groups is needed
2014, Brazil [19]	419	6–11 years	School	– Provided similar prevalence of dental caries values and dmf/DMF counts as the WHO criterion – Time spent on examining children did not differ between CAST and the WHO criterion – Presents a premorbidity stage of dental caries
2015, Brazil [20]	354	2–6 years 19–30 years	Dental clinic	– Authors provided no comments on the CAST instrument
2016, India [21]	465	5–6 years	Dental clinic	– Useful for primary teeth and in epidemiological surveys
2016, Poland [22]	332	6–7 years	School	– An easy-to-use and useful tool for epidemiological analysis of primary molars – Good level of intra-examiner reproducibility – Results obtained with DMF or ICDAS need to be compared – Caries activity is not recorded
2016, India [23]	508	6–12 years	Not clear	– Authors provided no comments on the CAST instrument
2017, Tanzania [24]	525	2–4 years	Field clinic	– Authors provided no comments on the CAST instrument
2017, India [25]	301	7–8 years	School	– Scores the whole spectrum of dental caries – Effective in epidemiological surveys – Further testing on various age groups is needed

8.3 How to Apply the CAST Instrument

The implementation of an epidemiological survey using the CAST instrument should be preceded by training and calibration sessions lasting approximately 4 days. One or more experienced examiner(s), who have previously been trained and calibrated to use CAST, should be responsible for training and calibrating new examiners.

Training sessions should include the rationale and characteristics of the CAST instrument and the examination protocol. During training, experienced examiner(s) should use pictures and extracted teeth as examples of different CAST codes to present clinical situations. Trainee examiners should perform several examinations on selected subjects (not included in the main study), which will be compared with the examinations performed by an experienced examiner. In the beginning, differences will certainly be found between examiners, but the differences will be discussed in order to reach consensus [26].

After training has been successfully completed, the calibration exercises begin. This includes the examination of 5–10 subjects with the same profile as those to be examined in the main study. If possible, the full range of clinical situations covered by the CAST instrument should be included [26]. The subjects should be examined independently by trainee examiners and by an experienced examiner. Differences between the examiners should be discussed and consensus reached. When a good agreement is achieved (at least 85%), a new group of 5–10 subjects should be examined, and the results compared between all examiners being trained (intra- and inter-examiner agreement) and then with an experienced examiner as the gold standard [15]. After calibration is completed, the examiners should be ready to use the CAST instrument properly and the study can begin.

The CAST instrument can be used inside and outside the dental clinic (i.e., schools and field situations), and the arrangement of the setting depends on the structure available in each place [15, 16, 19, 20]. All tooth surfaces should be cleaned with a toothbrush, toothpaste, and dental floss (if available) prior to the examination. The instruments required are a flat mouth mirror and a CPITN (Community Periodontal Index of Treatment Needs) probe. The mirror helps the examiner to look indirectly at the dental surfaces, and the probe assists in sensing the tooth surfaces and removing plaque. Additionally, gauzes and cotton rolls should be available to remove excess saliva. The use of compressed air is not indicated while applying the CAST instrument [26].

8.4 CAST Codes and the Level of Severity of the Disease

Considering that the calculation of the prevalence of dental caries within a population with the CAST instrument is based on the epidemiological concept of health/disease [19, 27], the dentition is categorized into five stages: healthy, premorbidity, morbidity, serious morbidity, and mortality (Table 8.3).

The health/disease approach facilitates the planning of adequate health policies and dental care and shows the effects of treatments performed in the population. Sound dentition requires maintenance care. The premorbidity stage is represented by enamel lesions (code 3) and requires maintenance and preventive care. Morbidity is represented by dentin lesions (codes 4 and 5) and requires sealants or restorative treatment. Serious morbidity (codes 6 and 7) requires endodontic treatment and restoration or extraction. Finally, mortality indicates tooth loss because of dental caries. Therefore, after dental care is provided, the category of the dentition will change (Fig. 8.1), decreasing the prevalence levels of dental caries, as is explained in the next section.

Table 8.3 CAST codes distributed according to the level of severity of the disease

	CAST 0	CAST 1	CAST 2	CAST 3	CAST 4	CAST 5	CAST 6	CAST 7	CAST 8
Healthy	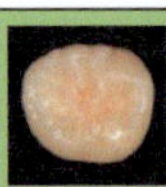	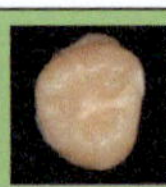	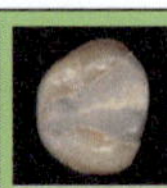						
Premor-bidity				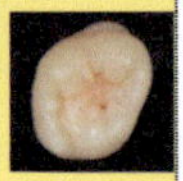					
Morbidity					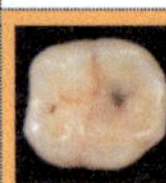	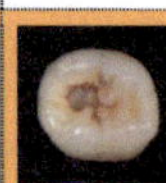			
Severe morbidity							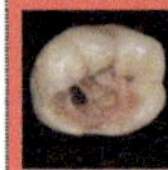	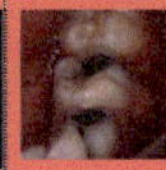	
Mortality									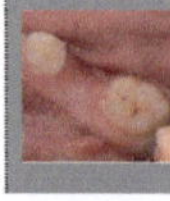

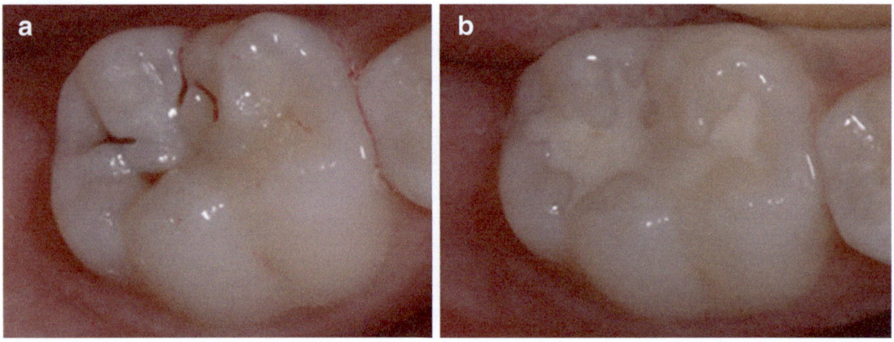

Fig. 8.1 (**a**) A second primary molar showing a maximum CAST score of 4 (morbidity stage); (**b**) The same tooth after dental treatment (ART restoration) showing a maximum CAST code of 2 (healthy stage)

8.5 Reporting CAST Results and Calculating the Prevalence of Dental Caries

A clear and readable way of reporting the results of an epidemiological survey is crucial to understanding the oral health status of those under investigation. Moreover, drawing conclusions from the prevalence statistics with respect to preventive and therapeutic interventions, cost–benefit analysis, design strategies, and the answers to certain research questions that will assist political and health policy decisions can only be done with straightforward reporting.

For decades, the dmf/DMF index was the gold standard for reporting the prevalence of dental caries worldwide. However, the index considers a restored tooth as a diseased tooth, as the "filling" component is included in the calculation of caries prevalence. To better illustrate this aspect, a hypothetical situation is used as an example: if 200 subjects are examined during an epidemiological survey and 80 present with a cavitated dentin lesion (d-component), the caries prevalence of this population is 40%. In the case where all these cavities are restored (f-component) and no new cavitated dentin carious lesions occur, the caries prevalence remains at 40%, even though there are no longer any diseased teeth. With the CAST instrument, a different way of dealing with caries prevalence is proposed: only those teeth that are diseased at the moment of the examination are counted, as is the case for other medical diseases.

CAST provides more accurate information about the different stages of carious lesions including not only enamel lesions but also the presence of abscesses/fistulas. Therefore, CAST does not need to be combined with another index. Information about the disease at the surface, tooth, and individual levels can be easily obtained. Finally, CAST codes can be converted into the DMF index, allowing comparison with past studies.

To illustrate how to report results using the CAST instrument, information obtained from a study performed in 2016 in a suburban area of Brazil's Federal District is used. The sample included 926 children (52.8% boys) aged between 6 and 8 years from six public schools.

In epidemiological studies, the results are usually presented using the tooth as the unit of observation. Therefore, after tabulating the data and checking for possible mistakes, all the surfaces of one tooth should be used to obtain the maximum CAST score per tooth. To create this score, the highest CAST code, excluding code 9, in one tooth is used, as shown in Fig. 8.2.

In the sample, 13,540 primary teeth and 3477 permanent teeth were examined. These teeth can be categorized by the maximum CAST score per tooth, using either

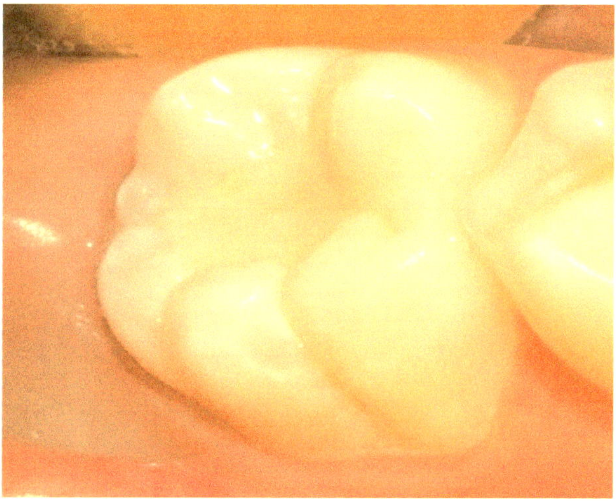

Fig. 8.2 A first permanent molar assessed with the CAST instrument showing the following codes: CAST code 2 (occlusal surface); CAST code 3 (buccal surface); CAST code 0 (mesial, lingual, and distal surfaces), resulting in a maximum CAST score of 3

frequency or percentage. Figure 8.3 presents the distribution of those teeth according to the maximum CAST score per tooth as a percentage.

The next step should be the calculation of caries prevalence. For this, the maximum score per subject is obtained. Analogous to obtaining the maximum CAST per tooth, the scores of all teeth present in the mouth (excluding code 9) are used to obtain the maximum CAST score per subject.

Using the same sample, the children were categorized by their maximum CAST score per subject (Fig. 8.4). A total of 926 children had primary teeth, and 453 children also had permanent teeth.

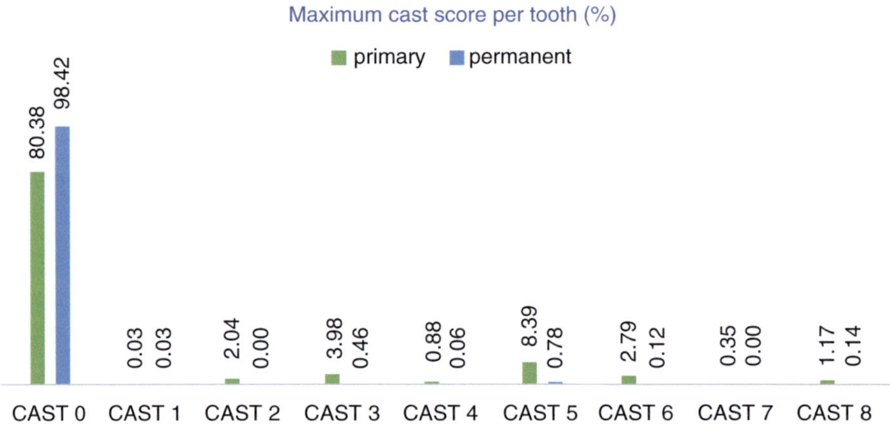

Fig. 8.3 Distribution of primary and permanent teeth according to the maximum CAST score per tooth (%)

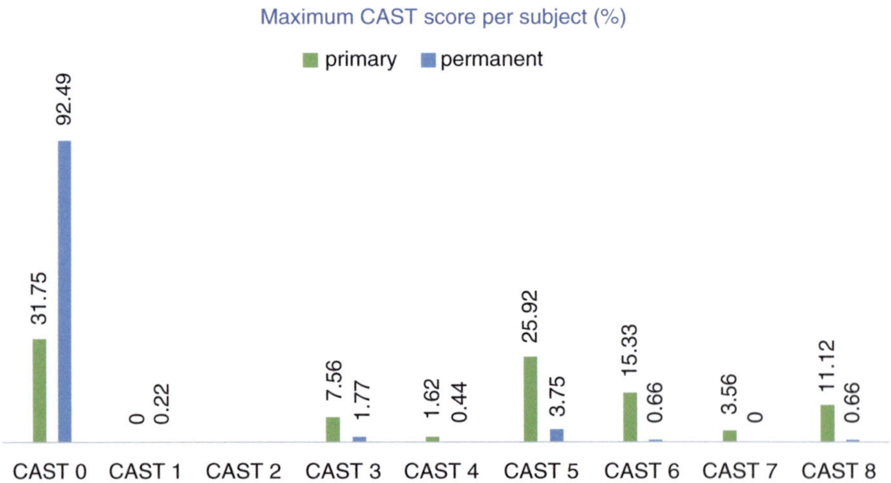

Fig. 8.4 Distribution of primary and permanent teeth according to the maximum CAST score per subject (%)

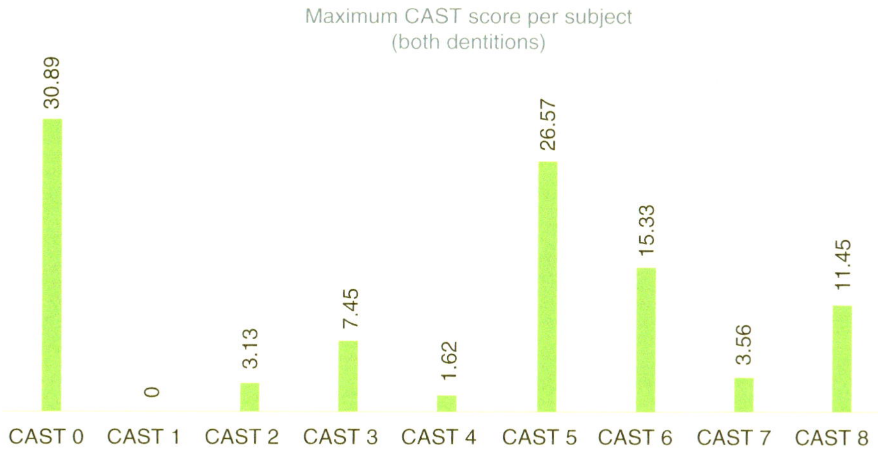

Fig. 8.5 Distribution of combined primary and permanent dentition according to the maximum CAST score per subject (%)

If the health/disease approach to presenting the results is preferred, the combination of both dentitions can be used to define one unique score per subject, as presented in Fig. 8.5.

In the current scenario, the percentage of healthy children was 34.02% (CAST code 0–2). The premorbidity, morbidity, and serious morbidity stages represent 7.45%, 28.19%, and 18.89% of this sample, respectively, while mortality represents 11.45% of these children. With this information, public health strategies can be developed to address the main concerns of this population. Considering our sample, we concluded that almost half the children need a restorative/pulp treatment or extraction (47%).

In an ideal scenario, these children will receive treatment, and their health/disease classification will then change. This approach allows comparison between "before and after" intervention, assisting policy makers in assessing the effectiveness of any oral health program implemented. In the present example, children initially included in the morbidity stage would receive restorative treatment, while those included in the serious morbidity stage would receive root canal treatment + restorative treatment or extraction. If we infer that half these children will move to CAST 2, while the other half move to CAST 8, the percentage of healthy children will increase from 34.12 to 71.65% (CAST 0 to CAST 2), leaving no children in the morbidity or serious morbidity stage. The mortality stage will then increase from 11.45 to 20.89% (Fig. 8.6).

Finally, the distribution of the population according to the maximum CAST score per subject allows dental caries prevalence to be calculated according to the dentition (primary or permanent). CAST considers only diseased subjects in the calculation of prevalence. Therefore, when only dentin carious lesions (CAST codes 4, 5, 6, and 7) are included, the prevalence of caries is 46.43% and 4.81% for primary and permanent dentitions, respectively. However, when enamel lesions are included, the prevalence increases to 53.99% and 6.58%, respectively, thereby

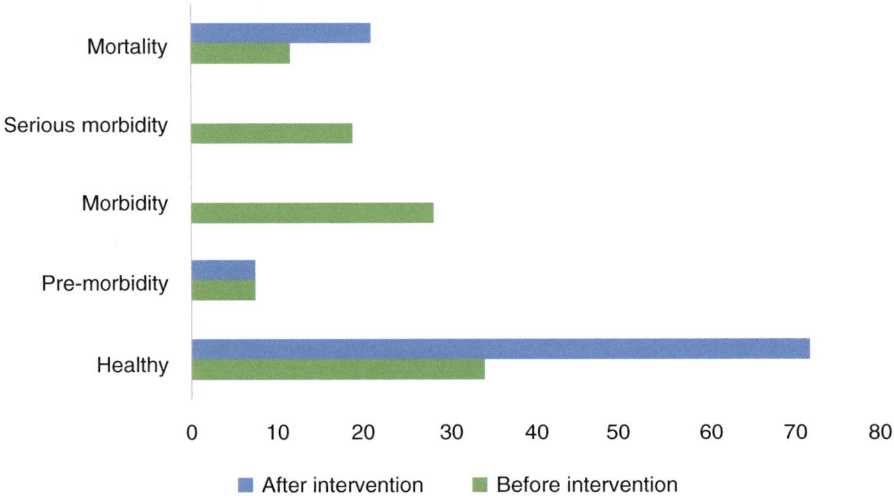

Fig. 8.6 Percentage of children categorized by health/disease allowing comparison between before and after intervention (%)

differentiating between the prevalence of dentin carious lesions (CAST codes 4–7) and enamel and dentin carious lesions (CAST codes 3–7). If a dmft/DMFT score from the CAST codes is needed to compare present results with those of previous studies, the dmft/DMFT score can be constructed. The d/D-component refers to codes 5–7, the m/M-component to code 8, and the f/F-component to code 2, resulting in a prevalence of 57.55% and 5.47% for primary and permanent dentition, respectively.

8.6 Concluding Remarks

The CAST instrument validation process was carried out using the Rand modified e-Delphi method and involved 56 epidemiologists from 24 different countries [14]. This methodology aimed to accommodate different cultural and social backgrounds, an important step in developing an instrument for worldwide use.

In terms of applicability, the CAST instrument provides more detailed information about the caries status of a population, without increasing the time spent during examinations in comparison with the WHO criterion [5]. Moreover, high levels of intra- and inter-examiner agreement have been reported in the literature.

The inclusion of enamel carious lesions and the identification of dentin carious lesions in three stages in one caries detection instrument eliminate the need for different indices to cover the whole spectrum of dental caries.

Finally, the organization of the CAST codes in hierarchical order facilitates the categorization of the disease according to severity levels (sound, premorbidity, morbidity, serious morbidity, and mortality) and, that in turn, provides a clear connection to the treatment needs of the population under investigation. Such a strategy assists policy makers in precisely planning oral health policies according to specific needs.

Summary table

CAST instrument				
For which surfaces/sites is it useful?	Occlusal (pits and fissures) **Y**	Proximal/ (approximal) **Y**	Smooth surface (buccal and lingual) **Y**	Root caries and which of the four surfaces? **N**
For which type of lesions is it valuable?	Primary coronal **Y**	Secondary coronal **Y**	Primary root caries **N**	Secondary root caries **N**
Type of dentition	Primary **Y**		Permanent **Y**	
Lesion severity	Enamel lesions **Y**		Dentinal lesions **Y**	
Sensitivity	Literature reported range as 90.9–96.6% [19]			
Specificity	Literature reported range as 86–100% [19]			
Perceived ease of use (PEOU)[a]	1. CAST is easy to use 2. It is easy to become skillful at using CAST 3. Learning to operate CAST is easy 4. CAST is flexible to interact with 5. My interaction with CAST is clear and understandable 6. It is easy to interact with CAST			
Advantages/ disadvantages	*Advantages* 1. Easy to apply 2. No need to use compressed air 3. Resources required to implement the study are simple 4. The codes are ordered hierarchically 5. Enamel lesions are included in only one code 6. Provides information about different stages of dentin lesions, including pulpal involvement 7. Provides information about teeth with functioning sealants and restorations 8. Easy to use with small and impaired children [15, 19, 23, 28] 9. Results obtained with CAST can be compared with those obtained with WHO criterion using dmf/DMF index 10. Time spent in examinations does not differ from that in WHO criterion 11. Prevalence of dental caries is calculated considering only teeth with a dentin lesion (codes 4–7) 12. Facilitates planning of adequate health policies and dental care planning 13. Allows assessment of the dental caries spectrum without the need to score an additional index, for example, enamel lesions or the consequences of untreated dentin lesions for soft tissues 14. Reporting data with CAST allows a more detailed approach, including the presentation of a premorbidity stage of dental caries and CAST severity scores *Disadvantages* 1. It is a new instrument, which needs studies to further test its performance in different age groups and at different levels of caries severity 2. It only includes coronal caries			
Time	Mean time for an examination is 66.3 s per child (6–11 years) [15]			
Cost	No data as to cost estimate has been published so far, but the cost appears to be relatively low. The examinations can be conducted almost anywhere, and no expensive equipment is required. The highest costs are represented by the dental examiner and recorder [27]			

[a]Davis (1989) [29]

All figures of this chapter are copyrighted to Prof. Dr. Soraya Coelho Leal, Department of Dentistry, University of Brasília, and were reproduced in this book under copyright's holder permission.

References

1. Casamassimo PS, Thikkurissy S, Edelstein BL, Maiorini E. Beyond the dmft: the human and economic cost of early childhood caries. J Am Dent Assoc. 2009;140:650–7.
2. Monse B, Heinrich-Weltzien R, Benzian H, Holmgren C, van Palenstein Helderman WH. PUFA—an index of clinical consequences of untreated dental caries. Community Dent Oral Epidemiol. 2010;38:77–82.
3. Cavavid AS, Lince CM, Jaramillo MC. Dental caries in the primary dentition of a Colombian population according to the ICDAS criteria. Braz Oral Res. 2010;24:211–6.
4. de Amorim RG, Figueiredo MJ, Leal SC, Mulder J, Frencken JE. Caries experience in a child population in a deprived area of Brazil, using ICDAS II. Clin Oral Investig. 2012;16:513–20.
5. World Health Organization (WHO). Oral health surveys. 5th ed. Geneva: World Health Organization; 2013. p. 125.
6. Klein H, Palmer CE. Studies on dental caries: VII. Sex differences in dental caries experience of elementary school children. Public Health Rep. 1938;53:1685–90.
7. Lagerweij MD, van Loveren C. Declining caries trends: are we satisfied? Curr Oral Health Rep. 2015;2:212–7.
8. Ismail AI, Sohn W, Tellez M, Amaya A, Sen A, Hasson H, Pitts N. The International Caries Detection and Assessment System (ICDAS): an integrated system for measuring dental caries. Community Dent Oral Epidemiol. 2007;35:170–8.
9. Nyvad B, Machiulskiene V, Baelum V. Reliability of a new caries diagnostic system differentiating between active and inactive caries lesions. Caries Res. 1999;33:252–60.
10. World Health Organization. The world health report 2008. Primary health care: now more than ever. Geneva: WHO; 2008.
11. Brazilian Ministry of Health: project oral health Brazil 2010—National Survey on Oral Health 2010. 2011. https://189.28.128.100/dab/docs/geral/apresentação_SB2010.pdf.
12. Shidara EK, McGlothlin JD, Kobayashi S. A vicious cycle in the oral health status of schoolchildren in a primary school in rural Cambodia. Int J Dent Hyg. 2007;5:165–73.
13. Frencken JE, Amorim RG, Faber J, Leal SC. The Caries Assessment Spectrum and Treatment (CAST) index: rational and development. Int Dent J. 2011;61:117–23.
14. de Souza AL, Sanden WJ, Leal SC, Frencken JE. The Caries Assessment Spectrum and Treatment (CAST) index: face and content validation. Int Dent J. 2012;62:270–6.
15. de Souza AL, Bronkhorst EM, Creugers NHJ, Leal SC, Frencken JE. The Caries Assessment Spectrum and Treatment (CAST) instrument: its reproducibility in clinical studies. Int Dent J. 2014;64:187–94.
16. Baginska J, Rodakowska E, Kierklo A. Status of occlusal surfaces of first permanent molars in 6-8-year-old children evaluated by the CAST and DMF indices. Eur J Paediatr Dent. 2014;2:107–12.
17. Baginska J, Rodakowska E, Milewski R, Kierklo A. Dental caries in primary and permanent molars in 7-8-year-old schoolchildren evaluated with Caries Assessment Spectrum and Treatment (CAST) index. BMC Oral Health. 2014;14:1–8.
18. Malik A, Shaukat MS, Qureshi A. Prevalence of dental caries using novel caries assessment index—CAST. J Dow Univ Health Sci. 2014;8:7–10.
19. de Souza AL, Leal SC, Bronkhorst EM, Frencken JE. Assessing caries status according to the CAST instrument and WHO criterion in epidemiological studies. BMC Oral Health. 2014;14:119.

20. Medeiros PBV, Otero SAM, Frencken JE, Bronkhorst E, Leal SC. Effectiveness of an oral health program for mothers and their infants. Int J Paediatr Dent. 2014;7(25):29–34.
21. Anchala K, Challa R, Vadaganadham Y, Kamatham R, Deepak V, Nuvvula S. Assessment of dental caries in primary dentition employing caries assessment spectrum and treatment index. J Orofac Sci. 2016;8:115–9.
22. Baginska J, Rodakowska E. Caries Assessment Spectrum and Treatment (CAST) index in the primary molars of 6- to 7-year-old polish children. Oral Health Prev Dent. 2016;14:85–92.
23. Kar S, Kundu G, Maiti S, Ghosh C, Bazmi B, Mukhopadhyay S. A comparative evaluation of dental caries status among hearing-impaired and normal children of Malda, West Bengal, evaluated with the Caries Assessment Spectrum and Treatment. J Indian Soc Pedod Prev Dent. 2016;34:306–9.
24. Mwakayoka H, Masalu JR, Namakuka Kikwilu E. Dental Caries and associated factors in children aged 2–4 years old in Mbeya City, Tanzania. J Dent (Shiraz). 2017;18(2):104–11.
25. Doneria D, Thakur S, Singhal P, Chauhan D, Jayam C, Uppal A. Comparative evaluation of Caries status in primary and permanent molars in 7–8-year-old schoolchildren of Shimla using Caries Assessment Spectrum and Treatment Index. Contemp Clin Dent. 2017;8(1):128–33.
26. Frencken JE, de Souza Hilgert AL, Bronkhorst EM, Leal SC. CAST Caries Assessment Spectrum and Treatment manual. 1st ed. Nijmegen: Radboud University Nijmegen; 2015. p. 48.
27. de Souza Hilgert AL. Caries Assessment Spectrum and Treatment (CAST): a new epidemiological instrument. Doctoral thesis. Nijmegen: Radboud University Nijmegen; 2015.
28. de Souza AL, Leal SC, Chaves SB, Bronkhorst E, Frencken JE, Creugers NHJ. The Caries Assessment Spectrum and Treatment (CAST) instrument: construct validation. Eur J Oral Sci. 2014;122:149–53.
29. Davis FD. Perceived usefulness, perceived ease of use, and user acceptance of information technology. MIS Q. 1989;13(3):319–40. https://doi.org/10.2307/249008.

Caries Detection Dyes

9

Marisa Maltz, Rodrigo Alex Arthur, and Clarissa Fatturi-Parolo

9.1 Introduction

Historically, the removal of all infected dentin was advised prior to placement of a restoration. The aim was to have dentin devoid of bacterial infection. Caries detection dyes were developed to guide the dentist in the removal of infected dentin. This chapter discuss the clinical use of detection dyes and the evidence behind.

9.2 Restorative Treatment: The Need for Carious Dentin Removal

The lack of carious activity control may lead to lesion progression from enamel to dentin. Bacteria are present within enamel carious lesion, and to a lesser extent on dentin tubules, even before cavitation [1]. Once the demineralization reaches dentin, the inorganic crystals might get lost. This leaves the organic part unprotected, the phosphoproteins readily dissolve although a minor part is still associated with collagens. Degradation of exposed collagenous organic matrix is also found as result of salivary- and host-derived metalloproteinases that are activated by the low pH induced by bacterial acid-end products [2]. The longer the cariogenic challenge lasts, the more porous the enamel subsurface will become, which creates conditions for surface breakdown and dentin exposure. The bulk of carious tissue consists of interconnecting forces between more or less disrupted collagen cross-linked with other proteins. As a result, the organic phase is not disintegrated and dissolved as the mineral and the remaining bulk of carious tissue is very well anchored to the cavity floor. In this scenario, dentin will be heavily exposed to bacterial infection and superficial tubular invasion occurs. At this point, and in response to progressing dentinal lesions,

M. Maltz (✉) · R. A. Arthur · C. Fatturi-Parolo
Department of Preventive and Social Dentistry, Faculty of Dentistry, UFRGS—Universidade Federal do Rio Grande do Sul, Porto Alegre, RS, Brazil

© Springer Nature Switzerland AG 2019

A. Ferreira Zandona, C. Longbottom (eds.), *Detection and Assessment of Dental Caries*, https://doi.org/10.1007/978-3-030-16967-1_9

different layers of carious dentin may be present and used to be classified as *infected dentin*, represented by superficial necrotic zone with bacterial invasion; and *affected dentin*, represented by an inner layer of dentin that is partially demineralized and contains minimal bacterial infection. It has been shown that the pattern of amino acid composition on both layers is similar to sound dentin, but affected dentin presented decreased collagen cross-links and increased precursors, yet preserving the network of organic matrix and odontoblastic process, while in the infected dentin both the cross-links and the precursors were decreased and the odontoblastic process disappeared [3]. This way, it is considered that molecular changes induced on affected dentin are reversible, which makes this layer able to be re-hardened, while the extend of changes found on collagen matrix of infected dentin layer makes it irreversibly demineralized [3].

Cavitated caries lesion can be controlled once the external biofilm is regularly removed. However, under certain conditions, cavitated carious lesions need to receive restorative management which aims to facilitate control of biofilm accumulation on carious sites, protect the pulp-dentin complex and restore function, esthetics, and form of the tooth. Carious tissue removal is then an important clinical step that precedes the placement of a restoration. This way, the main aspects involved in carious tissue removal are to create conditions for a long-lasting restoration, preserve healthy and remineralizable tissue, achieve a sufficient seal, maintain pulpal health, and maximize success of the restoration.

In order to achieve those goals, it has been traditionally accepted that carious tissues need to be completely removed from the surrounding cavity walls, but only the more disorganized and demineralized infected dentin layer should be removed from the cavity pulpal floor leaving the affected but repairable carious dentin on place. The rationale of this approach is to eliminate the presence of bacteria on the remaining dentin. Although the conventional restorative treatment demands a firm and clean cavity floor, it is been known that it is very difficult to achieve a dentin completely devoid of bacterial infection [4]. The most common criterion used to assess carious tissue removal is hardness. By means of an excavator, all necrotic and soft dentin is then removed from the surrounding walls until a hard dentin is left while a firm dentin (resistant to hand excavator) is left at the pulpal dentin floor [5].

The abovementioned clinical criterion for carious dentin removal may be subjective. Caries-detecting dyes were developed to guide the dentist to precisely differentiate between carious dentin and sound dentin during carious dentin removal. The rationale for the use of detection dyes is to avoid over-reduction of the remaining dentin underneath the carious lesion. Examples of caries disclosing dye products along with clinical technique, mode of action, and available evidence regarding their use are provided below.

9.3 Caries Disclosing/Detection Dyes

9.3.1 Products

Back to the early 1970s, the first developed caries disclosing dye was based on a solution of 0.5% basic red fuchsin in propylene glycol. It was suggested that this dye selectively red-stained the superficial- and heavily degraded-collagen carious

Table 9.1 Caries disclosing dye products

Dye	Manufacturer	Composition
Caries check	Nippon Shika, Japan	1% acid red or 1% brilliant blue in polypropylene glycol
Caries check red	Nishida Co., Japan	1% acid red 52 or brilliant blue dye in polypropylene glycol
Caries check blue	Nishida Co., Japan	1% acid red 52 or brilliant blue dye in polypropylene glycol
Caries detector	Kuraray Co.	1% acid red 52 in propylene glycol base
Caries finder	Danville materials	1% acid red 52 in propylene glycol base
Caries finder green	Danville materials	1% FD&C green dye in propylene glycol
Seek	Ultradent products	D&C red dye in 90% propylene glycol base
Sable seek	Ultradent products	FD&C dark green dye in 70% propylene glycol base
Snoop	Pulpdent Corporation	Dark blue dye in 47% propylene glycol and 47% water

dentin layer (*infected layer*) [6] and was able to identify infected dentin [7]. Yet, traces of viable bacteria were still detected at the deepest portion of carious lesions even after guided dentin carious removal [8]. Concerns were arisen regarding a potential carcinogenic effect of fuchsin and its use was replaced by acid red dye, which is a frequently used food component.

One of the first reports on the use of 1% acid red staining in propylene glycol base for selective carious tissue removal come from the study of Shimizu et al. [9]. Human extracted teeth with carious dentin were stained and both the depth of the staining and the depth of bacterial invasion were assessed. Authors concluded that it was possible to differentiate both layers of carious dentin and that the extent of bacterial invasion was closely comparable to the extent of the stained dentin, suggesting that the complete removal of stainable dentin would result in complete removal of infection. Since then, several studies were carried out to evaluate the use of this staining as an adjunct for carious tissue removal. Additionally, slight modifications on available commercial products were made over years. Table 9.1 presents caries disclosing dye products.

Despite the differences on composition amongst dye products, application mode is similar. Before application of dyes, carious cavity needs to be cleaned and air-dried. One drop of the dye solution is then applied to the lesion for 5 s (caries finder/caries finder green) or 10 s (caries detector, seek/sable seek, snoop, caries marker) and rinsed away with water. The infected dentin is red-stained (caries detector, caries finder), green-stained (caries finder green/sable seek) or dark blue stained (Snoop) and removed by an excavator or a round steel bur of low speed without irrigation. According to manufacturer's instructions, solution needs to be re-applied on cavities to identify residual infected dentin until cavity floor is no longer stainable.

9.3.2 Mode of Action

Overall, propylene glycol-based dyes were designed to stain only the outer layer of carious dentin since propylene glycol penetrates only loosened collagen fibers with broken intermolecular cross-links. There is a concern that the reddish-brown color of the interface between infected and affected dentin might impair the precise identification of both carious dentin layers by using a staining that provides a red background. Therefore, acid red has been replaced by green or blue dyes in some products [10].

9.3.3 Accuracy of Disclosing/Detection Dyes on Carious Tissue Removal

9.3.3.1 In Vitro Studies

Wariness regarding the use of dyes is reported in the literature as they have been found to be non-selective. There is some level of disagreement regarding the ability of dyes to stain and precisely identify bacteria on carious tissues. While some studies found that complete removal of stainable dentin results in almost complete removal of infection [9], others found that the deepest portion of carious lesions may still contain bacteria even after the removal of the stained carious tissue [8, 11]. Shimizu et al. [9] and Ganter et al. [12] showed that the cavity floor of the excavated dentin area after stained dentin removal was always deeper than the bacterial invasion [9, 12]. It has been suggested then that staining and bacterial penetration are independent phenomena, mostly because dye does not stain bacteria but the organic matrix

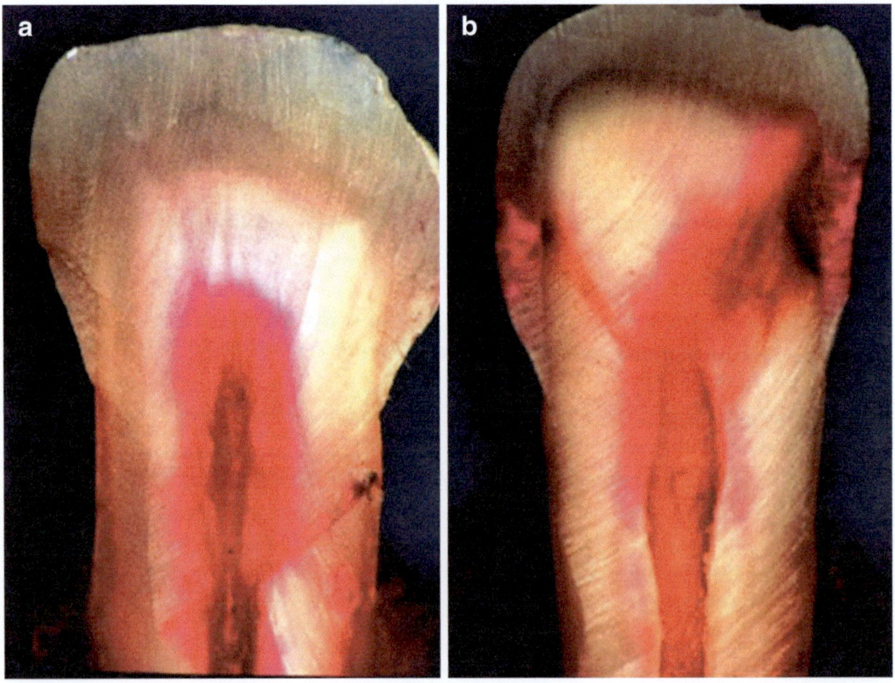

Fig. 9.1 Longitudinal ground sections of sound teeth (**a**) and non-cavitated enamel lesion (**b**) after application of 1% acid red dye. Circumpulpal deep dentine as well as demineralized enamel and dentine are stained by the dye. Courtesy of Dr. Sandra Henz (Federal University of Rio Grande do Sul)

of less mineralized dentin [11]. The circumpulpal dentin and the enamel–dentin junction of sound teeth are normally stained due to their higher proportion of organic matrix [13, 14]. Also, the porous non-cavitated lesions are disclosed by dye (Fig. 9.1).

De Almeida Neves et al. [15] evaluated the caries removal effectiveness comparing nine different methods for caries removal [15]. Over-excavation was observed when burs were combined with Caries Detector (CD). In this study, it was preferable to use the bur alone than combining with the CD in relation to sound dentin preservation. This way, dyes have presented high specificity but questionable sensitivity in relation to their capability on the identification of bacterial penetration on carious tissues [16]. In vitro and ex vivo studies are presented on Table 9.2 [8, 9,11, 13, 15–19, 28].

9.3.3.2 Clinical Studies

Clinical studies are the best reference to guide dental practice. Therefore, it is very important to evaluate the use of dyes in this context. Unfortunately, to our knowledge, there are few clinical trials on this subject (Table 9.3) [10, 20–27, 35]. Some studies recommend the use of the dye to help the caries removal procedures once the bacterial load was higher in the initial sample and lowest in unstained dentin following dye application [21]. However, concerns about the use of the dye arose once hard dentin was stained with the dye [20, 24]. When the use of dye was validated by microbiological methods, it was possible to observe that no differences in level of contamination between stained and non-stained sites were observed [22]. Subsequently, it has been concluded that dye staining and bacterial penetration are different phenomena [22]. Therefore, dye staining is a rather poor indicator for the presence or absence of carious dentin. For this same reason, caries excavation using dye indicators also does not ensure the elimination of bacteria [27]. Hosoya et al. [10] evaluated different caries detector dyes and recommended the use of caries check blue to circumvent the problem of inadvertent removal of caries-affected dentin. Their conclusion was granted once the fluorescence readings of residual dentin with caries check blue were higher than the other dyes evaluated, indicating a more conservative dentin removal [10]. Nevertheless, caution should be taken to interpret these findings once the validation criteria (DIAGNOdent readings) had important limitations [15]. Sensitivity and specificity are important measures of the diagnostic accuracy of a test. The sensitivity of a caries detector dye is defined as the proportion of samples with viable bacteria that will stain with the dye. The specificity of a dye is the proportion of samples without viable bacteria that will have a negative result (no-stain). In general, a minimal value of 70% is expected for both sensitivity and specificity when a diagnostic test is used. If values are lower than 70%, the diagnostic accuracy is compromised and the test should not be applied in clinical situations. Having this in mind, we can look up at the values of sensitivity and specificity for dye utilization in clinical practice (Summary Table). For Peskersoy et al. [25] the sensitivity for the caries detector was 65.1% and specificity of 37.6% [25]. As we can observe the sensitivity value is not good enough. The specificity is even lower than sensitivity for this study and it is related to the higher numbers of false positives when the dye is used to aid the caries removal. Therefore, the accuracy of the dye is questionable for clinical purposes. A summary of in vivo findings is presented on Table 9.3.

Table 9.2 In vitro and ex vivo studies of caries disclosing dyes

In vitro and ex vivo studies					
Reference	Dye	Sample	Validation method	Outcome	Results
Anderson et al. [8] Part 2	0.5% basic fuchsin in propylene glycol solution	$N = 10$ extracted teeth	Microbiological	Total viable count from stained and no stained dentin	The fuchsin-stained dentin always contained demonstrable bacteria, while six of the ten non-stained samples showed no growth Fuchsin-stained sample contained 1300 times more CFU/mg than the adjacent non-stained sample
Shimizu et al. [9]	1% acid red dye in propylene glycol	Extracted human teeth ($n = 20$) with dentine carious lesions	Histological	Depth of stained carious dentine and depth of bacteria invasion	– The use of dye clearly differentiates between infected (stainable) and affected (not stainable) dentine layers – Bacteria invasion was closely comparable and did not exceed the extent of stained carious tissue – The cavity floor of the excavated area was always deeper than the bacterial invasion
Boston and Graver [11]	1% acid red dye in propylene glycol (Sulforhodamine B, Sigma Chemical Co.)	Extracted human permanent posterior teeth with dentine carious lesions ($n = 20$)	Histological	Presence of bacteria on dentine tubules before and after carious removal	– 75% of the stained infected dentine harbored bacteria – The deepest portion of carious lesions may still contain bacteria even after stained carious tissue removal
Yip et al. [13]	0.5% basic red fuchsin 1% acid red dye in propylene glycol (Sulforhodamine B, Sigma Chemical Co.)	Extracted human primary ($n = 40$) and permanent ($n = 40$) posterior teeth with dentine carious lesions	Light microscopy and backscattered electron imaging (BSE)	Presence of staining and mineral density in the vicinity of circumpulpal area and EDJ before/after caries removal	– Both dyes were able to clearly differentiate between outer layer of carious dentine (heavily stained) from the inner layer – Sound dentine was stained by both dyes in the vicinity of circumpulpal dentine and along EDJ

Banerjee et al. [17]	Caries detector	Extracted human permanent molars ($n = 50$) with cavitated occlusal lesions	Confocal microscopy	Cavity extent after excavation guided by carious tissue staining compared to conventional excavation without staining based on hardness criterion and auto-fluorescence (AF) signal outline for carious dentine	– Greater quantity of dentine (up to 58%) was removed after excavation guided by carious tissue staining when compared to excavation based on AF of dentinal carious tissue
Boston and Liao [28]	Caries detector Caries finder green Sable seek Snoop	Extracted sound ($n = 12$) and with carious dentine ($n = 5$) human permanent posterior teeth	Histological	Intensity of staining at DEJ, circumpulpal area and main body of dentine	– All dyes were effective in distinguishing between the outer carious dentine layer (intensively stained) and the inner carious dentine layer (very lightly stained) – Some degree of false-positive staining was found for the studied sites
Yazici et al. [18]	Caries finder	Extracted human molars with carious dentine ($n = 40$)	Polarized light microscopy	Detection of residual caries by DIAGNOdent and detector dye after chemo-mechanical caries removal	Sensitivity of DIAGNOdent (0.6–0.7) was statistically higher than caries finder (0.4) Specificity of DIAGNOdent (0.83–0.91) was statistically similar to caries finder (1.0)
Lennon et al. [19]	Caries detector	Extracted human permanent molars with carious dentine ($n = 20$/group)	Confocal microscopy	Relative cavity size and quantity of remaining bacteria after excavation guided by carious tissue staining compared to conventional excavation without staining and FACE[a]	– No differences were found on the relative cavity size amongst the tested methods – Pulp exposure ($n = 2$) was found on caries detector group – FACE removed more heavily infected dentine than the other methods
Javaheri et al. [16]	Caries detector Caries check[b]	Extracted human posterior teeth with carious dentine ($n = 20$)	Histological	Bacterial presence into dentinal tubules in relation to stained/not stained samples	– Sensitivity: Caries detector: 74% Caries check: 71% – Specificity: Caries detector: 100% Caries check: 100%

(continued)

Table 9.2 (continued)

In vitro and ex vivo studies					
Reference	Dye	Sample	Validation method	Outcome	Results
De Almeida Neves et al. [15]	Caries detector	Extracted human molars with occlusal caries ($n = 63$)	Micro-CT	Caries removal effectiveness (CRE), by assessing relative volume of residual caries and mineral density at the cavity floor, and minimal invasiveness potential (MIP), by assessing the relative cavity size after caries removal, of the following caries removal techniques – Rotatory/oscillating instruments followed or not followed by the use of caries detector – Chemo-mechanical caries removal – Laser (Er-YAG)	• Laser-guided carious tissue removal presented the highest MIP • Rotatory/oscillating instruments presented more favorable CRE with some tendency towards over-excavation • Carious tissue removal by chemo-mechanical excavation aided by conventional metal excavators presented the best CRE and MIP • Lasers resulted in non-selective carious tissue removal • Rotatory/oscillating instruments may lead to over-excavation especially if it is guided by caries detection dye, whereas the sole use of tungsten-carbide burs resulted in a reduced risk for over-excavation • Chemo-mechanical methods were the most selective and able to preserve sound tissue

[a]Fluorescence Aided Caries Excavation

[b]It contains 1% acid red dye in polypropylene glycol

Table 9.3 Clinical studies of caries disclosing dyes

Clinical studies					
Reference	Dye	Sample	Validation method	Outcome	Results
Kidd et al. [20]	1% acid red in propylene glycol	100 cavities in need of operative treatment	No validation method Comparison of clinical appearance and staining	After caries removal Each tooth was divided and one half stained and another not stained, pulpal dentin and EDJ were analyzed	40/76 hard pulpal dentine were stained with the dye
Zacharia and Munshi [21]	1% acid red in propylene glycol	$N = 30$ teeth, carious lesions in dentin	Microbiological	Caries removal by visual and tactile criteria and, after that, dye application. Microbiological analysis (total CFU) from the initial caries dentine, stained carious dentine and non-stained carious dentin	The bacterial load was higher in the initial sample and lowest in unstained dentin following dye application
Kidd et al. [22]	1% acid red in propylene glycol	201 cavities in need of operative treatment from primary or secondary caries	Microbiological	Microbial load from initial dentine sample and from final dentine sample after complete caries removal (hard to probe and stain free) in stained and non-stained areas from EDJ	52% of the cavities showed staining areas at EDJ after complete caries removal Stained and unstained areas resulted in low number of bacterial growth No differences in level of contamination between stained and non-stained sites Acid red staining and bacterial penetration are not corresponding events
Maupomé et al. [24]	G1: 1% acid red in propylene glycol, G2: 8% povidone-iodine in water	221 cavities in dentin, G1 = 110 cavities and G2 = 111	Not applied	Dental students diagnosed the cavity as caries-free and after that the dye was applied. It was evaluated the percentage of the cavities that were stained or not stained after the clinical judgment as caries-free cavity	After dental caries removal by clinical judgment, 21.3% of the cavities stained with acid red and 15.4% of the cavities stained with povidone-iodine The relevance of these findings is limited since no validation method was performed

(continued)

Table 9.3 (continued)

Clinical studies					
Reference	Dye	Sample	Validation method	Outcome	Results
Ribeiro et al. [23]	Vide cárie, Inodom	38 children, G1: Complete caries removal using bur and dye, G2: partial caries removal from pulpal/axial wall	Not applied	Clinical evaluation, retention and marginal integrity of the restoration, radiographic evaluation, SEM evaluation from extracted teeth	Retention rate, marginal integrity, and pulpal symptoms identical in both groups
Maltz et al. [27, 35]	1% acid red in propylene glycol	Complete caries removal (CCR) aided by dye ($n = 60$) × incomplete caries removal and seal (ICR-seal) ($n = 32$)	Microbiological	The counts of anaerobic, aerobic, mutans streptococci, and Lactobacilli samples were obtained from the initial demineralized dentine, after CCR and after ICR-seal	The counts of anaerobic, aerobic, mutans streptococci, and
Hosoya et al. [10]	Caries check blue (CCB) × caries check (CC) × caries detector (CD)	Experimental groups (and number of teeth) were primary- CCB [34], primary-CC [33], primary-CD [31], permanent-CCB [33], permanent-CC [23], and permanent-CD [26]	DIAGNOdent readings and clinical parameters such as color and hardness	Correlation coefficients between DIAGNOdent reading and the clinical parameters	The correlation coefficients between the DIAGNOdent reading and the clinical parameters of color and hardness of the caries-infected dentin were low both in primary and young permanent teeth The fluorescence readings of residual dentin using DIAGNOdent after caries removal guided by acid red in caries check blue were higher than those when caries was removed using CD and CC, indicating that less dentin was removed Caries check blue might be useful, especially in permanent teeth to circumvent the problem of inadvertent removal of caries-affected dentin

Peskersoy et al. [25]	Caries detector (CD)	273 patients with 451 black II (OM/OD) cavities	FACE	CD x conventional visual assessment and tactile probing method × FACE	CD: Sensitivity 65.1% and specificity 37.6% CD stained demineralized dentin areas close to the pulp chamber in 6.7% of the cavities (that had been diagnosed as sound using the FACE) CD could not stain the carious areas of 94 cases (22.6%) that the FACE diagnosed as partially excavated caries
Singhal et al. [26]	1% acid red solution in propylene glycol for group C	$N = 42$ primary molars with acute carious lesions in inner half of dentine and vital pulp, group A: Partial caries removal using hand instruments atraumatic restorative treatment (ART) only; group B: Partial caries removal using bur; group C: Complete caries removal using bur and caries detector dye	Microbiological	Initial and 3 weeks sealing period	The difference in microbial count observed between the three groups at baseline disappeared at the end of the 3 weeks follow-up

Limitation of Validation Methods Used to Assess the Accuracy of Caries Disclosing Dyes on Carious Removal

What would be the ideal caries excavation? It would be the one that removes the irreversible and most contaminated destroyed tissue leaving a potentially remineralizable cavity floor. So, if we want to study caries removal how we could measure if what we were doing is right? To answer to this question, a validation criterion for caries removal should be established. Microbiological and histological data are the validation methods most used to assess the accuracy of caries disclosing dyes. In Tables 9.2 and 9.3 it is stated, for each of the selected studies, the validation criteria applied to judge a cavity as caries-free or not. Microbiological and confocal microscopy data give us the bacterial load related to caries excavation. Although microbiological validation can be used in both in vitro and in vivo *studies*, the histological evaluation can only be applied for in vitro studies. On the other hand, the use of DIAGNOdent to assess the endpoint of caries excavation is doubtful [15] and the correlation coefficients between the DIAGNOdent reading and the clinical parameters of color and hardness of the caries-infected dentin were low [10].

The above validation methods have been questioned once recent studies suggest it is not necessary to remove all carious dentin before the restoration is placed because, over time, sealing of carious dentin results in lower levels of infection than traditional dentin caries removal. Maltz et al. [27] compare the microbiological infection (through culture) after conventional carious dentin removal (hardness criteria plus dye—CCR) with partial carious dentin removal (PCR) that has been sealed for 6 months. Sealing of carious dentin results in lower levels of infection than traditional dentin caries removal [27]. The microbial load after PCR-seal was lower than the microbial load after CCR using dye. Similar results have been observed by Singhal et al. [26]. They showed that the difference in microbial count at baseline observed between the three different dentin caries removal methods (atraumatic restorative treatment, partial caries removal using bur, and complete caries removal using bur and caries detector dye) disappeared at the end of the 3 weeks follow-up.

9.4 What Is the Impact of Caries Detector/Disclosing Dyes Use on Clinical Practice?

Some degree of false-positive staining has been found for sound enamel, sound dentin, in the vicinity of circumpulpal dentin and along EDJ [13, 28, 29] which could also lead to unnecessary sound dentin removal leading to increased risk of pulpal exposures in deep carious lesions [13, 17, 19] (Fig. 9.2). There is also a concern that the dentin overstaining might be related to low molecular weight of propylene glycol-based solution, which makes it more prone to penetrate deeper into porous carious dentin. However, its replacement by a higher molecular weight carrier, such as polypropylene glycol, did not result in an enhanced sensitivity [16]. Yet, the use of caries disclosing dyes has shown low sensitivity on the detection of

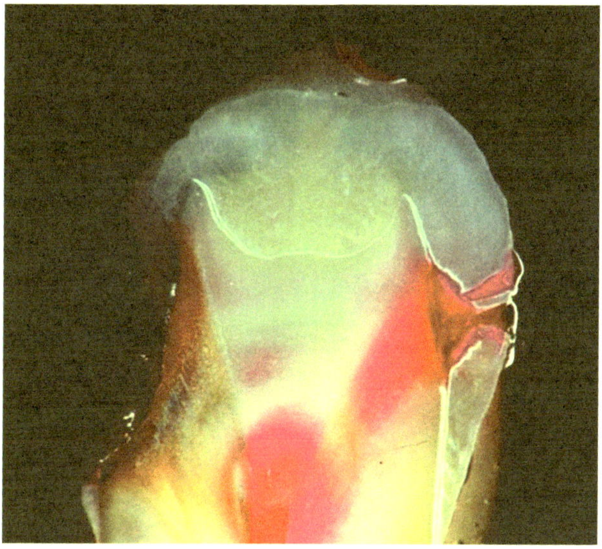

Fig. 9.2 Deep caries lesion and circumpulpar dentine stained by acid red. Note that the disclosed carious tissue (lesion) and the sound circumpulpar dentine are very close which can lead to pulp exposure during excavation procedure guided by staining. Courtesy of Dr. Sandra Henz (Federal University of Rio Grande do Sul)

remaining dentin caries on cavity floor after carious tissue removal [18]. This way, a recent systematic review and network meta-analysis has suggested that the available evidence is not sufficient to support any conclusion regarding the clinical use of guided dentin carious tissues excavation methods, such as the one performed with the aid of disclosing dyes [30].

Another concern regarding the use of disclosing dyes is the difficulty in removing the staining in the esthetic restorations. Additionally, the effect of caries detector/disclosing dyes on the mechanical properties of adhesive materials has been questioned. It has been reported by some studies that the use of dyes does not alter the dentin-to-composite shear bond strengths for total-etch or self-etching bonding systems [31]. On the other hand, a negative effect of dyes on adhesive bonding strength of total-etch bonding systems has been reported [32]. It has been suggested that dyes remain trapped in the remaining dentin affecting the adhesion mechanism between restorative materials and tooth [32]. It is important though to emphasize that all available data on the effect of dyes on adhesive restorations come from in vitro studies. There is not any clinical report on the long-term survival rate of adhesive restorations placed on cavities after caries detector/disclosing also dyes use. This way, the effect of dyes on bonding properties of adhesive restoration remains unclear. Another concern in the literature is the possibility of the dye to stain the restorative material [33].

The use of a dye seems to have limited clinical application. Clinical studies with real validated outcomes for bacterial contamination (cultured based, FACE) show us that dye presented a low specificity and sensitivity. Therefore, the clinical application of dye to aid caries removal is limited. Therefore, there is a lack of substantive scientific evidence with good quality supporting the use of caries-detecting dyes.

9.5 Is It Really Necessary to Have a Complete Clean Cavity Before the Placement of a Restoration?

In caries removal, dentists have to face the risks of leaving infected dentin in the cavity or removing dentin unnecessarily. What the literature would indicate as best choice? To answer this question, three aspects have to be considered. (a) Studies have shown that during a caries removal process it is impossible to leave a cavity without bacteria [4] even with the use of disclosing dyes [27]. (b) The view that cavity sealing modifies bacterial growth and drastically reduces the presence of cariogenic bacteria is an important observation in many clinical studies. When the bacterial contamination with partial or total caries removal is compared after sealing, no difference in the bacterial load is observed [26, 27]. This means that, irrespectively from the initial bacterial load in dentin, the reduction of bacteria load is similar after sealing. (c) Sealing of carious dentin did not interfere with pulp vitality or restoration survival [34–36].

9.6 Concluding Remarks

Based on available evidence we can conclude that leaving bacteria underneath restoration is inevitable once we usually leave infected dentin both in the conventional treatment (hardness criteria) and/or using disclosing dyes. Furthermore, bacteria underneath restoration did not hamper restoration survival. Therefore, the use of dyes to disclose carious tissue that should be removed seems not to be an essential procedure during the restoration process.

Summary table

Bitewing radiography	Caries detection dyes			
Which surfaces/ sites is it useful for	Occlusal (pits and fissures)	Proximal/ (approximal)	Smooth surface (buccal and lingual)	Root caries (buccal, lingual, and approximal)
	Y	**Y**	**Y**	**Y**
What type of lesions is valuable for	Primary coronal	Secondary coronal	Primary root caries	Secondary root caries
	Y	**Y**	**Y**	**Y**
What type of dentition	Primary		Permanent	
	Y		**Y**	
Lesion severity	Enamel lesions		Dentinal lesions	
	N		**Y**	
Sensitivity	Literature reported range in 0.4–0.6			
Specificity	Literature reported range in 0.3–1.0			
Perceived Ease Of Use (PEOU)[a]	Dye is easy to use			
Advantages/ disadvantages	*Advantages*			
	1. No advantages			
	Disadvantages			
	1. It would lead to excessive dentin removal, may affect the adhesive properties for restorations, may cause discoloration in some dental materials, extra step in the clinical section			

Time	Quick to apply (10 s) but difficult to remove all stain prior to restoration (time depends on the operator skills and size of the cavity preparation). Approximate time: 10 s–10 min
Cost	Approximate cost per unit and any disposables: $40

[a]Davis (1989)

References

1. Parolo C, Maltz M. Microbial contamination of noncavitated caries lesions: a scanning electron microscopic study. Caries Res. 2006;40(6):536–41.
2. Chaussain-Miller C, Fioretti F, Goldberg M, Menashi S. The role of matrix metalloproteinases (MMPs) in human caries. J Dent Res. 2006;85(1):22–32.
3. Kuboki Y, Ohgushi K, Fusayama T. Collagen biochemistry of the two layers of carious dentin. J Dent Res. 1977;56(10):1233–7.
4. Banerjee A, Yasseri M, Munson M. A method for the detection and quantification of bacteria in human carious dentine using fluorescent in situ hybridisation. J Dent. 2002;30(7–8):359–63.
5. Innes NP, Frencken JE, Bjørndal L, Maltz M, Manton DJ, Ricketts D, et al. Managing carious lesions: consensus recommendations on terminology. Adv Dent Res. 2016;28(2):49–57.
6. Fusayama T, Terachima S. Differentiation of two layers of carious dentin by staining. J Dent Res. 1972;51(3):866.
7. Sato Y, Fusayama T. Removal of dentin by fuchsin staining. J Dent Res. 1976;55(4):678–83.
8. Anderson MH, Loesche WJ, Charbeneau GT. Bacteriologic study of a basic fuchsin caries-disclosing dye. J Prosthet Dent. 1985;54(1):51–5.
9. Shimizu C, Inokoshi S, Bushita M, Hosoda H, Fusayama T. Caries detector for pulpless teeth. Oper Dent. 1983;8(3):94–8.
10. Hosoya Y, Taguchi T, Arita S, Tay FR. Clinical evaluation of polypropylene glycol-based caries detecting dyes for primary and permanent carious dentin. J Dent. 2008;36(12):1041–7.
11. Boston DW, Graver HT. Histological study of an acid red caries-disclosing dye. Oper Dent. 1989;14(4):186–92.
12. Ganter P, Al-Ahmad A, Wrbas KT, Hellwig E, Altenburger MJ. The use of computer-assisted FACE for minimal-invasive caries excavation. Clin Oral Investig. 2014;18(3):745–51.
13. Yip HK, Stevenson AG, Beeley JA. The specificity of caries detector dyes in cavity preparation. Br Dent J. 1994;176(11):417–21.
14. Boston DW, Graver HT. Histobacteriological analysis of acid red dye-stainable dentin found beneath intact amalgam restorations. Oper Dent. 1994;19(2):65–9.
15. de Almeida Neves A, Coutinho E, Cardoso MV, Lambrechts P, Van Meerbeek B. Current concepts and techniques for caries excavation and adhesion to residual dentin. J Adhes Dent. 2011;13(1):7–22.
16. Javaheri M, Maleki-Kambakhsh S, Etemad-Moghadam S. Efficacy of two caries detector dyes in the diagnosis of dental caries. J Dent (Tehran). 2010;7(2):71–6.
17. Banerjee A, Kidd EA, Watson TF. In vitro validation of carious dentin removed using different excavation criteria. Am J Dent. 2003;16(4):228–30.
18. Yazici AR, Baseren M, Gokalp S. The in vitro performance of laser fluorescence and caries-detector dye for detecting residual carious dentin during tooth preparation. Quintessence Int. 2005;36(6):417–22.
19. Lennon AM, Attin T, Buchalla W. Quantity of remaining bacteria and cavity size after excavation with FACE, caries detector dye and conventional excavation in vitro. Oper Dent. 2007;32(3):236–41.
20. Kidd EA, Joyston-Bechal S, Smith MM, Allan R, Howe L, Smith SR. The use of a caries detector dye in cavity preparation. Br Dent J. 1989;167(4):132–4.
21. Zacharia MA, Munshi AK. Microbiological assessment of dentin stained with a caries detector dye. J Clin Pediatr Dent. 1995;19(2):111–5.

22. Kidd EA, Joyston-Bechal S, Beighton D. The use of a caries detector dye during cavity preparation: a microbiological assessment. Br Dent J. 1993;174(7):245–8.
23. Ribeiro CC, Baratieri LN, Perdigão J, Baratieri NM, Ritter AV. A clinical, radiographic, and scanning electron microscopic evaluation of adhesive restorations on carious dentin in primary teeth. Quintessence Int. 1999;30(9):591–9.
24. Maupomé G, Hernández-Guerrero JC, García-Luna M, Trejo-Alvarado A, Hernández-Pérez M, Díez-de-Bonilla J. In vivo diagnostic assessment of dentinal caries utilizing acid red and povidone-iodine dyes. Oper Dent. 1995;20(3):119–22.
25. Peskersoy C, Turkun M, Onal B. Comparative clinical evaluation of the efficacy of a new method for caries diagnosis and excavation. J Conserv Dent. 2015;18(5):364–8.
26. Singhal DK, Acharya S, Thakur AS. Microbiological analysis after complete or partial removal of carious dentin using two different techniques in primary teeth: a randomized clinical trial. Dent Res J (Isfahan). 2016;13(1):30–7.
27. Maltz M, Henz SL, de Oliveira EF, Jardim JJ. Conventional caries removal and sealed caries in permanent teeth: a microbiological evaluation. J Dent. 2012;40(9):776–82.
28. Boston DW, Liao J. Staining of non-carious human coronal dentin by caries dyes. Oper Dent. 2004;29(3):280–6.
29. Maltz M, Henz S, Volkveiss A, Campos C. Morphological and ultrastructural evaluation of the specificity of caries detector dye in the identification of carious dentine. In: Karger, editor. 45th Orca Congress; Stockholm, Sweden: Karger; 1998. p. 294.
30. Schwendicke F, Göstemeyer G, Gluud C. Cavity lining after excavating caries lesions: meta-analysis and trial sequential analysis of randomized clinical trials. J Dent. 2015;43(11):1291–7.
31. Kazemi RB, Meiers JC, Peppers K. Effect of caries disclosing agents on bond strengths of total-etch and self-etching primer dentin bonding systems to resin composite. Oper Dent. 2002;27(3):238–42.
32. Singh UP, Tikku A, Chandra A, Loomba K, Boruah LC. Influence of caries detection dye on bond strength of sound and carious affected dentin: an in-vitro study. J Conserv Dent. 2011;14(1):32–5.
33. Harorli O, Barutcigil Ç, Akgül N, Bayindir Y. Caries detector dyes: do they stain only the caries. J Restorat Dent. 2014;2(1):20–6.
34. Carvalho JC, Dige I, Machiulskiene V, Qvist V, Bakhshandeh A, Fatturi-Parolo C, et al. Occlusal caries: biological approach for its diagnosis and management. Caries Res. 2016;50(6):527–42.
35. Maltz M, Garcia R, Jardim JJ, de Paula LM, Yamaguti PM, Moura MS, et al. Randomized trial of partial vs. stepwise caries removal: 3-year follow-up. J Dent Res. 2012;91(11):1026–31.
36. Alves LS, Giongo FCMS, Mua B, Martins VB, Barbachan E, Silva B, Qvist V, et al. A randomized clinical trial on the sealing of occlusal carious lesions: 3–4-year results. Braz Oral Res. 2017;31:e44.

Fluorescence-Aided Caries Excavation: FACE

10

Áine M. Lennon and Wolfgang Buchalla

10.1 Introduction

Caries excavation is an integral part of restorative therapy. The manner in which caries is removed has a direct influence on whether a healthy pulp can be preserved or not. Furthermore, it determines how much dental hard tissue is lost or preserved during cavity preparation. Both aspects influence restoration stability and longevity. The first step in caries excavation is the identification of tissue that needs to be removed. This is most commonly done using a dental probe to test hardness while assessing color visually at the same time. Unfortunately, neither hardness nor staining is a highly accurate method to identify the presence of, or more importantly quantify, bacteria in dentin. The question as to how much infected dentin must be removed and how much may be allowed to remain is more important today than ever. It could be that we can be much more conservative in the removal of dentin in the future. But, an accurate diagnosis of where the bacteria in dentin are, and also in what quantity is indispensible in order to make an informed decision on what and how much we excavate. Highly accurate methods have long been available as gold standards for use in the laboratory. Since the introduction of the FACE (Fluorescence-Aided Caries Excavation) method, a tool has become available which can identify the presence of bacteria in dentin in vivo with accuracy similar to laboratory methods. This allows precise differentiation between infected and noninfected dentin, allowing maximum preservation of tissue. Another useful feature is that most resin-based tooth-colored restorative materials which are indistinguishable from tooth substance in white light can be readily differentiated from enamel or dentin using the fluorescence technique. This in turn also helps to conserve healthy tooth substance because it is not mistakenly removed when removing restorative materials.

Á. M. Lennon (✉) · W. Buchalla
Department of Conservative Dentistry and Periodontology, University Hospital Regensburg, Regensburg, Germany
e-mail: aine.lennon@ukr.de

© Springer Nature Switzerland AG 2019

A. Ferreira Zandona, C. Longbottom (eds.), *Detection and Assessment of Dental Caries*, https://doi.org/10.1007/978-3-030-16967-1_10

10.2 History

The use of visible fluorescence in carious dentin to identify residual caries was initially described in 2002 [1]. The first commercially available devices for FACE excavation using a separate handheld light source and filter glasses appeared on the market in Europe in 2012 and have been in use clinically since then (SiroInspect, Dentsply Sirona, Germany). A new dental handpiece whereby the light source is integrated into the handpiece allowing fluorescence to be observed directly during excavation, Fluoresce™ HD is now available in Europe and the United States from Lares Dental, Chico, CA, USA.[1]

10.3 What is FACE?

During FACE excavation the cavity is illuminated with a violet light (405 nm) and observed through a high-pass filter glass (Fig. 10.1). The high-pass filter blocks the violet excitation light and allows higher wavelengths or fluorescent light through. This causes infected dentin to fluoresce red, while noninfected dentin fluoresces green (Fig. 10.4). We use the naturally occurring fluorescence of carious dental hard tissue to identify infected dentin during excavation. This fluorescence is emitted by fluorophores either naturally present in dental hard tissue (green fluorescence) or produced by active oral bacteria (red fluorescence). Importantly, there is no need for the use of dyes.

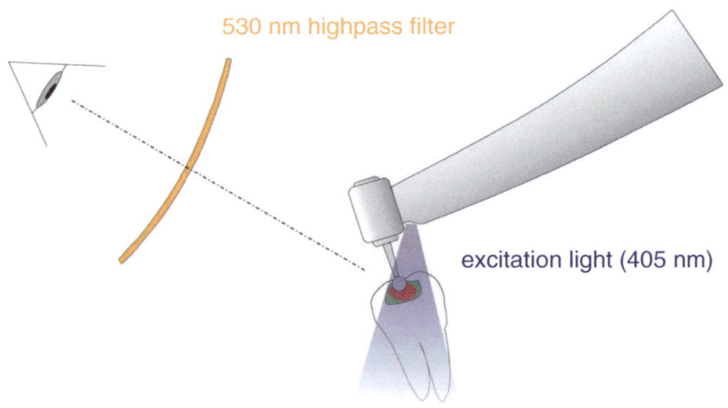

Fig. 10.1 During FACE excavation the cavity is excited with violet light and observed through a high-pass filter

[1] Available in the USA pending FDA clearance to market.

The excitation light is either handheld separately from the handpiece or, more conveniently, integrated into the dental handpiece used for excavation so that the cavity is illuminated by the excitation light during excavation.

10.4 What Causes the Red Fluorescence?

Spectral analyses of carious dentin have shown that red fluorescence in carious dentin is strongest when excited at 405 nm. This excitation peak corresponds very well with the known Soret peaks for porphyrins and therefore it has been presumed that porphyrins are responsible for the red fluorescence [2]. More recently, porphyrins have been extracted directly from carious dentin [3] and from caries bacteria [4] using HPLC proving that porphyrins are indeed present in carious tissue and cause its red fluorescence.

10.5 What Do We Need to Excavate, What Can We Leave Behind?

Initial caries in the enamel can be treated noninvasively. But as soon as there is cavitation into dentin, a niche is formed which cannot be cleaned by the patient. A cariogenic biofilm develops rather undisturbed within the cavitation and the proportion of acidogenic microorganisms increases. Under these conditions caries lesions quickly spread deeper into the tooth and a restoration is required to stop lesion progression. How much carious dentin needs to be removed in order to arrest caries and prevent further spread of the lesion and further destruction of tooth substance? The answer differs depending on whether we are talking about the area close to the pulp or that at the enamel–dentin junction.

The traditional approach is to remove infected dentin as completely as possible and then place a restoration so that the patient can again clean the tooth surface. In this case FACE can be very useful because infected areas are readily identified and inadvertent removal of healthy dentin can be avoided. As compared with using tactile hardness as a criterion, complete removal of red fluorescing dentin is less invasive, because bacteria-free but still softened dentin areas are conserved.

If the lesion is so deep that removing all of the infected dentin would risk or result in a pulp exposure, it has been shown that it is better to leave a layer of infected dentin over the pulp [5]. This is reffered to as selective caries excavation. In this case FACE helps identify the layer of infected dentin in order to aid its complete removal in the periphery, while it informs the dentist whether or not the dentin left close to the pulp is infected or not. This way, pulpal integrity can be assured with a high likelihood of long-term preservation of pulp vitality. Still, using FACE, bacterially invaded dentin should be removed from the periphery as well as from enamel margins in order to promote a tightly sealed and well-anchored adhesive restoration.

Using the FACE excitation light, it is also possible to differentiate between tooth substance and various tooth-colored dental materials, which can be very difficult to identify in white light. This prevents inadvertent removal of tooth substance during the preparation of previously restored teeth.

Taken together, we need to remove enough infected dentin to allow placement of a restoration with excellent cavity seal so that any bacteria remaining in the cavity are cut off from their carbohydrate supply and at the same time avoid removing the layer of dentin directly over the pulp chamber even if this is infected.

10.6 Clinical Technique

There are two different "FACE" instruments available on the market at the moment. The first is a handheld light source (SiroInspect, Dentsply Sirona, Germany). In this case, the light is held by an assistant while the dentist removes the red fluorescing areas using a slow-speed handpiece. In the newer version, the excitation light is integrated directly into the fiber optics of the handpiece used during excavation (Fluoresce™ HD, Lares Dental, Chico, CA, USA).

10.7 Clinical Case

Approximal caries in tooth 24, mirror image (Fig. 10.2).

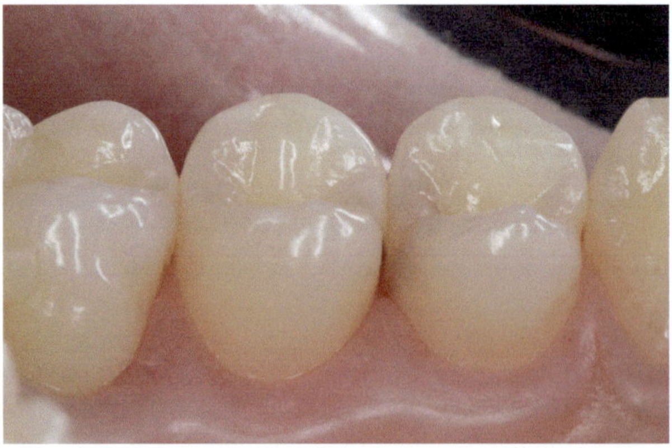

Fig. 10.2 Preoperative photograph of tooth 24 (mirror image) with distal caries. Copyright Prof. Wolfgang Buchalla

10.7.1 Access Cavity Preparation

Generally, an access cavity in enamel needs to be prepared using a diamond bur so that the extent of the lesion in dentin can be assessed. This step is the same as for conventional caries excavation (Fig. 10.3). This can be done using a conventional high-speed handpiece and diamond bur (Fig. 10.4).

10.7.2 Diagnosis and Removal of Carious Dentin

At this stage, the extent of the lesion in dentin is checked, by illuminating the cavity with the violet excitation light. Bacterially infected areas in dentin are easy to differentiate from yellow-green fluorescing noninfected areas (Fig. 10.4) [6]. Along the dentin–enamel junction, strongly red fluorescing areas are the areas with high bacterial infiltration and should be removed. Carious dentin is removed using the slow-speed handpiece and round burs as in conventional excavation. If preferred, a hand excavator can be used as well.

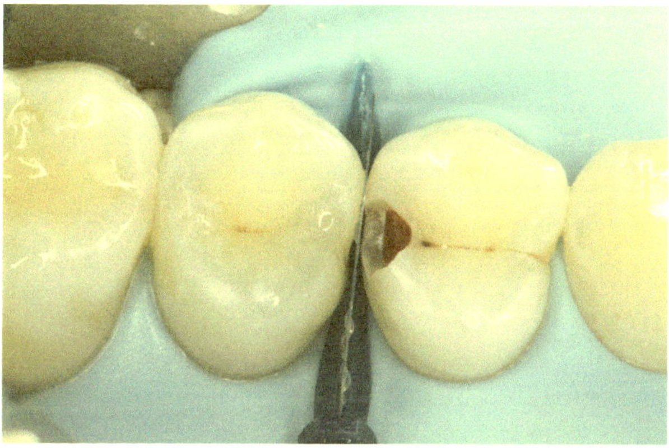

Fig. 10.3 After preparation of an access cavity. Caries in dentin is exposed. Copyright Prof. Wolfgang Buchalla

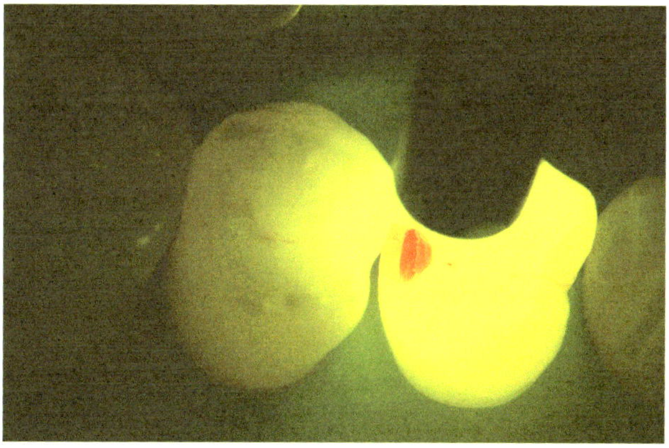

Fig. 10.4 Using FACE the cavity is excited with violet light and observed through a high-pass filter. Infected dentin fluoresces red, while healthy dentin fluoresces yellow-green. Copyright Prof. Wolfgang Buchalla

10.7.2.1 Endpoint of Excavation

The operator can choose to remove infected dentin completely or to allow some to remain.

In areas, which are not close to the pulp, red fluorescing dentin can be completely removed. The carious tissue is removed layer by layer using a round bur until the cavity floor is yellow-green fluorescing. Eliminating infected tissue is preferable to achieve both a good seal and reliable adhesive anchorage in the new restoration. By removing bacterially infected tissue the load of lippopolysacharides (LPS) and lipoteichoic acids (LTA) can be reduced. LPS and LTA are known to interfere with pulp homeostasis, leading to pulpal inflamation. It is not necessary to probe the cavity floor to check for hardness. Usually, after complete removal of red fluorescing dentin, the dentin left behind is still soft. This tissue, histologically described as the inner layer of carious dentin, while demineralized, is not infected and not irreversibly denatured [7]. This layer has the ability to remineralize via minerals from the pulp and is worth preserving.

On the other hand, when close to the pulp, complete removal of red fluorescing dentin should be avoided. In these cases a small amount of infected dentin should be left (Fig. 10.5) to avoid an inadvertent pulp exposure. The infected dentin should be covered with calcium hydroxide or hydraulic calcium silicate cement because of its bioactive properties and in order to protect pulpal cells from cytotoxic effects of monomeric substances from, e.g., dental adhesives [8, 9]. In most cases it is possible to retain pulp vitality using this method.

Another approach is to complete the caries removal in a second step. Quite often there is hardly any red fluorescence found when the cavity is opened for the second time. This indicates that the bacteria, which were left behind the first time, are no longer active. For this reason, two-step excavation is no longer generally recommended.

10.7.3 Restoration

The use of FACE for excavation does not result in any special requirements regarding the restoration placed. The clinician is free to choose any suitable restoration for the cavity prepared. In this case, a composite restoration was placed (Fig. 10.6). However, particularly when leaving some bacterially infected dentin in the cavity, an adhesive restoration provides a more reliable seal than other, nonadhesive approaches.

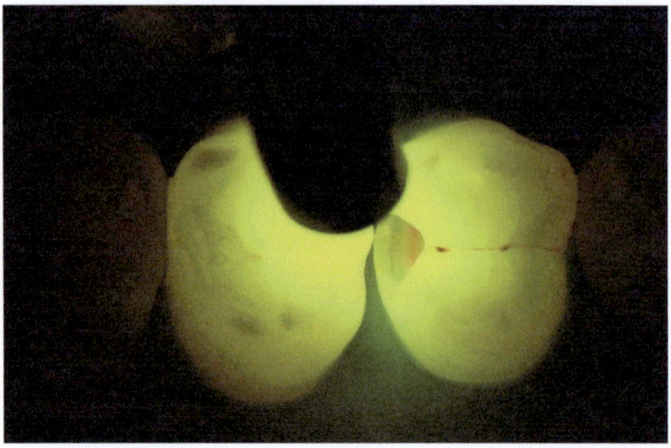

Fig. 10.5 Red fluorescing dentin has been removed along the dentin–enamel junction. In the cavity floor, a small amount of red fluorescing dentin has been left behind. Copyright Prof. Wolfgang Buchalla

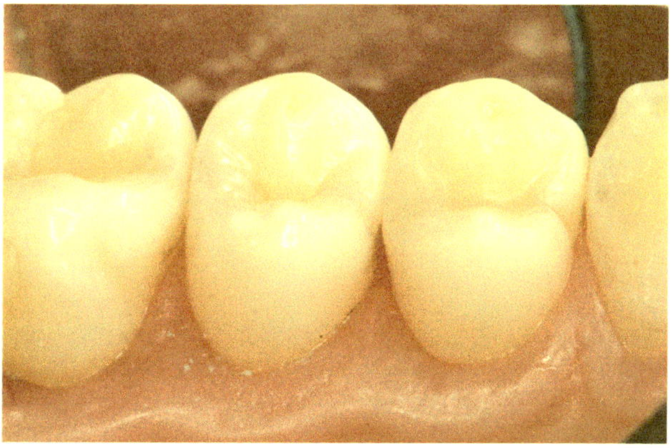

Fig. 10.6 Tooth 24 following placement of a composite restoration. Copyright Prof. Wolfgang Buchalla

Summary table

FACE				
Which surfaces/ sites is it useful for	Occlusal (pits and fissures) **Y**	Proximal/ (approximal) **Y**	Smooth surface (buccal and lingual) **Y**	Root caries **Y**
What type of lesions is valuable for	Primary coronal **Y**	Secondary coronal **Y**	Primary root caries **Y**	Secondary root caries **Y**
What type of dentition	Primary **Y**		Permanent **Y**	
Lesion severity	Enamel lesions Can be used		Dentinal lesions **Y**	
Sensitivity	Literature reported range in 94%			
Specificity	Literature reported range in 83%			
Perceived Ease Of Use	1. FACE is very easy to use 2. Some experience is required to become skillful at using FACE 3. Learning to operate FACE is easy 4. FACE is flexible to interact with 5. Interacting with FACE is clear and understandable, but can be confounded by other factors (red-green color blindness, blood) 6. It is very easy to interact with FACE			
Advantages/ disadvantages	*Advantages* 1. Suitable for both permanent and primary teeth 2. Suitable for all surfaces 3. Easy to use 4. No dyes needed 5. Other useful features: identifying resin-based tooth-colored restorative materials *Disadvantages* 1. Cost associated with the device 2. Special device or handpiece needed			
Time	Time needed depends on the complexity of the lesion to be excavated but usually less than for conventional excavation			
Cost	Fluoresce™ HD LED fiber optic low speed motor Lares Dental, Chico, CA, USA (Available in the United Kingdom) £595 Siroinspect Set, Dentsply Sirona Germany 660€			

10.8 Concluding Remarks

Fluorescence aided caries excavation (FACE) is based on the principle that infected dentin fluoresces red while dentin, which is not bacterially invaded, fluoresces green. The red fluorescence is caused by bacterial porphyrins.

References

1. Lennon AM, Buchalla W, Switalski L, Stookey GK. Residual caries detection using visible fluorescence. Caries Res. 2002;36:315–9.
2. Buchalla W, Lennon AM, Attin T. Comparative fluorescence spectroscopy of root caries lesions. Eur J Oral Sci. 2004;112:490–6.
3. Buchalla W, Attin T, Niedmann Y, Niedmann PD, Lennon AM. Porphyrins are the cause of red fluorescence of carious dentine: verified by gradient reversed-phase HPLC. Caries Res. 2008;42:223.
4. Fyrestam J, Bjurshammar N, Paulsson E, Johannsen A, Östman C. Determination of porphyrins in oral bacteria by liquid chromatography electrospray ionization tandem mass spectrometry. Anal Bioanal Chem. 2015;407:7013–23.
5. Bjørndal L, Fransson H, Bruun G, Markvart M, Kjaeldgaard M, Näsman P, Hedenbjörk-Lager A, Dige I, Thordrup M. Randomized clinical trials on deep carious lesions: 5-year follow-up. J Dent Res. 2017;96:747–53.
6. Buchalla W, Lennon AM. Die fluoreszenzunterstützte Kariesexkavation—Funktionsprinzip und Empfehlungen für den Gebrauch. Dtsch Zahnarztl Z. 2015;2:110–20.
7. Fusayama T, Kurosaki N. Structure and removal of carious dentin. Int Dent J. 1972;22:401–11.
8. Schweikl H, Buchalla W, Krifka S. Cell responses to cariogenic microorganisms and dental resin materials-crosstalk at the dentin-pulp interface? Dent Mater. 2017;33:514–24.
9. Schweikl H, Widbiller M, Krifka S, Klement J, Petzel C, Bolay C, Hiller K-A, Buchalla W. Interaction between LPS and a dental resin monomer on cell viability in mouse macrophages. Dent Mater. 2016;32:1492–503.

Part III

Additional Detection Methods as Aid to Caries Lesion Diagnosis

Conventional Bitewing Radiographs

11

Falk Schwendicke and Gerd Göstemeyer

11.1 Introduction

Clinical, i.e. visual-tactile detection is able to detect accessible caries lesions with high accuracy, as has been discussed in other chapters of this book (Chaps. 3, 5–8). However, such detection has a limited sensitivity for proximal, non-accessible lesions. This chapter will review the use of bitewing radiographs to complement visual-tactile caries detection.

11.2 Background

If interproximal lesions are not detected for long enough, i.e. remain untreated and active, i.e. progressing, they will eventually cavitate, i.e. lose surface integrity. In this case, non- or micro-invasive treatment involving e.g. fluoride, sealants or caries infiltration is no longer possible; and invasive (restorative) interventions are needed. This is in any case unfortunate given the irreversible character of any restorative intervention, putting the tooth on a path of repeated (and increasingly costly) re-interventions given the limited (mean) lifespan of any intervention (also termed the cycle of restorations or "death spiral") [1–3]. For proximal restorations, initiating this cycle or spiral is especially problematic, as any restorative intervention will need to sacrifice large amounts of sound tissue, as access is usually provided through the (intact) marginal ridge, but also as proximal restorations show lower survival than restorations placed on other (more accessible and hence controllable) surfaces [4, 5]. Thus, the aim of contemporary caries detection is to detect lesions early enough for allowing to manage them non- or micro-invasively (see Chap. 22). For making sound treatment decisions, it is further required to have some kind of information about the surface status (cavitated

F. Schwendicke (✉) · G. Göstemeyer
Charité–Universitätsmedizin Berlin, Freie Universität Berlin, Humboldt-Universität zu Berlin, and Berlin Institute of Health, Berlin, Germany
e-mail: falk.schwendicke@charite.de; gerd.goestemeyer@charite.de

© Springer Nature Switzerland AG 2019

A. Ferreira Zandona, C. Longbottom (eds.), *Detection and Assessment of Dental Caries*, https://doi.org/10.1007/978-3-030-16967-1_11

yes/no), as cavitated lesions are (in line with the description above) treated differently than non-cavitated ones. The ideal detection method complementing visual-tactile caries detection should provide information on both aspects, the presence of the lesion and its depth/surface status.

Bitewing radiography is a method which, at least in parts, fulfils this requirement. If the beam projection is correct (i.e. near parallel to the oro-vestibular axis), then proximal coronal caries lesions are well detectable, and their extent can be assessed. For proximal lesions, bitewing radiography has a sensitivity of around 0.2–0.3 for early lesions (e.g. extending only into enamel, not dentin), i.e. around 20–30% of all present lesions are detected (it can be assumed that very early lesions, mainly in the outer enamel half histologically, will usually be missed); sensitivity increases to 0.4–0.6 for more advanced (dentin) lesions or even cavitated lesions. The specificity is around or above 0.9, i.e. around 10% of all detected lesions are in reality sound surfaces [6].

In summary, for early proximal coronal lesions, bitewing radiography thus carries a risk of under-detection (around 70–80% of lesions are missed); while for advanced lesions, this risk is significantly lower. Specificity is high. Given that bitewing detection is usually performed in repeated intervals (e.g. every 12–24 months), one should consider that the risk of under-detection decreases with each examination cycle, while that of over-detection increases. In most populations these days, with most lesions progressing only slowly (as discussed in other chapters of this book, Chaps. 3, 5–7), the described sensitivity and specificity is suitable to detect most lesions early enough without carrying the risk of many false positive detections [7]. There are no studies assessing the accuracy of bitewings for detecting proximal root lesions. One can assume the accuracy to be comparable with that for proximal coronal lesions (note that there is no enamel involvement). One aspect to consider is the cervical beam-out artefact detected on dental root surfaces close to the alveolar ridge; this should not be confused with root caries.

Proximal lesions detected on radiographs can be scored according to their depth, and a wide range of scoring systems is available [8], for example discriminating the outer and inner enamel half and dentin (sometimes termed as D1-D4 for Decayed 1-4, or R1-4 for Radiographically decayed 1-4), or discriminating the outer and inner enamel half (E1, E2) and the outer, middle and inner dentin third (D1-3). This relatively fine staging allows to describe lesions in sufficient detail and also relates to treatment decisions: E1-D1 lesions will be mainly managed non-restoratively given their surface status (see below), while D2 and D3 will usually be managed by placing restorations; however, carious tissue removal will differ between D2 and D3 given their different proximity to the pulp [9]. Examples of these lesion stages are given in Fig. 11.1. Such scoring can also be used to monitor lesions with time (Fig. 11.2), to confirm or refute that a lesion truly shows clinically relevant activity (in addition to the clinical lesion activity determination, as described in other chapters of this book, Chaps. 3, 5–7).

Bitewing radiography does only seldomly allow for the detection of surface cavitation (sometimes, a cavitation can also be detected on a radiograph, but especially for lesions in doubt, this is not likely). However, from a number of observational studies, summarized in a recent review [10], the most likely cut-off from which onwards cavitation is likely might be determined. However, when inspecting the studies included in this review, it becomes clear that the surface cavitation probability varies widely: in low-risk patients only a third of lesions radiographically extending into dentin was found to be cavitated; in high-risk patients (e.g. those with orthodontic appliances),

17		16		15		14		13		23		24		25		26		27	
	D1	D2	E2	E1									E1		E2	E2	D2	D1	

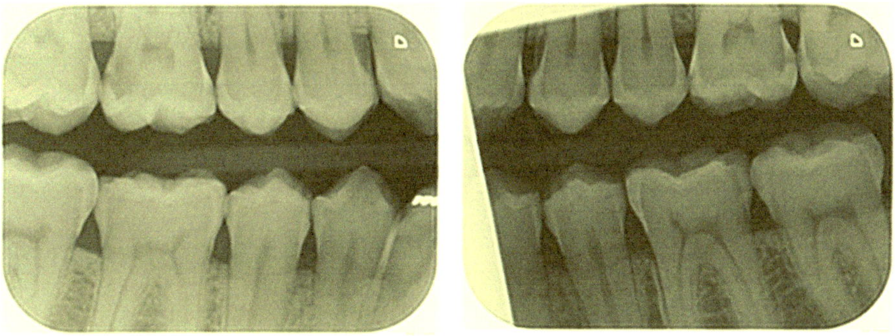

	E2														E2	E2	D1		
47		46		45		44		43		33		34		35		36		37	

Fig. 11.1 Scoring of lesions according to lesion depth. E1/2 lesions into outer/inner enamel half, D1-3 lesions into outer/middle/inner dentin third

this number was near to 100%. Most studies found that around half of the lesions radiographically extending into the outer dentin were cavitated. It should be noted that most studies are more than 25–30-year-old; lesion progression rates seem to be slower nowadays in most populations (at least in rich countries) [11], which may mean that the probability of cavitation of lesions in outer dentin is even lower today (note that this is somewhat speculative). Considering this uncertainty, dentists should thus always strive to double-check findings based on radiographs (i.e. confirm a presumed cavitation) and, if in doubt, apply non-restorative treatments (applying non- or micro-invasive therapy does no harm, while the option to restore in the future remains) (see Chap. 22). Double-checking of the surface status can be performed via gentle probing with a cow-horn ended instrument (without any force, as this may lead to cavitation of demineralized, but surface-intact enamel). Alternatively, a separation of suspect proximal spaces using orthodontic rings can be performed; this then allows direct inspection (as discussed in another chapter of this book, Chap. 2).

For detection of lesions on other (than proximal) surfaces, radiographs are less suitable or common. For example, smooth surfaces are not detectable on two-dimensional images given their overlap and projection (a buccal lesion in a pit on a lower molar may look like a deep occlusal lesion on a radiograph, for instance). Generally, radiograph artefacts due to overlapping need to be carefully considered when interpreting radiographs (e.g. metal elements like orthodontic appliances or retainers, see Fig. 11.1). For occlusal lesions, the sensitivity is similar to that of proximal lesions, while the specificity is lower. Hence, bitewing radiography comes with a higher risk of false positive detections on occlusal surfaces. Moreover, lesions are usually significantly under-scored, i.e. lesions "just" extending into the dentin on a radiograph are clinically oftentimes deeper (Fig. 11.3). There is currently debate as to how to manage these lesions best [9, 12–14].

17	16	15	14	13	23	24	25	26	27
O: D1	E2					E2	E2	O: D1	

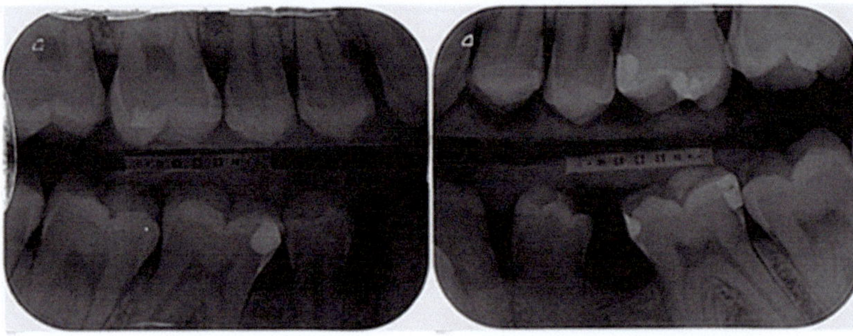

E2									
47	46	45	44	43	33	34	35	36	37

17	16	15	14	13	23	24	25	26	27
O: D2	D1					E2	E2	O: D1	

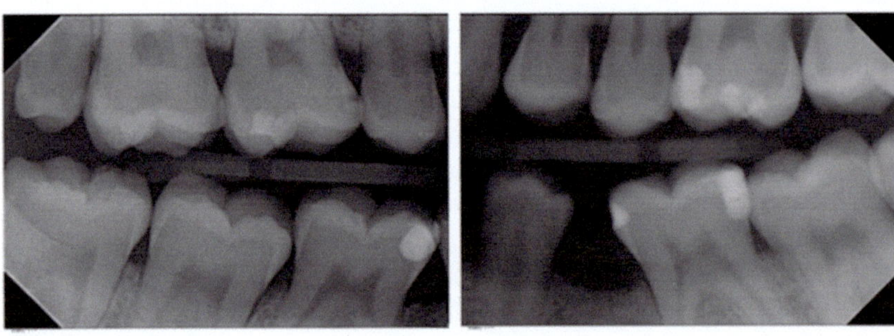

E2									
47	46	45	44	43	33	34	35	36	37

Fig. 11.2 Radiographs allow monitoring and detecting progressing (active) lesions. The upper set of bitewings was taken in 2014 at this 25-year-old male, the lower set in 2017. The patient showed progression of the lesion at the UR6 from E2 to D1; the interproximal gingiva was bleeding and there was plaque stagnation (i.e. also signs of lesion activity). Note that no individualized bitewing holder was used, as the patient changed his dentist and visited the clinic with the old digital radiographs being provided. Hence, the radiographs are not fully standardized. Caution is needed when interpreting the lesion progression. Consequently, the lesion was managed micro-invasively, with only very limited risk of harm in case of a misdiagnosis (i.e. the lesion being inactive). Abbreviation: *o* occlusal, E1/2 lesions into outer/inner enamel half, D1-3 lesions into outer/middle/inner dentin third, *o* occlusal lesions

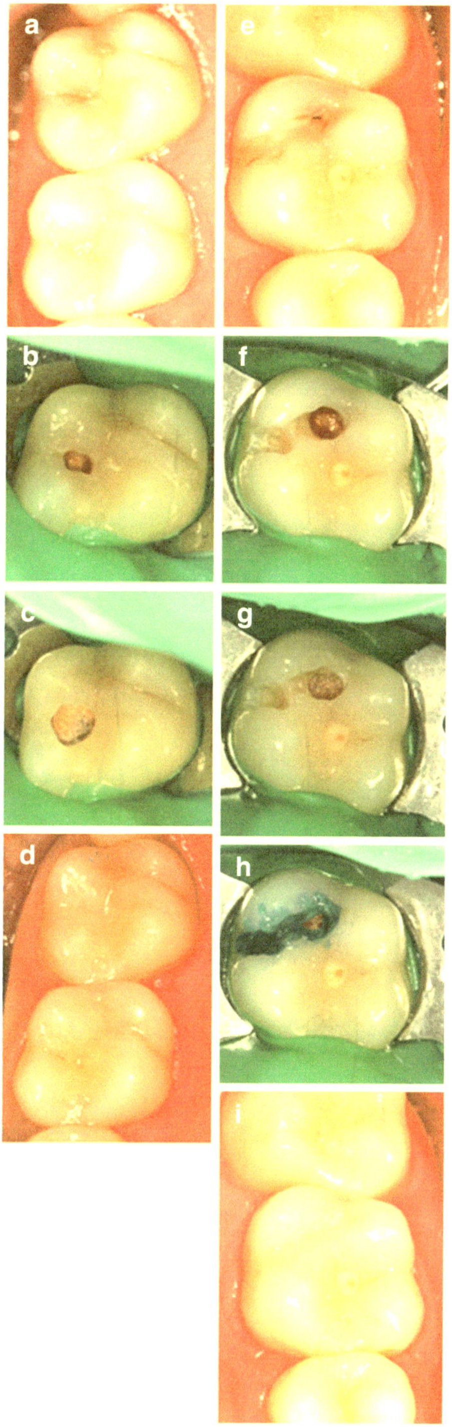

Fig. 11.3 Radiographic and clinical lesion depth. The occlusal lesions from Fig. 11.2 extending into the outer third of the dentin at the UR7 (left) and UL6 (right) are clinically barely detectable (**a**, **e**). When opening them up (**c**, **f**, **g**), there is a clear dentin involvement and soft, carious dentin. The lesions were minimally-invasively treated using composite (**d**, **h**, **i**)

Bitewing radiography is also a major detection aid for secondary caries detection. However, it is—again—mainly suitable for proximal lesions, when the lesion is located "within" the beam (in this case, both coronal and root secondary lesions are well detectable). For secondary lesions, sensitivity is around 0.50–0.60 and specificity around 0.80, which is similar to other detection aids (like laser-fluorescence) and much better than tactile assessment (probing) [15].

Besides the risks of artefacts and under- or over-detection (something all detection methods are, to some extent, marred with), a major drawback of bitewing radiography is ionizing radiation. This limits the repeatability and, generally, the application in young children. Dentists should follow the rules of radiation protection (reducing the radiation to dose to as low as reasonably possible) and should be restrictive in their indication of bitewing radiography. Last, bitewing radiographs should be planned and taken not in regular, standardized intervals but risk-adjusted. Caries risk assessment is discussed in other chapters of this book (Chaps. 7 and 22).

11.3 Clinical Application

A number of rules should be followed when indicating, taking or interpreting bitewing radiographs.

1. Use an optimal projection, aiming to have the beam being directed right into the proximal space, i.e. parallel to the oro-buccal tooth axis.
2. Standardize bitewing radiographs or, optimally, use individualized bitewing holders (e.g. Icon X-ray Holder, DMG, Hamburg, Fig. 11.4). For individualizing these holders, patients bite into a fixation mass (wax or hard-curing silicone), which allows to place the holder in the exact same position again when another bitewing is taken. Note that this only works in adults, i.e. not in children (exfoliation, growth) or during orthodontic treatment (tooth movement). Using these holders ensures the exact same projection, enabling more valid comparison of lesions with time (otherwise, changes in the projection will automatically lead to some lesions being found "progressing" or "regressing").
3. Record findings on an appropriate scale, allowing useful staging and deducing treatment decisions from the resulting diagnosis.
4. Determine cavitation status clinically not only based on probabilities (i.e. a lesion extending into the outer dentin on a radiograph is cavitated in around 50% of the cases), but confirm it clinically (gentle probing, tooth separation using orthodontic rings).
5. Integrate the uncertainty of any diagnosis based on radiographs into your decision-making. If in doubt, non-restorative interventions should be chosen [7, 16].

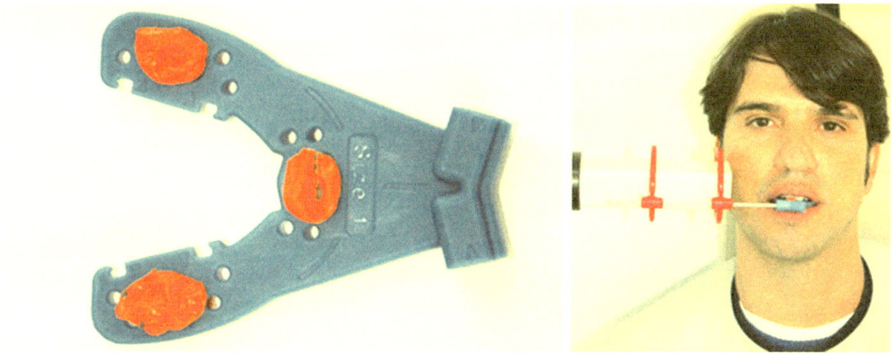

Fig. 11.4 Bitewing holders can be individualized (left part), which allows standardize re-takes in the future given the identical position of the cone and the image to each other and the dentition, respectively. This is useful for monitoring lesions

Summary table

Bitewing radiography				
Which surfaces/sites is it useful for	Occlusal (pits and fissures)	Proximal/ (approximal)	Smooth surface (buccal and lingual)	Root caries (all surfaces)
	Y	**Y**	**N**	(**Y**) if proximal location
What type of lesions is valuable for	Primary coronal	Secondary coronal	Primary root caries	Secondary root caries
	Y	**Y**, if proximal location	**Y**, if proximal location	**Y**, if proximal location
What type of dentition	Primary		Permanent	
	Y		**Y**	
Lesion severity	Enamel lesions		Dentinal lesions	
	Y (mainly for proximal)		**Y**	
Sensitivity proximal[a]	Early lesions 0.24–0.43, advanced lesions 0.36–0.45, cavitated lesions 0.61–0.64			
Specificity proximal[a]	Early lesions 0.89–0.97, advanced lesions 0.94–0.95, cavitated lesions 0.90–0.98			
Sensitivity occlusal[a]	Early lesions 0.35–0.41, advanced lesions 0.56			
Specificity occlusal[a]	Early lesions 0.78–0.80, advanced lesions 0.87–0.95			
Perceived Ease Of Use (PEOU)	Accuracy increases with experience			
Advantages/ disadvantages	*Advantages* 1. Rather sensitive, also for early proximal lesions 2. Can be applied in a clinical setting but also useful for research purposes 3. Allow monitoring if taken standardized or using individualized holder *Disadvantages* 1. Cannot with certainty make determinations as to surface status (cavitation) 2. Low sensitivity if not within beam, i.e. smooth surfaces 3. Ionizing radiation 4. Require ion source and equipment			
Time	Approx. 5 min for taking bitewings, another 5 min for full evaluation			

[a]Mean value ranges from different pooled study types in [6]

11.4 Concluding Remarks

Visual detection of caries lesions has low sensitivity on non-accessible (mainly proximal) surfaces, especially for early (non-cavitated) lesions. To successfully manage these lesions, such early detection is needed. Bitewing radiography has a sensitivity of around 0.4 for detecting these lesions, with high specificity (0.9 or above). Similar values can be found for occlusal lesions (0.4/0.8), or for detecting proximal secondary lesions (0.5/0.8), while on smooth (buccal, lingual) surfaces, bitewing radiography is not useful. Bitewings also allow monitoring lesions over time, especially when using individualized holders. Detections from bitewing radiographs should, if possible, be confirmed using other detection methods. Bitewing radiography is a useful caries detection aid, with some limitations as to its accuracy, but more so its applicability in many settings, and its repeatability (given the release of ionizing radiation) in short intervals for caries detection.

References

1. Schwendicke F, Meyer-Lueckel H, Stolpe M, Dorfer CE, Paris S. Costs and effectiveness of treatment alternatives for proximal caries lesions. PLoS One. 2014;9:e86992.
2. Brantley C, Bader J, Shugars D, Nesbit S. Does the cycle of rerestoration lead to larger restorations? J Am Dent Assoc. 1995;126:1407–13.
3. Qvist V. Longevity of restorations: the 'death spiral'. In: Fejerskov O, Kidd EAM, editors. Dental caries: the disease and its clinical management. Oxford: Blackwell Munksgaard; 2008. p. 444–55.
4. Demarco FF, Correa MB, Cenci MS, Moraes RR, Opdam NJ. Longevity of posterior composite restorations: not only a matter of materials. Dent Mater. 2012;28:87–101.
5. Opdam NJ, van de Sande FH, Bronkhorst E, Cenci MS, Bottenberg P, Pallesen U, Gaengler P, Lindberg A, Huysmans MC, van Dijken JW. Longevity of posterior composite restorations: a systematic review and meta-analysis. J Dent Res. 2014;93:943–9.
6. Schwendicke F, Tzschoppe M, Paris S. Radiographic caries detection: a systematic review and meta-analysis. J Dent. 2015;43:924–33.
7. Schwendicke F, Paris S, Stolpe M. Detection and treatment of proximal caries lesions: milieu-specific cost-effectiveness analysis. J Dent. 2015;43:647–55.
8. Innes N, Schwendicke F. Dentists' thresholds for restorative intervention in carious lesions: systematic review and meta-analysis. J Dent Res. 2017;96(5):501–8.
9. Schwendicke F, Frencken JE, Bjorndal L, Maltz M, Manton DJ, Ricketts D, Van Landuyt K, Banerjee A, Campus G, Domejean S, Fontana M, Leal S, Lo E, Machiulskiene V, Schulte A, Splieth C, Zandona AF, Innes NP. Managing carious lesions: consensus recommendations on carious tissue removal. Adv Dent Res. 2016;28:58–67.
10. Wenzel A. Radiographic display of carious lesions and cavitation in approximal surfaces: advantages and drawbacks of conventional and advanced modalities. Acta Odontol Scand. 2014;72:251–64.
11. Reda S, Elhennawy K, Meyer-Luckel H, Paris S, Schwendicke F. Industry sponsorship in trials on fluoride varnish or gels for caries prevention. Community Dent Oral Epidemiol. 2017;45:289–95.
12. Fontana M, Platt JA, Eckert GJ, Gonzalez-Cabezas C, Yoder K, Zero DT, Ando M, Soto-Rojas AE, Peters MC. Monitoring of sound and carious surfaces under sealants over 44 months. J Dent Res. 2014;93:1070–5.

13. Hesse D, Bonifacio CC, Mendes FM, Braga MM, Imparato JC, Raggio DP. Sealing versus partial caries removal in primary molars: a randomized clinical trial. BMC Oral Health. 2014;14:58.
14. Bakhshandeh A, Qvist V, Ekstrand K. Sealing occlusal caries lesions in adults referred for restorative treatment: 2–3 years of follow-up. Clin Oral Investig. 2012;16:521–9.
15. Brouwer F, Askar H, Paris S, Schwendicke F. Detecting secondary caries lesions: a systematic review and meta-analysis. J Dent Res. 2016;95:143–51.
16. Schwendicke F, Stolpe M, Meyer-Lueckel H, Paris S. Detecting and treating occlusal caries lesions: a cost-effectiveness analysis. J Dent Res. 2015;94:272–80.

12 Digital Bitewing Radiographs

Gerd Göstemeyer and Falk Schwendicke

12.1 Introduction

In this chapter we will discuss the advantages and disadvantages of digital radiography technologies compared with conventional radiography for the scope of caries lesion detection. We will further give an outlook on future developments in digital radiography, which might improve accuracy of detection and analysis of caries lesions.

12.2 Background

Intraoral radiography is still the most commonly used imaging technique in dentistry [1, 2]. Amongst the various types of intraoral radiographs for different indications, bitewing radiographs are most suitable for the detection and assessment of caries lesions. While the clinical application of bitewing radiography itself has basically not changed over decades, introduction of digital radiography into dentistry has changed some modalities regarding processing and assessment of the obtained images. Digital radiography in general is assumed to have a number of advantages compared to conventional radiography. These are: reduced time and material costs, lower radiation dose, better image quality and easier access, storage and transport (between practices, etc.) of the obtained radiographs [2, 3]. However, there are some factors which should be considered when using digital radiography in order to obtain the best possible outcome regarding diagnosis, workflow and patient safety (Table 12.1).

G. Göstemeyer (✉) · F. Schwendicke
Charité–Universitätsmedizin Berlin, Freie Universität Berlin, Humboldt-Universität zu Berlin, and Berlin Institute of Health, Berlin, Germany
e-mail: gerd.goestemeyer@charite.de; falk.schwendicke@charite.de

© Springer Nature Switzerland AG 2019

A. Ferreira Zandona, C. Longbottom (eds.), *Detection and Assessment of Dental Caries*, https://doi.org/10.1007/978-3-030-16967-1_12

Table 12.1 Comparison of advantages and disadvantages between digital and conventional bitewing radiography

	Digital radiography	Conventional radiography
Accuracy	+/– No difference in accuracy for bitewings radiographs + Future developments in image processing and analysis might improve accuracy	+/– No difference in accuracy for bitewings radiographs
Image analysis	+ Advanced image processing and analysis available – Image analysis can introduce bias on the user's part	– No direct digital analysis—images can not be changed once processed
Radiation dose	+/– The dose for an image is reduced, but overall effective dose reduction for patient is not clear	– Higher dose per image
Handling	+ Conventional film processing not required + Image is immediately available – Placement of image sensor in mouth can lead to retakes	+ Due to smaller dimensions of film more comfortable for patients – Image is available after film processing – Time- and material effort required for film processing
Archival storage/data protection/data transmission	+ Transmission via networks or internet is possible + Long storage periods without quality reduction	– Transmission of films is more time-consuming – Possible degradation of film over time
Cost	+ Lower maintenance costs	– Higher maintenance costs (mainly due to time- and material-costs required for film processing)

For dental applications, there are two different techniques available for digitally recording radiographs: The first group are solid-state sensors, which can be based on charge-coupled device (CCD) or complementary metal oxide semiconductor technology (CMOS). These sensors are built of chips, which are situated on silicon crystal plates. When exposed to radiation the silicon crystals convert absorbed radiation energy into light. The chip in the sensor is recording the amount of emitted light [2]. After exposure these sensors can transfer image data directly to a computer by use of a cord or by sending radio waves containing the recorded data to a receiver, which is connected to a computer. The second group are photostimulable storage phosphor plate systems that use film-like plates [2]. When exposed to radiation, the phosphor layer stores energy by exciting electrons, which are then being trapped in the phosphor crystal lattice. In a second illumination process, which is induced by visibly wavelength laser, the stored energy is being released from the crystals. By recording the amount of energy release on the different locations of the plate, the image is generated. This scanning procedure can take between a few seconds to several minutes depending on type of scanner and image quality [2].

For digital bitewing radiography both recording techniques seem equivalent regarding accuracy and diagnostic value of the obtained images [4]. However, it has been stated that given their increased thickness, the existence of a cable in some systems and the reduced effective radiation field, solid-state sensors might have some disadvantages for use in bitewing radiography compared with phosphor plate systems [5]. Sensors might also result in an increased number of retakes of images due to positioning errors [6]. With the recent developments of new sensors with thinner geometries and larger effective image areas, however, this possible disadvantage might not be particularly relevant anymore.

The geometries of phosphor plate systems correspond to those of conventional films and therefore, there is no relevant difference in handling between these digital systems and conventional analogue films. However, in contrast to solid-state sensors, images taken on phosphor plate systems are not immediately available, as these films have to be read by a laser-scanning device. This process is more time consuming and needs additional equipment.

The evidence on accuracy between digital vs. conventional bitewing-radiographs for proximal caries detection is ambiguous: Older studies found inferior accuracy for detection of proximal enamel caries lesions for digital compared with conventional radiographs [5]. However, more recent studies found digital radiography to be as accurate as conventional films for detection and assessment of both occlusal and proximal caries lesions in permanent [3, 7–9] as well as primary teeth [10, 11]. It should be noted that these data are mostly based on in vitro investigations.

Radiation dose reduction is one frequent reason to implement digital radiography. Such dose reduction has been reported to lie between 30 and 80% compared to conventional radiographs [2, 12, 13]. However, the effective dose reduction for the patient is frequently not as large as suggested; it could be shown that the number of radiographs taken by dentists is increased when using digital devices (average radiographs per week: phosphor plate system users 42.8, solid-state system users 48.4, conventional film 32.5). The reasons for this are not fully clear; it might be that the easier handling and reduced time efforts needed for digital versus analogue radiograph play a role; also an increased number of positioning errors of the digital recording devices has been reported [2, 13]. Consequently, the radiation exposure but also time and cost for obtaining an accurate radiograph may not necessarily be lower with digital instead of analogue radiography [2]. Another study found that both digital imaging techniques (plate and sensors) require less radiation exposure than conventional films to obtain acceptable radiographs. However, in the same study it was also found that observers preferred images taken on phosphor-plates using a high radiation exposure [14]. The dynamic range as well as the range of radiation exposure in phosphor-plate systems is wider compared with solid-state sensors or films and conventional films. These receptors therefore can tolerate a larger variation in radiation dose while still producing an acceptable image. This can be seen as an advantageous property of these systems, as it results in less retakes of images due to incorrect radiation exposure [2]. In summary, digital radiography allows for obtaining images with the same quality as conventional radiographs by use of lower radiation doses. However, it mostly depends on the operator whether patients can effectively benefit from this dose reduction.

Another often stated advantage of digital radiography is the reduced time needed for obtaining an image. Images of solid-states sensors are directly available after radiation exposure. While the saved time using phosphor plate systems is lower than that for solid-state sensors, the time needed remains lower than that for processing conventional films [2]. There are, however, very limited data regarding the time needed for image post-processing or retakes of the digital image (which seem to be more often performed in digital radiography, as discussed). It seems reasonable to conclude that switching from conventional to digital radiography will result in saving of time [2].

Due to the larger dimensions of solid-state sensors, patients more frequently report discomforts when using sensors instead of analogue films. Thinner and more flexible phosphor-plate systems may be more comfortable for the patient. For bitewing examinations, it could be demonstrated that 76% of patients perceived a solid-state sensor more unpleasant than a conventional film [15]. As discussed, this might result in a higher occurrence rate of positioning errors, especially in children [2, 16].

Storing and dissemination of digital radiographs is more convenient when using digital instead of conventional analogue radiographs, which need physical space for storage. However, if the obtained radiographic digital images are being saved in a compressed format (e.g. JPEG) image data can get lost [2]. A study performed in 1996 has demonstrated that the accuracy of proximal caries detection on digital bitewing radiographs can be reduced depending on the compression rate of the image [17]. In contrast, a more recent study found moderate compression rates not to impair diagnosis of caries lesions [18]. It might be that the resolution obtained with up-to-date digital radiographic devices has increased and hence, the information loss due to compression is nowadays limited. Nonetheless, given that data space is inexpensive, it seems reasonable to store digital radiographs in an uncompressed format for clinical but also forensic reasons [2].

With the introduction of digital radiography various new methods became available, which potentially can facilitate the clinical workflow and improve accuracy of diagnosis. By use of computer-aided image processing various parameters on the digital image can be adjusted. A simple but effective way to recognize image details more easily is the ability to zoom in and out. Adjusting other parameters such like brightness, density or contrast can optimize image quality. While these adjustments can improve diagnostic value of the radiograph, they can also lead to biased diagnoses [19]. Hence, standard image optimizing tools like standard gamma correction should be used [12]. Other image processing tools involve inversion of the grey scale, which results in a so-called "negative image" and edge-enhancement, which converts contrast gradients into a texture that is visible as a shape. Both tools are designed to make details on the radiographs better detectable for the human eye [12].

A more advanced image analysis tool, which is valuable for distinguishing changes on radiographs over time, is digital subtraction radiography [5, 20]. By subtracting corresponding pixels on subsequent radiographs from the same projection, unchanged anatomical background structures will disappear and changes between both radiographs become more noticeable (Fig. 12.1) [2, 12]. By recording these changes between two subsequent bitewing radiographs this method is useful to detect and also to assess activity status of caries lesions. This method has been shown to have a higher inter-observer agreement for evaluation of lesion status (arrest/progression) over time compared with comparison between conventional bitewings [2, 21].

Despite the availability of more sensitive radiographic diagnostic tools offered by digital radiography, there is still a high variability in interpretation of radiographs and a weak correlation between clinical and radiographic findings. The main reason for this is the subjectivity of interpretation of radiographic findings by the observer

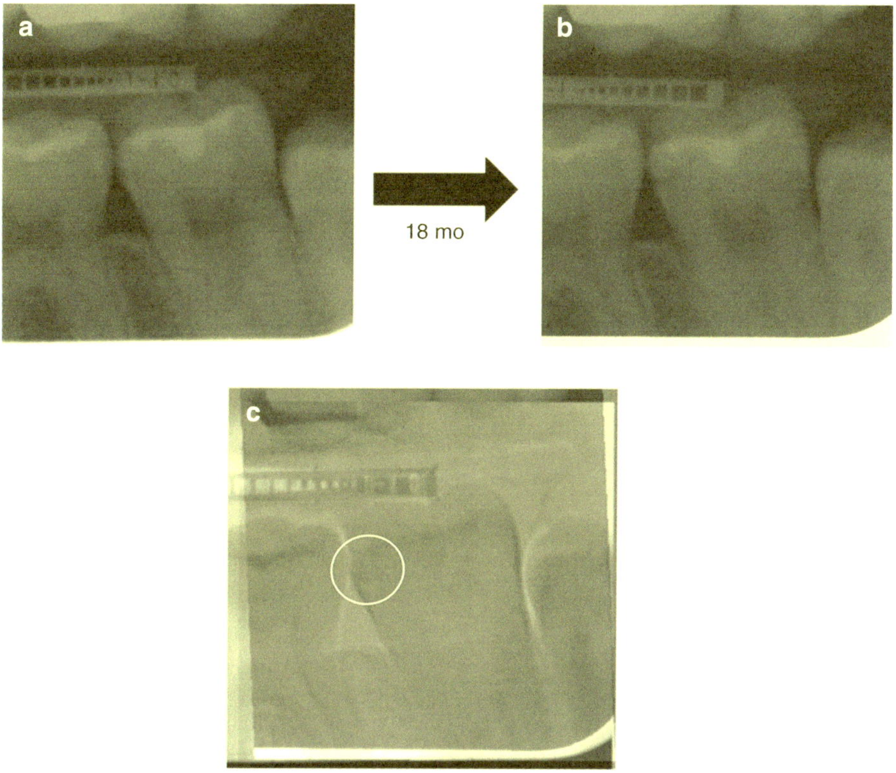

Fig. 12.1 Digital radiographs and digital subtraction of radiographs showing progression of a caries lesion: (**a**) Baseline situation showing a caries lesion extending into the outer third of dentin (D1-lesion) on the mesial surface of a lower second molar. (**b**) Bitewing radiograph taken 18 month later. (**c**) Digital subtraction between the two radiographs. The darker area in the lesion area (white circle) reveals lesion progression within the 18-month interval. (Source: Prof. Sebastian Paris, Charité-University, Berlin)

[2, 19]. Computer-aided detection and analysis of radiographs aims to overcome this by applying statistical or rule-based models to describe sound or pathologic structures. Given the numerous approaches that can be used to manage early caries lesions available today, such models which are able to accurately detect caries lesions at early stages are highly demanded [19]. However, commercially available programmes are currently, at best, as accurate as human observers [2].

A relevant question for treatment decision for proximal caries lesions is whether the lesion is cavitated or not (see Chap. 22). Neither visual inspection nor bitewing radiographs are able to clearly discriminate between cavitated and non-cavitated lesions in most situations. By use of three-dimensional radiographic imaging technology with cone beam computed tomography (CBCT), cavitated lesions can be detected more accurately compared with standard methods [1, 22]. However, use of this technology for detection and assessment of carious lesions has some limitations compared to bitewing radiography: it is more time and cost-consuming, it is more prone to artefacts resulting from the mathematical reconstruction of the images if metallic restorations are present and it provides a high radiation dose to the patients (compared to bitewing radiation, the dose from a CBCT of the same region would be 10–100 times higher) [1]. However, if cone beam examination has been performed for other clinical reasons, proximal surface cavities might also be assessed [1, 22].

12.3 Concluding Remarks

There are a number of aspects, which should be clinically considered if performing caries diagnosis using digital bitewing radiographs:

1. While first generation digital radiographic devices were inferior, digital bitewing radiography is now at least as accurate as conventional films. New developments in image processing and analysis might further improve accuracy of detection and analysis of caries lesions.
2. Radiation dose for a single radiograph is reduced in digital instead of conventional radiography. However, due to behaviour change of the operator when using digital systems, the effective radiation dose reduction for the patients is frequently not as high as assumed. Regardless of the imaging type, the radiation dose should be as low as reasonably possible.
3. Digital radiography has advantages over conventional radiography in other practical aspects: it is less time consuming, allows for digital adjustment in order to improve image quality and can be stored and transferred more easily.
4. Computer-aided detection and analysis seem promising for reducing observer related subjectivity of interpretation of radiographs. However, the currently available technology does not provide a more accurate diagnosis than a human observer.
5. CBCT may be helpful to assess surface cavitation status of proximal caries lesions. While this technology should, however, not be applied solely for caries diagnosis (mainly due to an increased radiation exposure), teeth on CBCT images obtained for other reasons should be assessed for caries lesions, too.

Summary table

Digital bitewing radiography				
Which surfaces/ sites is it useful for	Occlusal (pits and fissures)	Proximal/ (approximal)	Smooth surface (buccal and lingual)	Root caries (all surfaces)
	Y	**Y**	**N**	**(Y)** if proximal location
What type of lesions is valuable for	Primary coronal	Secondary coronal	Primary root caries	Secondary root caries
	Y	**Y**, if proximal location	**Y**, if proximal location	**(Y)** if proximal location

Digital bitewing radiography		
What type of dentition	Primary Y	Permanent Y
Lesion severity	Enamel lesions Y (mainly for proximal)	Dentinal lesions Y
Sensitivity proximal[a]	Similar to conventional bitewing radiographs: Early lesions 0.24–0.43, advanced lesions 0.36–0.45, cavitated lesions 0.61–0.64	
Specificity proximal[a]	Similar to conventional bitewing radiographs: early lesions 0.89–0.97, advanced lesions 0.94–0.95, cavitated lesions 0.90–0.98	
Sensitivity occlusal[a]	Similar to conventional bitewing radiographs: early lesions 0.35–0.41, advanced lesions 0.56	
Specificity occlusal[a]	Similar to conventional bitewing radiographs: early lesions 0.78–0.80, advanced lesions 0.87–0.95	
Perceived Ease Of Use (PEOU)	Accuracy increases with experience	
Advantages/ disadvantages	*Advantages* 1. Rather sensitive, also for early proximal lesions 2. Can be applied in a clinical setting but also useful for research purposes 3. Allows monitoring if taken standardized or using individualized holder 4. Possible to digitally adjust the image in order to improve image quality 5. Computer-aided detection and analysis seem promising for reducing observer related subjectivity of interpretation of radiographs 6. Potential for decrease of radiation if the number of images is not increased *Disadvantages* 1. Cannot with certainty make determinations as to surface status (cavitation) 2. Low sensitivity if not within beam, i.e. smooth surfaces 3. Ionizing radiation 4. Require ion source and equipment	
Time	Approx. 5 min for taking bitewings, another 5 min for full evaluation	

[a]Mean value ranges from different pooled study types in [23]

References

1. Wenzel A. Radiographic display of carious lesions and cavitation in approximal surfaces: advantages and drawbacks of conventional and advanced modalities. Acta Odontol Scand. 2014;72(4):251–64.
2. Wenzel A, Moystad A. Work flow with digital intraoral radiography: a systematic review. Acta Odontol Scand. 2010;68(2):106–14.
3. Neuhaus KW, et al. Traditional lesion detection aids. Monogr Oral Sci. 2009;21:42–51.
4. Hintze H. Diagnostic accuracy of two software modalities for detection of caries lesions in digital radiographs from four dental systems. Dentomaxillofac Radiol. 2006;35(2):78–82.
5. Wenzel A. Bitewing and digital bitewing radiography for detection of caries lesions. J Dent Res. 2004;83 Spec No C:C72–5.
6. Bahrami G, Hagstrom C, Wenzel A. Bitewing examination with four digital receptors. Dentomaxillofac Radiol. 2003;32(5):317–21.
7. Crombie K, et al. Comparing the performance of storage phosphor plate and insight film images for the detection of proximal caries depth. SADJ. 2009;64(10):452, 454–6, 458–9.
8. Minston W, et al. Comparison of diagnostic performance on approximal caries detection among Swedish and Chinese senior dental students using analogue and digital radiographs. Swed Dent J. 2013;37(2):79–85.

9. Muchhal M, et al. Spanning the horizon of accuracy of different intraoral radiographic modalities: a systematic review. J Contemp Dent Pract. 2017;18(12):1206–12.
10. Nuvvula S, et al. Diagnostic accuracy of direct digital radiography and conventional radiography for proximal caries detection in primary teeth: a systematic review. J Indian Soc Pedod Prev Dent. 2016;34(4):300–5.
11. Dias da Silva PR, et al. Accuracy of direct digital radiography for detecting occlusal caries in primary teeth compared with conventional radiography and visual inspection: an in vitro study. Dentomaxillofac Radiol. 2010;39(6):362–7.
12. van der Stelt PF. Better imaging: the advantages of digital radiography. J Am Dent Assoc. 2008;139(Suppl):7S–13S.
13. Berkhout WE, Sanderink GC, Van der Stelt PF. Does digital radiography increase the number of intraoral radiographs? A questionnaire study of Dutch dental practices. Dentomaxillofac Radiol. 2003;32(2):124–7.
14. Berkhout WE, et al. The dynamic range of digital radiographic systems: dose reduction or risk of overexposure? Dentomaxillofac Radiol. 2004;33(1):1–5.
15. Bin-Shuwaish M, et al. Estimation of clinical axial extension of class II caries lesions with ultraspeed and digital radiographs: an in-vivo study. Oper Dent. 2008;33(6):613–21.
16. Russo JM, Russo JA, Guelmann M. Digital radiography: a survey of pediatric dentists. J Dent Child (Chic). 2006;73(3):132–5.
17. Wenzel A, et al. Impact of lossy image compression on accuracy of caries detection in digital images taken with a storage phosphor system. Oral Surg Oral Med Oral Pathol Oral Radiol Endod. 1996;81(3):351–5.
18. Schulze RK, Richter A, d'Hoedt B. The effect of wavelet and discrete cosine transform compression of digital radiographs on the detection of subtle proximal caries. ROC analysis. Caries Res. 2008;42(5):334–9.
19. Analoui M, Stookey GK. Direct digital radiography for caries detection and analysis. Monogr Oral Sci. 2000;17:1–19.
20. Neuhaus KW, et al. Novel lesion detection aids. Monogr Oral Sci. 2009;21:52–62.
21. Wenzel A, Anthonisen PN, Juul MB. Reproducibility in the assessment of caries lesion behaviour: a comparison between conventional film and subtraction radiography. Caries Res. 2000;34(3):214–8.
22. Sansare K, et al. Should cavitation in proximal surfaces be reported in cone beam computed tomography examination? Caries Res. 2014;48(3):208–13.
23. Schwendicke F, Tzschoppe M, Paris S. Radiographic caries detection: a systematic review and meta-analysis. J Dent. 2015;43:924–33.

13 Caries Detection with Dental Cone Beam Computed Tomography

Jeffery B. Price

13.1 Introduction

Dental cone beam computed tomography (CBCT) was first described in 1998 by Mozzo et al. [1] and in 1999 by Arai's group [2]. The primary indication for the use of dental CBCT was for dental implant planning; however, today practitioners are using CBCT technology on a routine basis not only for dental implantology treatment planning, but also for evaluation of endodontically involved teeth, localizing impacted teeth, evaluation of craniofacial asymmetries, and other growth and development disturbances as well as various types of dento-maxillofacial pathoses. During the course of evaluating these patients using dental CBCT examinations, dental caries is sometimes diagnosed as an incidental finding. The purpose of this chapter is to evaluate how well CBCT technology performs at this task. It should be remembered that currently, diagnosis of dental caries is not considered a primary indication for the use of dental CBCT since bitewing radiographs can provide diagnostic information at a lower radiation dose than does dental CBCT [3] (see Chaps. 11 and 12 for bitewing radiographs).

13.2 Principles of Dental CBCT

A comprehensive review of the principles of dental CBCT is beyond the context of this chapter. Many existing sources provide excellent reviews of the basics of computed tomography in general [4–6] as well as the specifics of dental CBCT [7–9]. The following specific principles and relationships are included in this chapter since these may be limiting factors for the reliable use of dental CBCT in the diagnosis of caries.

J. B. Price (✉)
University of Maryland School of Dentistry, Baltimore, MD, USA
e-mail: jbprice@umaryland.edu

© Springer Nature Switzerland AG 2019

A. Ferreira Zandona, C. Longbottom (eds.), *Detection and Assessment of Dental Caries*, https://doi.org/10.1007/978-3-030-16967-1_13

The name "cone beam computed tomography" derives from the "cone" shape of the primary X-ray beam. The X-ray beam in dental CBCT has a distinctive cone or pyramidal shape rather than having X-ray photons that travel parallel with one another such as those in the original conventional computed axial tomography, or "CAT" scanning that was developed in the 1970s by Sir Godfrey Hounsfield and Allan M. Cormack, who were awarded the 1979 Nobel Prize in Physiology or Medicine [10]. This cone beam configuration is seen in Fig. 13.1b. As this beam rotates around the region of interest, the default program for many dental CBCT machines is to acquire approximately 200 raw projection images which cover an arc of at least 180°; some companies allow optional programming by the user to allow capture of raw data in a complete 360 circle [11]. Let us look at how the shape of the primary X-ray beam combined with the total arc travelled may affect caries diagnosis (Fig. 13.2). If a machine only rotates ~180° on an arc around the object of interest, a shadow zone will be created around the imaged object [12] (Fig. 13.3). The shadow zone is an area in which there is a lack of radiographic signal that reaches the receptor, resulting in areas that lack anatomic information from which to generate an image. If the arc of travel is 180°, the shadow zone includes the top, bottom, and opposite areas of the imaged object. If the arc of travel is 360°, the shadow zone is much smaller, consisting of just the top and bottom areas, resulting in greater anatomic coverage [12]. The result is that using an imaging program with a full arc of 360° travel by the gantry will result in images with more anatomically accurate and reliable information; however, in routine dental CBCT, there will still be areas in the

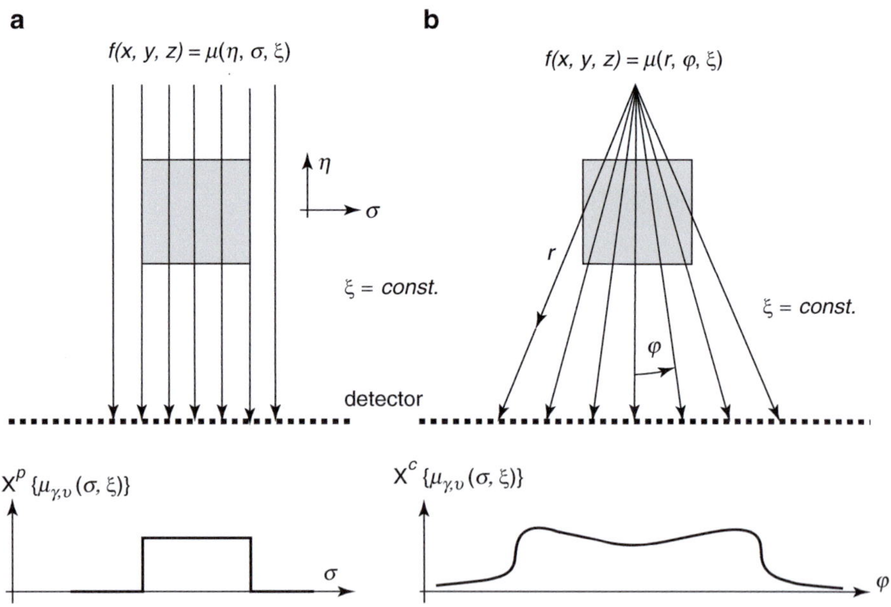

Fig. 13.1 Difference between parallel-beam and cone-beam geometry. (**a**) The parallel line integrals can easily be converted into a surface integral, (**b**) this cannot so easily be done with cone-beam geometry (Fig. 8.28 from T. Buzug's Computed Tomography From Photon Statistics to Modern Cone Beam CT book, a Springer book published in 2008, all can be found in Chapter 8, as noted below)

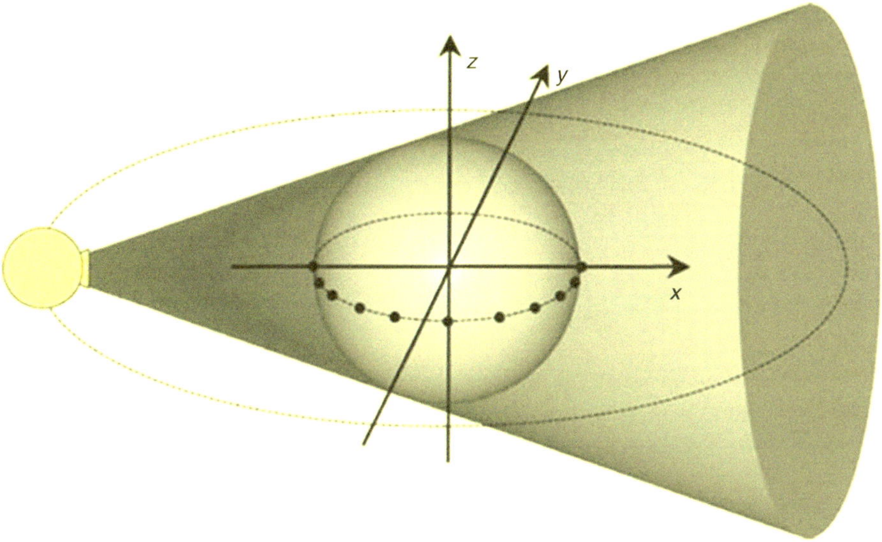

Fig. 13.2 In cone-beam geometry those object points for which the Radon space is complete are located within the plane defined by the X-ray source trajectory. For a spherical object this applies to all those points within the circle that results from a section of the trajectory plane through the sphere. Some outermost points with a complete set of Radon values are exemplarily shown on the front hemisphere of the spherical object (Fig. 8.44 from T. Buzug's Computed Tomography From Photon Statistics to Modern Cone Beam CT book, a Springer book published in 2008, all can be found in Chapter 8, as noted below)

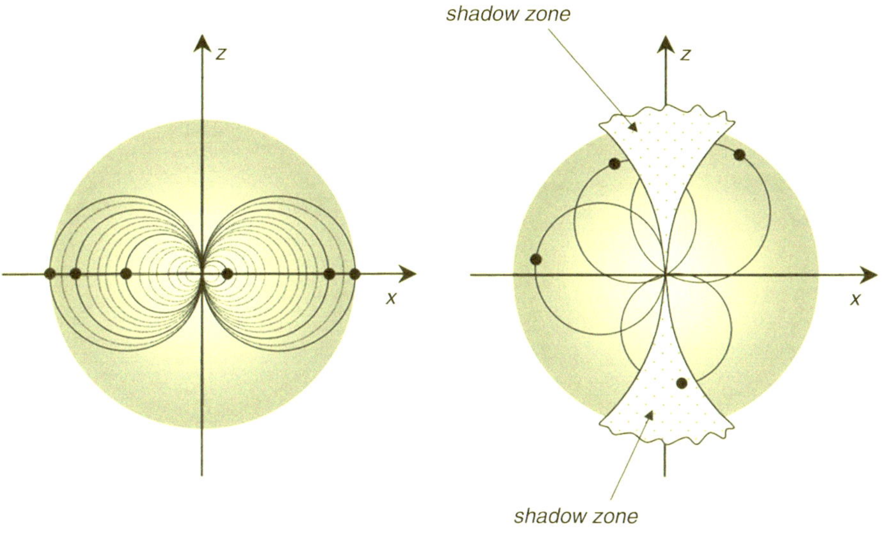

Fig. 13.3 Location of the practically available Radon value in the (x, z) plane. *Left*: As the set of Radon space value is complete for points in the (x, y) plane and the corresponding Radon value for each individual point are located on a spherical surface, the sections again result in *circles*. *Right*: Data are missing in the three-dimensional Radon space for points above and below the (x, y) plane. The Zone in which data are missing is called the *shadow zone* (Fig. 8.43 from T. Buzug's Computed Tomography From Photon Statistics to Modern Cone Beam CT book, a Springer book published in 2008, all can be found in Chapter 8, as noted below)

volume that are not fully imaged (Figs. 13.4 and 13.5). This problem is solved in multi-slice CT (MSCT) imaging by using helical path scanning; however, helical scanning negates one of the main advantages of dental CBCT, which is maintaining radiation doses at a low level [12].

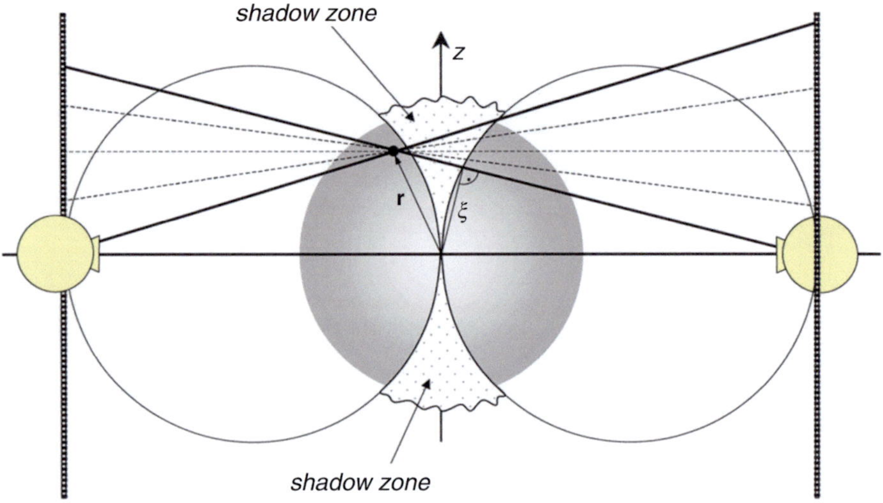

Fig. 13.4 There are points in the Radon space, of the cyclic source orbit in a plane, for which the necessary integration over the surface cannot be carried out. The points assigned in the spatial domain may then not be correctly reconstructed. The Radon value for which the integration surface does not intersect the X-ray source orbit are missing. The missing zone in the Radon space is again the *shadow zone* (Fig. 8.45 from T. Buzug's Computed Tomography From Photon Statistics to Modern Cone Beam CT book, a Springer book published in 2008, all can be found in Chapter 8, as noted below)

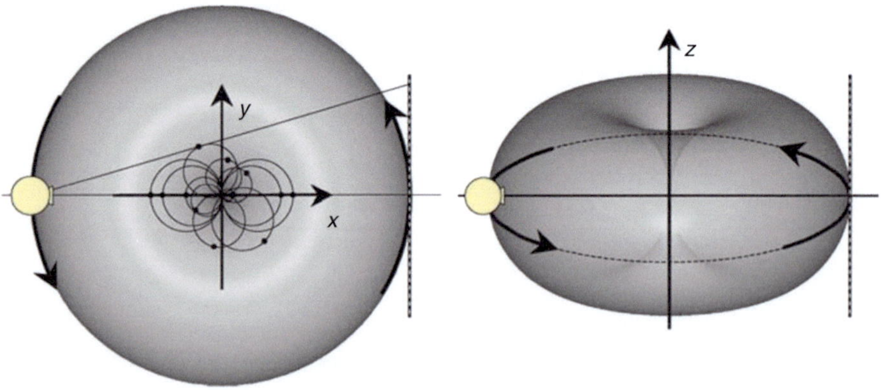

Fig. 13.5 In the Radon space of the cyclic source orbit those points that can theoretically be measured are located within a torus. Nevertheless, it is in fact not possible to measure all theoretically available points of the Radon space with a detector of finite size (Fig. 8.46 from T. Buzug's Computed Tomography From Photon Statistics to Modern Cone Beam CT book, a Springer book published in 2008, all can be found in Chapter 8, as noted below)

13.3 Scatter Radiation, Contrast Resolution, and Diagnosis of Caries

Most researchers agree that scatter radiation in dental CBCT prevents the use of CT numbers to quantitatively evaluate bone and tooth mineral density thereby forcing clinicians to rely on more subjective evaluations such as gray scale values [13]. When using dental CBCT, clinicians are able to distinguish biologic materials with densities similar to bone, dentin and enamel very well; in addition, we can determine the boundaries between tissues of dissimilar densities, such as between the airway and parapharyngeal soft tissues, with very good accuracy. A significant limitation is seen however when attempting to accurately diagnose details in low-density objects, such as soft tissues or dental caries, especially when the caries is adjacent to high-density objects, such as dental restorations, that emit scatter radiation and other artifacts.

Many authors have researched how well CBCT machines perform at diagnosing dental caries. Most of the existing research indicates that the diagnostic efficacy of dental CBCT and intraoral digital radiography when used to detect primary proximal caries, in the absence of nearby dental restorations for CBCT imaging, is very similar [14–22]. When diagnosing primary occlusal caries, dental CBCT may have a slight advantage over intraoral imaging; however, due to image artifacts related to occlusal enamel thickness, further investigations are needed [20, 23].

Several authors have evaluated the difficulties in diagnosing recurrent caries, mainly on the interproximal surfaces. Most authors have reported limited reliable and predictable diagnosis of recurrent caries using dental CBCT technology [3, 24–31] although it appears to be the case that the higher the density of the restorative material, the greater the amount of x-ray scatter, resulting in a less reliable diagnostic outcome. Recurrent caries can be detected on dental CBCT with varying degrees of success; however, the following are a few of the questions that still need to be considered. How predictable and reliable is diagnosing recurrent caries on CBCT? How large does the recurrent carious lesion need to be before it can be diagnosed? How does the type of restoration adjacent to the recurrent carious lesion affect the clinician's ability to detect the lesion on dental CBCT? What are the optimal scanning factors, such as X-ray energy (kVp), mA, time, number of basis projections, etc.

13.4 Radiographic Technique

In this section we will illustrate some of the various ways that carious lesions are manifested in dental CBCT images using case reports. We will begin with primary caries and end with recurrent caries.

The first case represents primary enamel and dentinal caries involving the interproximal surfaces of the premolar teeth of a 15-year-old male patient who presented with a chief complaint of previous trauma to his maxillary anterior teeth. The attending endodontist ordered a CBCT examination to evaluate the maxillary left central incisor for a vertical root fracture and other associated pathoses. Incidental findings included interproximal carious lesions involving the maxillary right second premolar and the mandibular left second premolar as seen in Fig. 13.6. These carious lesions were then managed as part of the patient's overall treatment plan after the initial endodontic care.

The next case is an example of a recurring clinical problem that practitioners faces—how best to manage defective lingual pits of maxillary incisors? The patient is a 54-year-old male who was imaged with dental CBCT to evaluate his chronic maxillary sinusitis condition. As we see in Fig. 13.7, the lingual pits were not previously restored and did not appear to be carious clinically; however, one of the incidental findings on the CBCT images was the presence of low densities, i.e., radiolucencies, within the dentin lingual to the pulp chambers of the maxillary lateral incisors. As

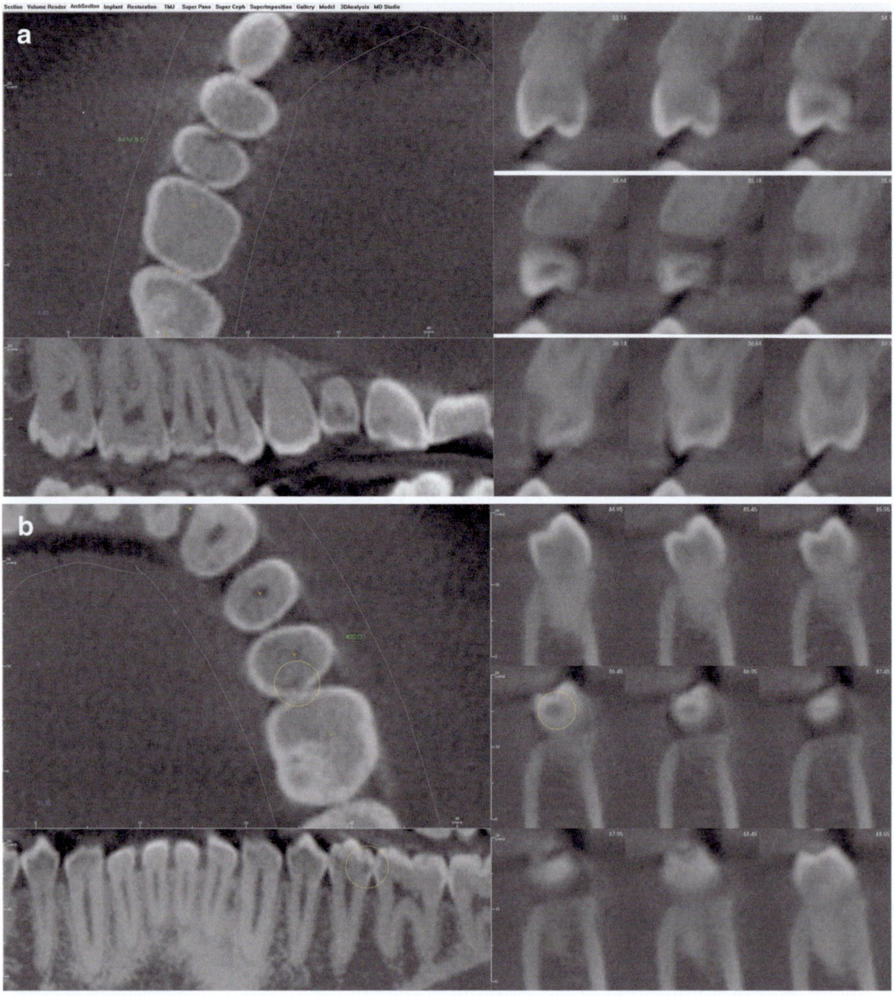

Fig. 13.6 (**a**) Low-density lesions representing dental caries noted on the mesial and distal surfaces of the maxillary right second premolar, (**b**) Low-density lesion representing dental caries noted on the distal surface of the mandibular left second premolar (Courtesy of Dr. Robert Block)

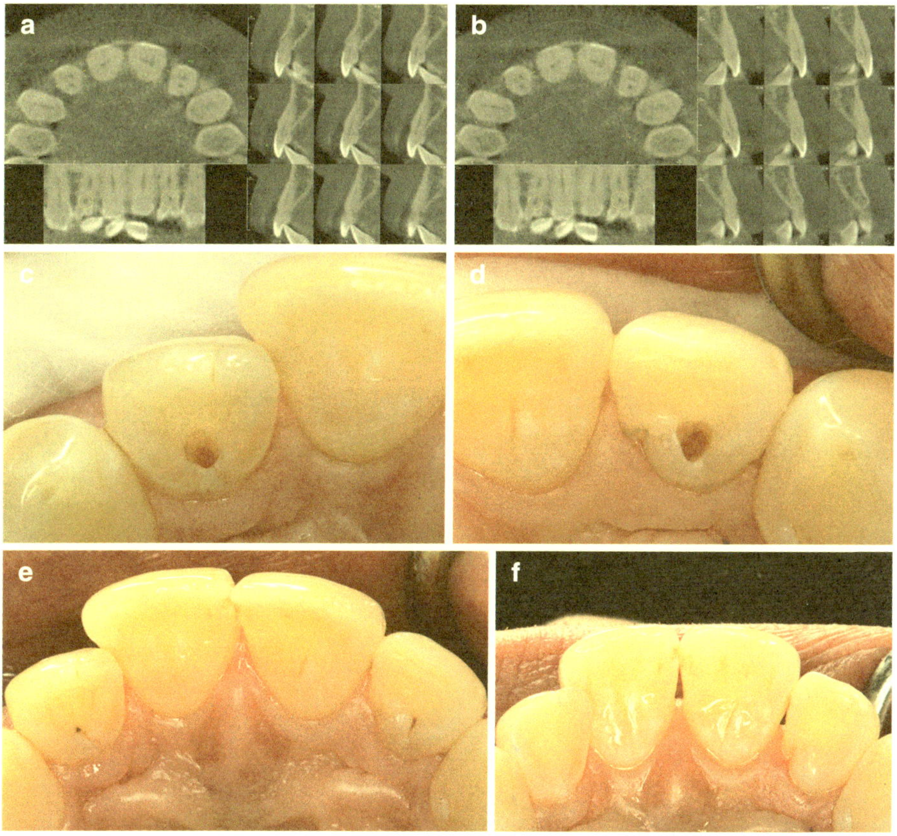

Fig. 13.7 (**a**, **b**) Sectional CBCT views of maxillary lateral incisors with low-density lesions lingual to the pulp chambers, (**c**, **d**) maxillary right and left lateral incisors after initial preparation with evidence of remaining caries, (**e**, **f**) clinical view of maxillary lateral incisors pre-op and post-op (Courtesy of Dr. Sahar Damghani)

confirmed during the clinical treatment, these low densities represented carious lesions (see Fig. 13.7c, d), which were restored before further extension could occur.

The third radiographic case illustrated in Fig. 13.8 involves recurrent caries along the gingival margin of a Class II molar composite adjacent to a more dense Class II amalgam restoration. This is a very challenging scenario in which to diagnose caries using dental CBCT technology due to the X-ray scatter and beam hardening artifacts that are commonly seen adjacent to metal restorations in CBCT images. As the periapical radiograph illustrates, there is a deep recurrent carious lesion apical to the existing MO composite in the maxillary second molar. The efficacy of dental CBCT often times depends on how well the clinician can manipulate the viewer software and whether the clinician can obtain proper views of the region of interest, in this case, a view of the recurrent carious lesion. Figure 13.8b presents nine static sagittal views that are 0.5 mm thick and taken from the center of the tooth; however, in the clinical setting, a clinician can scroll the full width of the tooth in whatever thickness desired,

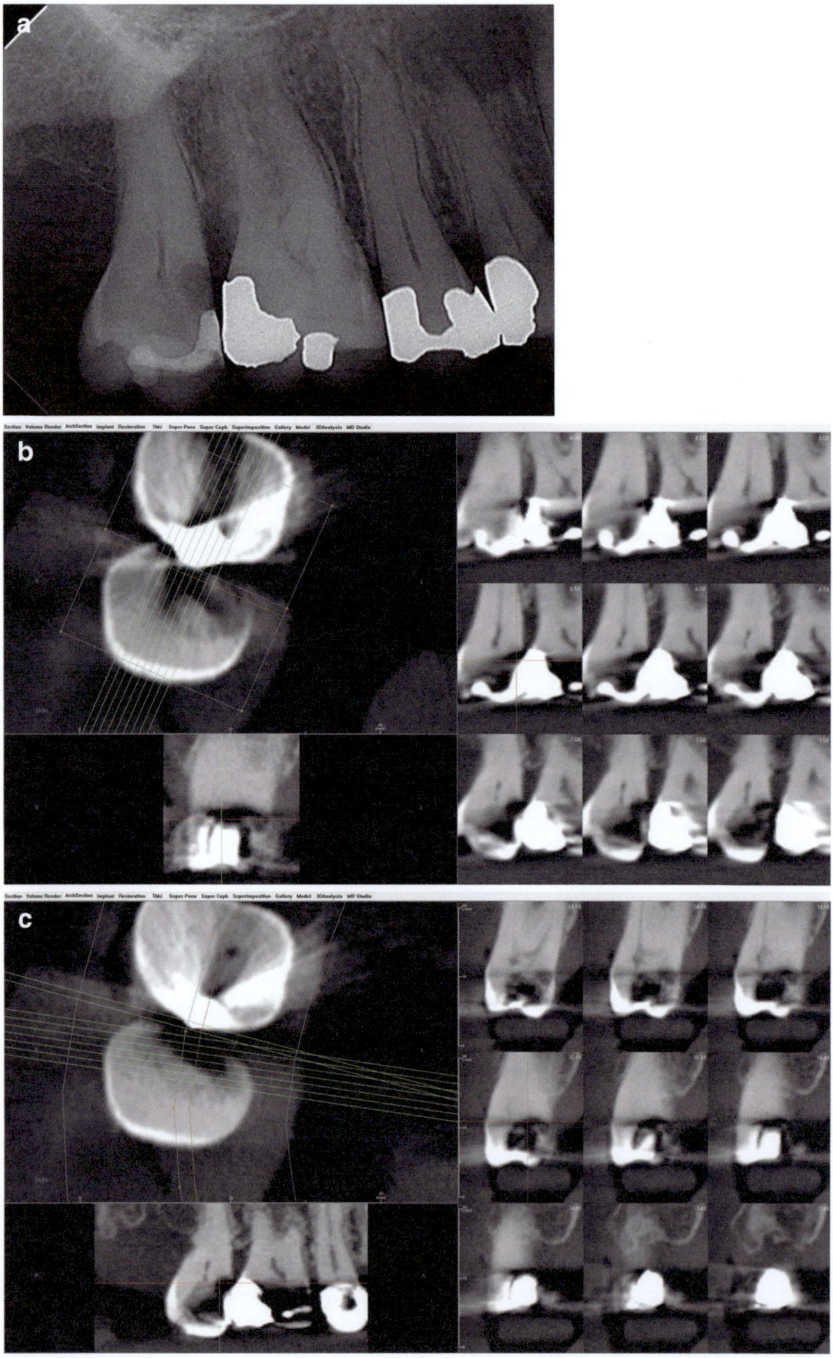

Fig. 13.8 (**a**) Periapical of the maxillary right second molar with an existing MO composite restoration and extensive mesial recurrent carious lesion, (**b**) CBCT sections with nine sectional images in the sagittal dimension, allowing for optimal viewing of the recurrent carious lesion, (**c**) CBCT sections with nine sectional images in the cross-sectional or coronal, dimension, which allows for less than optimal viewing of this recurrent carious lesion (Courtesy of Valley Endodontics & Microsurgery)

limited only by the software. In addition, axial and cross-sectional views can be used as well to examine the tooth and lesion. This advantage of evaluating the tooth and lesion in any desired direction can be helpful in many cases; however, the limiting factors of X-ray scatter and beam hardening artifacts remain a major limitation when attempting to rely solely on dental CBCT for diagnosing recurrent caries.

These radiographic cases confirm that dental CBCT can provide excellent diagnostic information regarding the presence of dental caries, when used on patients who do not have existing restorations. Furthermore, when used in conjunction with intraoral radiographs, such as bitewings and periapicals, dental CBCT images, when available, can provide very helpful information on the amount, depth, and configuration of carious lesions.

13.5 Concluding Remarks

This chapter has provided a review of some of the technical and physical limitations of dental CBCT when used in the diagnosis of dental caries. From a technical standpoint, primary interproximal caries without adjacent dental restorations can be diagnosed from dental CBCT's at least as well as from conventional intraoral bitewing radiographs; however, the increased enamel thickness encountered on occlusal surfaces may interfere with the reliability of dental CBCT during the diagnosis of occlusal caries. Using CBCT for the diagnosis of interproximal recurrent caries does not appear to be as predictable or as reliable as for the diagnosis of primary interproximal caries, although when available and used as an adjunct, dental CBCT can provide helpful diagnostic information. The accuracy and reliability of diagnosing recurrent dental caries using dental CBCT technology should improve as increased research in the area of X-ray beam filters, dual energy sources, X-ray scatter reduction and devices to compensate for patient motion come to market in the future. In addition, proper training and experience in the proper use of CBCT viewing software is very important and may be underestimated by many clinicians.

Finally, due to the increased radiation associated with the use of dental CBCT when compared to conventional bitewing radiography, dental CBCT cannot be recommended as a primary radiographic technique for diagnosing dental caries. The diagnosis of dental caries on dental CBCT images should only be performed during a review for "incidental findings" which means that under normal conditions the primary reason for ordering a dental CBCT would not be to detect dental caries.

Summary table

Caries diagnosis using CBCT				
Which surfaces/sites is it useful for	Occlusal (pits and fissures)	Proximal/ (approximal)	Smooth surface (buccal and lingual)	Root caries and which of the four surfaces?
	Y	**Y**	**Y**	**Y-all**

<table>
<tr><td rowspan="2">What type of lesions is valuable for</td><td>Primary coronal</td><td>Secondary coronal</td><td>Primary root caries</td><td>Secondary root caries</td></tr>
<tr><td>Y</td><td>Y, but caution</td><td>Y</td><td>Y, but caution</td></tr>
<tr><td rowspan="2">What type of dentition</td><td colspan="2">Primary</td><td colspan="2">Permanent</td></tr>
<tr><td colspan="2">Y, but limited due to radiation dose</td><td colspan="2">Y</td></tr>
<tr><td rowspan="2">Lesion severity</td><td colspan="2">Enamel lesions</td><td colspan="2">Dentinal lesions</td></tr>
<tr><td colspan="2">Y</td><td colspan="2">Y</td></tr>
<tr><td>Sensitivity</td><td colspan="4">Literature reported range
2D imaging: 0.31–0.33
CBCT imaging: 0.44–0.61</td></tr>
<tr><td>Specificity</td><td colspan="4">Literature reported range
2D imaging: 0.93–0.96
CBCT imaging: 0.89–0.95</td></tr>
<tr><td>Perceived Ease Of Use (PEOU)[a]</td><td colspan="4">1. The main factor regarding CBCT is that at current radiation dose levels, use of CBCT for caries diagnosis is limited to incidental findings only and not for a primary indication for diagnosis of dental caries
2. Dental CBCT requires a significant learning curve due to the time demands of learning CBCT principles and acquisition skills as well as the software associated with volume manipulation
3. Finally, the experience and skill to perceive the difference between caries and X-ray scatter artifacts requires time and effort to develop</td></tr>
<tr><td rowspan="4">Advantages/ disadvantages</td><td colspan="4">Advantages</td></tr>
<tr><td colspan="4">1. Caries diagnosis can be performed on CBCT images exposed primarily for other purposes; therefore, no additional radiographic dose to the patient is required</td></tr>
<tr><td colspan="4">Disadvantages</td></tr>
<tr><td colspan="4">1. (1) at the current time, the risk of exposure to excess radiation generally exceeds the benefit gained by the diagnostic information gained by ordering a CBCT ONLY for caries diagnosis; (2) the clinician must learn the new skill of properly manipulating a CBCT viewer in order to obtain the required diagnostic information</td></tr>
<tr><td>Time</td><td colspan="4">The time to open the viewer software, download the CBCT volume, draw a panoramic curve for each arch, evaluate the interproximal surfaces for a full complement of teeth; and, document the findings will require a minimum of 20–30 min, assuming that the volume has been reviewed by either an oral radiologist or the ordering clinician for pathology</td></tr>
<tr><td>Cost</td><td colspan="4">The added cost should be minimal, since caries diagnosis is an incidental finding on the CBCT; and, therefore, was ordered for a different primary reason. However, fees for CBCT examinations range from approximately $200 for limited volumes to greater than $500 for maxillofacial volumes, depending on the geographic location and type of practice, although some clinicians absorb the fee for the scan into the overall case fee for comprehensive care. Purchasing a dental CBCT machine (100,000 cost) solely for diagnosing caries in 75,000 to not recommended</td></tr>
</table>

[a]Davis (1989)

References

1. Mozzo P, Procacci C, Tacconi A, Martini PT, Andreis IA. A new volumetric CT machine for dental imaging based on the cone-beam technique: preliminary results. Eur Radiol. 1998;8(9):1558–64.
2. Arai Y, Tammisalo E, Iwai K, Hashimoto K, Shinoda K. Development of a compact computed tomographic apparatus for dental use. Dentomaxillofac Radiol. 1999;28(4):245–8.
3. Sousa Melo SL, Belem MDF, Prieto LT, Tabchoury CPM, Haiter-Neto F. Comparison of cone beam computed tomography and digital intraoral radiography performance in the detection of artificially induced recurrent caries-like lesions. Oral Surg Oral Med Oral Pathol Oral Radiol. 2017;124(3):306–14. (2212-4411 (Electronic)).
4. Kalender WA. Computed tomography fundamentals, system technology, image quality, applications. Erlangen: Publicis Publishing; 2011. 372 p.
5. Buzug T. Computed tomography from photon statistics to modern cone-beam CT. Heidelberg: Springer; 2008. 521 p.
6. Bushberg JT, Seibert JA, Leidholdt J, Edwin M, Boone JM. The essential physics of medical imaging [kindle edition]. Philadelphia: Lippincott Williams & Wilkins, a Wolters Kluwer business; 2012.
7. Miles DA. Atlas of cone beam imaging for dental applications. 2nd ed. Illinois: Quintessence Publishing; 2012.
8. Sarment DP. Cone beam computed tomography: oral and maxillofacial diagnosis and applications. Ames: Wiley Blackwell; 2014. 296 p.
9. Scarfe WC, Farman AG. What is cone-beam CT and how does it work? Dent Clin N Am. 2008;52(4):24.
10. The Nobel Prize in Physiology or Medicine 1979 was awarded jointly to Allan M. McCormack and Godfrey N. Hounsfield for the development of computer assisted tomography; [Website]. NobelPrize.org: Nobel Foundation; 1979 [cited 2017]. https://www.nobelprize.org/nobel_prizes/medicine/laureates/1979/.
11. Nemtoi A, Czink C, Haba D, Gahleitner A. Cone beam CT: a current overview of devices. Dentomaxillofac Radiol. 2013;42(8):20120443. (0250–832X (Print)).
12. Buzug T. Chapter 8.6 Approximate 3D reconstructions in cone-beam geometry. In: Computed tomography: from photon statistics to modern cone-beam CT. Berlin: Springer; 2008. p. 366–401.
13. Pauwels R, Nackaerts O, Bellaiche N, Stamatakis H, Tsiklakis K, Walker A, et al. Variability of dental cone beam CT grey values for density estimations. Br J Radiol. 2013;86(1021):20120135.
14. Tsuchida R, Araki K, Okano T. Evaluation of a limited cone-beam volumetric imaging system: comparison with film radiography in detecting incipient proximal caries. Oral Surg Oral Med Oral Pathol Oral Radiol Endod. 2007;104(3):412–6.
15. Kalathingal SM, Mol A, Tyndall DA, Caplan DJ. In vitro assessment of cone beam local computed tomography for proximal caries detection. Oral Surg Oral Med Oral Pathol Oral Radiol Endod. 2007;104(5):699–704.
16. Haiter-Neto F, Wenzel A, Gotfredsen E. Diagnostic accuracy of cone beam computed tomography scans compared with intraoral image modalities for detection of caries lesions. Dentomaxillofac Radiol. 2008;37(1):18–22.
17. Akdeniz BG, Grondahl HG, Magnusson B. Accuracy of proximal caries depth measurements: comparison between limited cone beam computed tomography, storage phosphor and film radiography. Caries Res. 2006;40(3):202–7.
18. Young SM, Lee JT, Hodges RJ, Chang TL, Elashoff DA, White SC. A comparative study of high-resolution cone beam computed tomography and charge-coupled device sensors for detecting caries. Dentomaxillofac Radiol. 2009;38(7):445–51.

19. Zhang ZL, Qu XM, Li G, Zhang ZY, Ma XC. The detection accuracies for proximal caries by cone-beam computerized tomography, film, and phosphor plates. Oral Surg Oral Med Oral Pathol Oral Radiol Endod. 2011;111(1):103–8.
20. Kayipmaz S, Sezgin OS, Saricaoglu ST, Can G. An in vitro comparison of diagnostic abilities of conventional radiography, storage phosphor, and cone beam computed tomography to determine occlusal and approximal caries. Eur J Radiol. 2011;80(2):478–82.
21. Senel B, Kamburoglu K, Ucok O, Yuksel SP, Ozen T, Avsever H. Diagnostic accuracy of different imaging modalities in detection of proximal caries. Dentomaxillofac Radiol. 2010;39(8):501–11.
22. Wenzel A, Hirsch E, Christensen J, Matzen LH, Scaf G, Frydenberg M. Detection of cavitated approximal surfaces using cone beam CT and intraoral receptors. Dentomaxillofac Radiol. 2013;42(1):39458105.
23. Kamburoglu K, Murat S, Yuksel SP, Cebeci AR, Paksoy CS. Occlusal caries detection by using a cone-beam CT with different voxel resolutions and a digital intraoral sensor. Oral Surg Oral Med Oral Pathol Oral Radiol Endod. 2010;109(5):e63–9.
24. Charuakkra A, Prapayasatok S, Janhom A, Pongsiriwet S, Verochana K, Mahasantipiya P. Diagnostic performance of cone-beam computed tomography on detection of mechanically-created artificial secondary caries. Imaging Sci Dent. 2011;41(4):143–50.
25. Murat S, Kamburoglu K, Isayev A, Kursun S, Yuksel S. Visibility of artificial buccal recurrent caries under restorations using different radiographic techniques. Oper Dent. 2013;38(2):197–207.
26. Kulczyk T, Dyszkiewicz Konwinska M, Owecka M, Krzyzostaniak J, Surdacka A. The influence of amalgam fillings on the detection of approximal caries by cone beam CT: in vitro study. Dentomaxillofac Radiol. 2014;43(7):20130342.
27. Bilgin MS, Aglarci OS, Erdem A. Posttreatment diagnosis of caries under fixed restorations: a pilot study. J Prosthet Dent. 2014;112(6):1364–9.
28. Aglarci OS, Bilgin MS, Erdem A, Ertas ET. Is it possible to diagnose caries under fixed partial dentures with cone beam computed tomography? Oral Surg Oral Med Oral Pathol Oral Radiol. 2015;119(5):579–83.
29. Shahidi S, Zadeh NK, Sharafeddin F, Shahab S, Bahrampour E, Hamedani S. An in vitro comparison of diagnostic accuracy of cone beam computed tomography and phosphor storage plate to detect simulated occlusal secondary caries under amalgam restoration. Dent Res J. 2015;12(2):161–6.
30. Vedpathak PR, Gondivkar SM, Bhoosreddy AR, Shah KR, Verma GR, Mehrotra GP, et al. Cone beam computed tomography- an effective tool in detecting caries under fixed dental prostheses. J Clin Diagn Res. 2016;10(8):Zc10–3.
31. Kasraei S, Shokri A, Poorolajal J, Khajeh S, Rahmani H. Comparison of cone-beam computed tomography and intraoral radiography in detection of recurrent caries under composite restorations. Braz Dent J. 2017;28(1):85–91.

Fibre-Optic Transillumination: FOTI

14

Richard Hogan, Iain A. Pretty, and Roger P. Ellwood

14.1 Introduction

From as early as the late 1800s, transillumination (TI) of teeth has been advocated as a diagnostic method for caries detection and assessment [1]. The introduction of fibre-optic light guides led to renewed academic interest and a series of research publications to support the method [2].

With very little experience or specialized training required, transillumination optically increases the contrast between sound and carious changes in tooth structure. The simplest form of this enhanced visual method—mirror-reflection of the overhead operating light—is familiar to many clinicians and integrated easily into everyday practice [2].

Fibre-optic transillumination (FOTI) expands upon this method through use of high intensity white light directed tangentially (usually perpendicularly) to the tooth surface(s) of interest. This allows the clinician to detect differences in the normal optical properties of teeth more readily than with ambient operating illumination through optical contrast enhancement [3].

Visual methods of caries detection rely upon the phenomenon of light scattering due to optical disruption of the light path [4]. In general, differences in porosity of the enamel or colour of dentin affect the light scattering or absorption properties of the tooth. When the light comes from an outside source, particularly after drying the tooth, any porous areas of the enamel will back scatter light making the lesions appear white. In contrast for FOTI, when light is shone through the tooth, light is backscattered into the tooth so areas of porosity appear dark on a lighter background. These differences are summarised in Table 14.1.

The technology underpinning FOTI is simple and has been available for many years [5]; however, its usefulness should not be underestimated. Visually, transillumination

R. Hogan (✉) · I. A. Pretty · R. P. Ellwood
Colgate-Palmolive Dental Health Unit, Division of Dentistry, The University of Manchester, Manchester, UK
e-mail: Richard.Hogan@postgrad.manchester.ac.uk

© Springer Nature Switzerland AG 2019

A. Ferreira Zandona, C. Longbottom (eds.), *Detection and Assessment of Dental Caries*, https://doi.org/10.1007/978-3-030-16967-1_14

Table 14.1 Differences in light scatter between FOTI and visual assessment

FOTI	Visual (White Light)
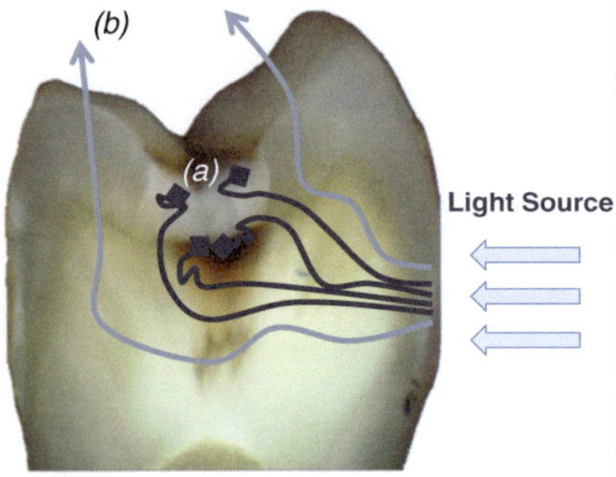	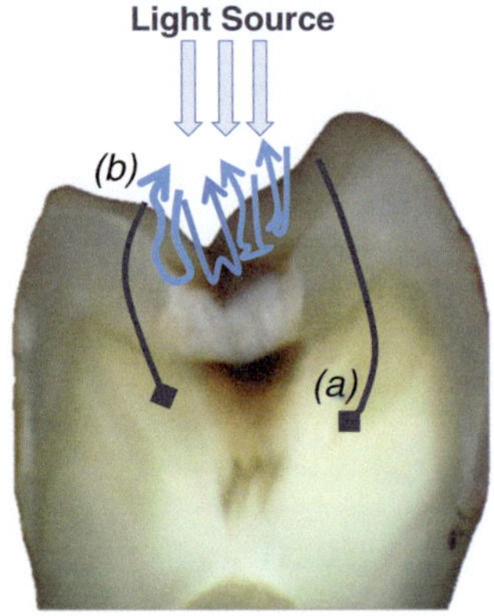
▪ Lesion scatters more light	▪ Lesion backscatters more light
▪ More photons absorbed, less light escapes (*a*)	▪ More photons reflected by lesion *(b)*
▪ Lesion appears **dark** on light background	▪ Lesion appears **light** on dark background
▪ Dentin lesions often appear orange	▪ Dentin lesions appear as grey shadows

of enamel lesions results in a grey, opaque appearance within the tooth, easily distinguishable from the usually translucent enamel layer. With dentin lesions, an orange-brown or bluish shadow within the tooth will often be observed; this finding is of significance during depth determination and differentiation between enamel and dentin lesions [6]. Previous work involving general dental practitioners demonstrated a trend for the participants to detect more interproximal and occlusal lesions when using FOTI as a supplement to their normal clinical routine. Additionally, a qualitative assessment from the same study indicated that the technology was well received by the participating clinicians who viewed it as a useful additional tool for caries detection [7]. The information derived from the use of FOTI facilitates three-dimensional localisation of the lesion aiding minimal cavity preparation when required.

The research surrounding the use of FOTI varies significantly in relation to the sensitivity and specificity of the method. A recent systematic review found sensitivity scores of 21–96% and specificity scores of 74–88% for detection of non-cavitated lesions using FOTI [8], whilst an earlier review presented sensitivity scores of 4–74% and specificity scores of 85–100% [9]. The wide range for sensitivity and specificity, as with most visual methods, is due to the experience of the clinician, the subjective nature of FOTI assessment and the thresholds used. A high specificity is desirable for a diagnostic device that might lead to restorative treatment or other intervention, although, using this method some earlier lesions that might require preventive treatment may be missed due to lower sensitivity.

Evidence suggests FOTI to be as valid as radiographic investigation (depending on lesion type) and that in combination with direct visual evidence-based caries indices (see Chap. 3—The Visual Signs of Caries Chaps. 5–8), the diagnostic yield is increased [5]. For this reason, it is important to view FOTI as an adjunct detection method, best employed in combination with robust visual assessment, and as an additional tool in deciding whether radiographic investigation is justified [6, 10–12]. A comparison of visual, FOTI and Micro-CT images can be found in Table 14.2,

Table 14.2 Comparison of ICDAS scores 0–6 with corresponding FOTI image and micro-CT scan

Code	ICDAS criteria	FOTI criteria	Visual	FOTI	Micro-CT
0	Sound—No change in enamel after prolonged air drying	No shadow or stained area	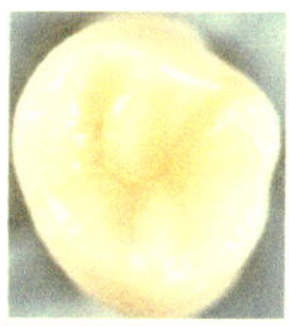	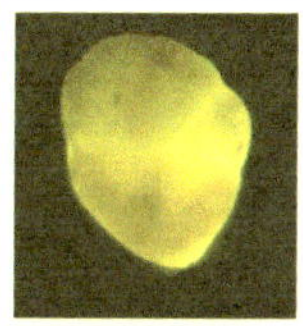	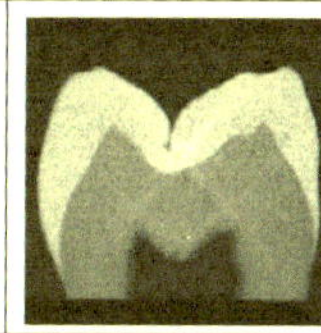
0	Stained—No evidence of white opacity on periphery of stain	Stain remains the same width when trans illuminated	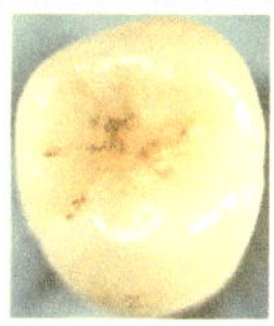	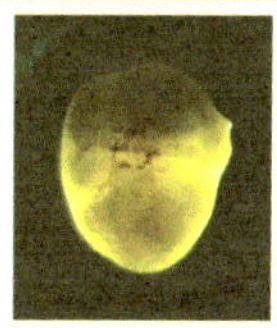	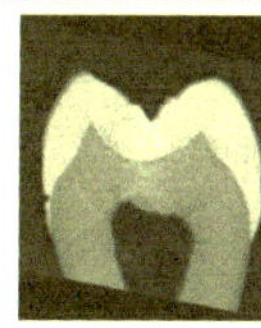
1	First visual change in enamel, visible after prolonged air drying	Visually sound tooth but thin grey shadow into enamel when transilluminated OR Stained lesion widens when trans illuminated OR ICDAS 1 visual lesion which remains the same when transilluminated	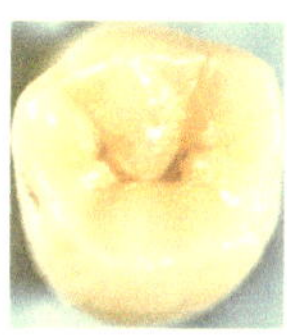	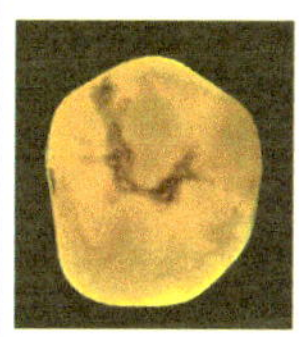	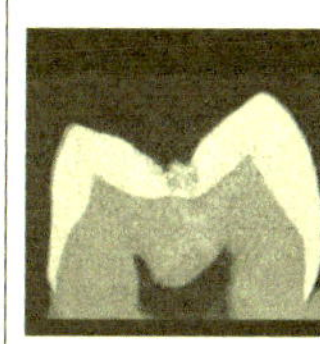
2	Distinct visual change in enamel, opacity and/or discolouratio n visible wet and dry	Wide grey shadow into enamel when trans illuminated Extends to EDJ for proximal lesions	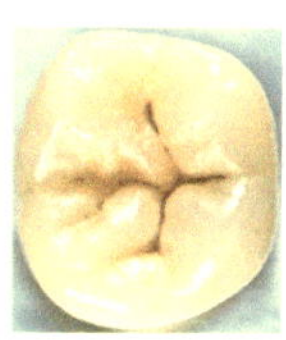	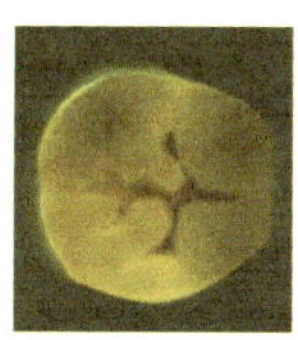	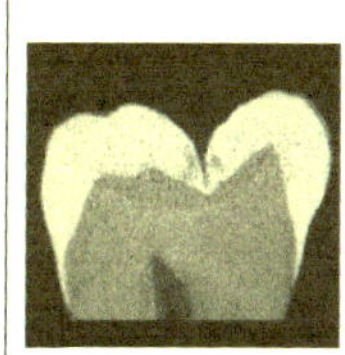
3	Localised enamel breakdown with opaque and/or discoloured enamel	Wide dark grey shadow into enamel with no evidence of dentin shadow	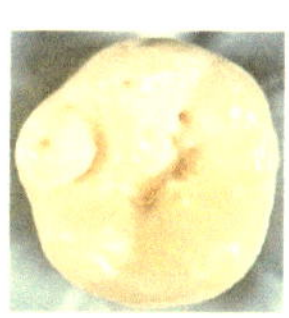	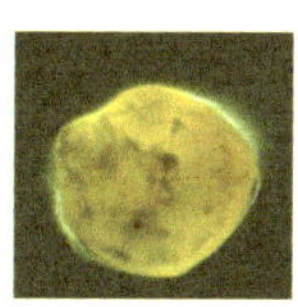	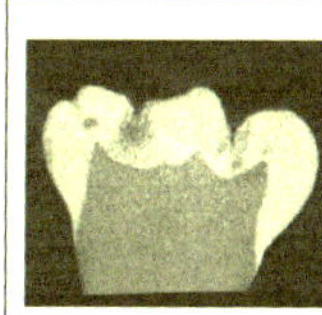

(continued)

Table 14.2 (continued)

4	Underlying dentin shadow	Orange/brown or bluish/black dentin shadow 4a - <2 mm in width 4b - >2 mm in width	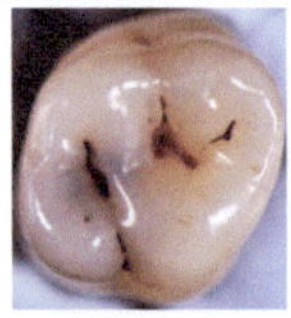	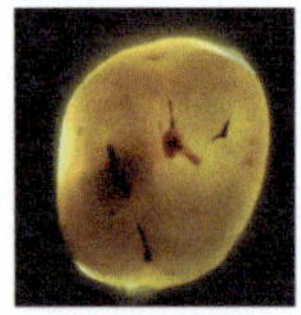	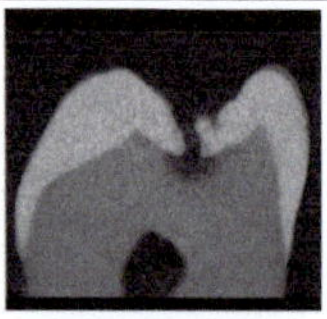
5	Distinct cavity with visible dentin	Shadow as described above and/or transilluminatio nlight is blocked, >2 mm in width	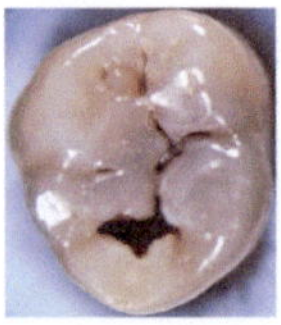	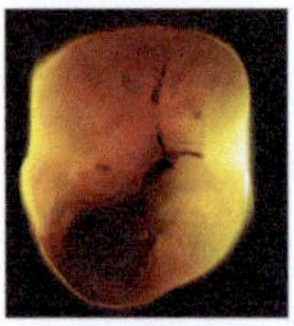	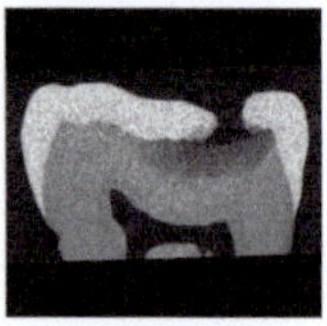
6	Extensive cavity with visible dentin	Large area of frank cavitation with likely pulpal involvement	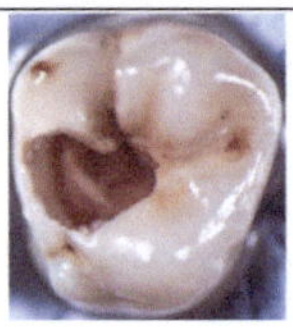	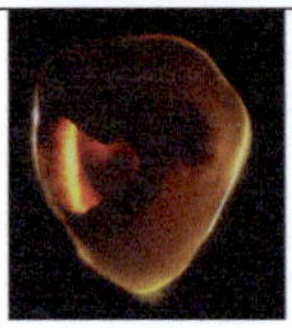	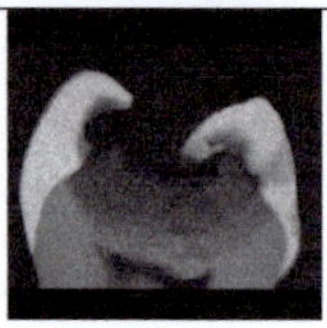

with both the ICDAS visual criteria (Chap. 6) and corresponding FOTI criteria listed. As discussed, use of this combined scoring system may increase the value of any diagnostic output gained through use of FOTI and should be recorded in the patient's records for purposes of follow-up investigation. The method can be particularly useful in discriminating between lesions into dentin or those confined to enamel [5]. It should be noted that the higher of the ICDAS visual or FOTI codes takes precedence if using these methods in combination.

FOTI offers a non-invasive, non-irradiating method of caries detection with no limitation on the frequency of use. Additionally, the learning curve is short, the equipment economical, and the time consumption low [4, 12]. One drawback of this method is the qualitative nature of any findings, which require subjective interpretation by the user, although, this is common to many of the frequently used caries detection and assessment methods. With no continuous and recordable output, longitudinal monitoring using FOTI is complex and as with any visual scoring system, clinically significant changes are potentially required before they are identified by a scoring system [5, 13, 14].

In an effort to overcome this limitation, a move was made to digitalise the process, resulting in the development of digital fibre-optic transillumination (DIFOTI). DIFOTI utilises a CCD sensor, effectively replacing the human eye with a grey scale camera, which allows for image capture and storage [15]. Whilst this improvement has obvious benefits in relation to longitudinal lesion monitoring through image storage, the captured images do still require subjective interpretation by the operator [13]. DIFOTI has been shown to be as valid as radiographic investigation for all lesions, with suggestions of superior performance in the detection of early enamel lesions [14, 15].

More recently, DIFOTI technology has been developed further through use of near-infrared light. This technology retains the benefit of image capture and storage but offers deeper penetration of light into the tooth structure, highlighting carious changes more clearly than traditional white light transillumination. Additionally, near-infrared light is less confounded by stain; reducing the risk of false-positives in relation to caries diagnosis [16, 17]. This technology is discussed further at the end of this chapter (see Sect. 14.3).

Whilst this chapter refers to the usefulness of transillumination in relation to caries detection, FOTI and DIFOTI can add additional value to detection of other conditions and peri-operatively for other procedures. Briefly, these methods can be utilised in the detection of crown and root fractures [18], although some operator experience is required to ensure cracks are not erroneously labelled as carious lesions [5]. Transillumination also offers some benefit during endodontic treatment; light shone perpendicularly into an access cavity can aid in location of canal orifices [18]. These additional applications merit consideration during any decision making around adoption of FOTI into clinical practice.

To date, visual assessment supplemented with radiographic investigation remains the mainstay of caries examinations. Despite successful use in research for many years [5, 6], methods employing transillumination are rarely utilised in practice or taught in dental schools [7]. In recent years, the availability and affordability of digital dental devices have increased significantly; more than ever, clinicians are, rightly, excited by novel methods capable of supplementing their clinical practice. Whilst these technologies merit enthusiasm, this should not come at the expense of proven methods using the simplest of techniques [12]. Using only light, FOTI and DIFOTI are capable of improving caries detection for all lesions, on all teeth, and across all surfaces. When the additional uses for other conditions are considered, it would seem every clinician stands to improve his or her clinical practice through adoption of this method.

14.2 Clinical Technique

14.2.1 FOTI Technique

With all device-related techniques, it is important to follow manufacturer-specific guidance to ensure correct usage, however, this section will describe generally the method used for most FOTI devices. It is recommended to use FOTI probes with tip sizes of 3 mm or less for all teeth to provide a more focussed beam, improving the definition of any visible changes. The dental operating light and any headlamp should be switched off and, if possible, the room lights should also be switched off or dimmed to further reduce interference from ambient light. The teeth, as for all visual methods of caries detection, should be clean and dry (see Chap. 2)—cleaning should include plaque removal from all coronal surfaces, including the interproximal areas; drying should include use of the air-syringe and isolation from saliva should be maintained.

For anterior teeth, place the FOTI probe tip on the cervical aspect of the buccal surface of one of the upper incisors, just above the gingival margin, and observe the tooth from the palatal direction using a mouth mirror. Steadily move the FOTI tip back and forth along the line of the cervical margin in both mesial and distal directions and into the embrasure. Keep the tip at right angles to the buccal surface, paying close attention to each of the interproximal surfaces in turn. It is important to change the angulation of the light source to provide a comprehensive three-dimensional perspective of any caries lesion, as well as to investigate other conditions such as enamel dysplasia, intrinsic staining and coronal tooth fractures (Fig. 14.1).

The differences in transparency and colour of the enamel and dentin should be clear; it should, therefore, be readily apparent if any grey shadows are present in enamel and how far these shadows extend towards, or past, the enamel-dentin junction. An orange or bluish shadow deep in the tooth is indicative of penetration into dentin.

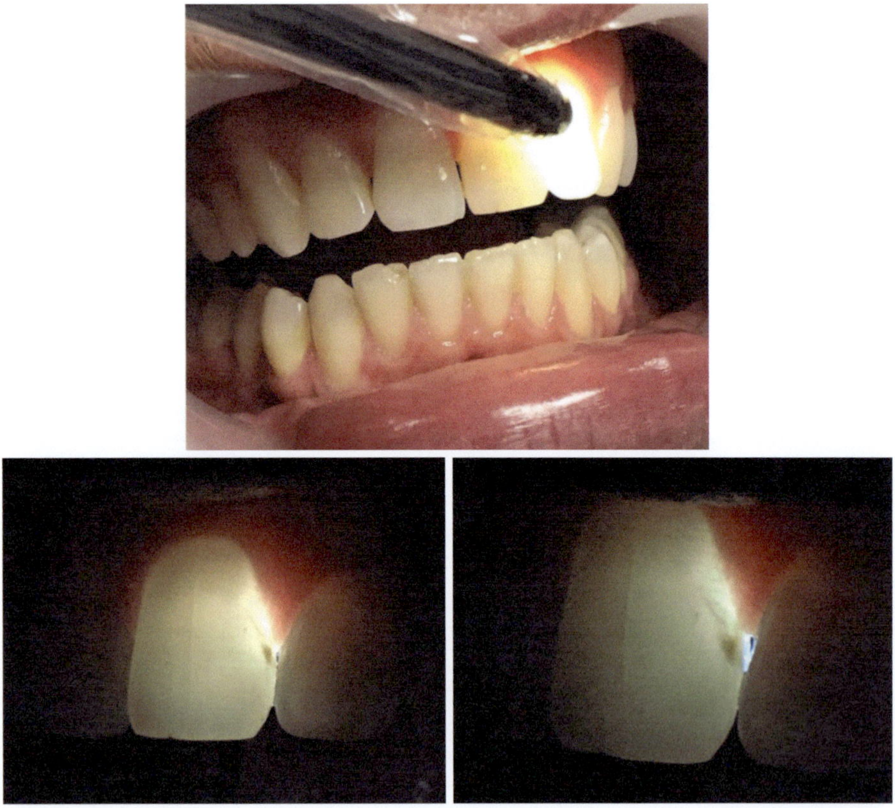

Fig. 14.1 Correct placement of FOTI probe for anterior caries detection (top), transilluminated central incisor with evidence of interproximal caries (bottom, left), example of changed angulation of FOTI tip on same central incisor resulting in altered contrast and highlighting potential craze line in enamel (bottom, right)

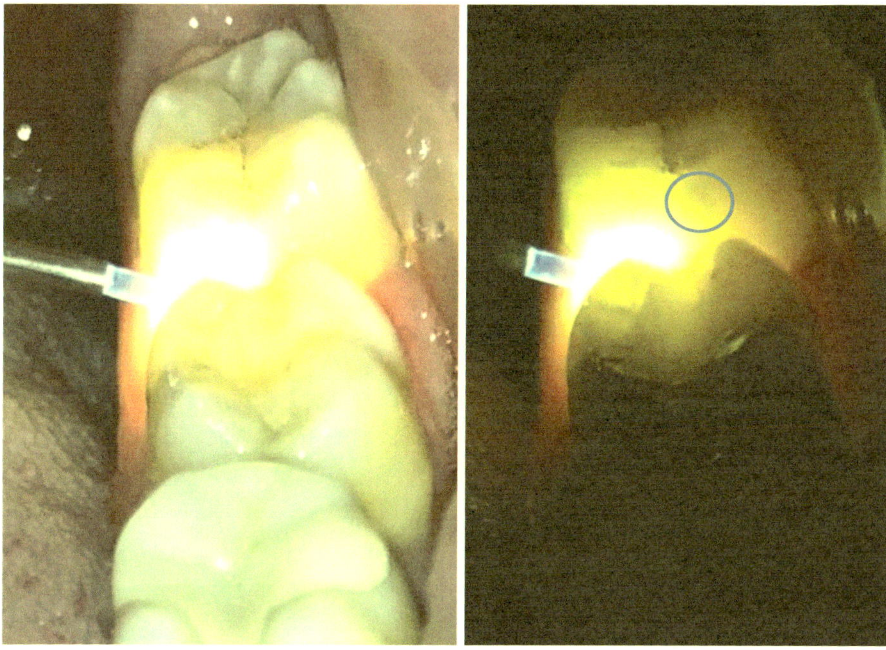

Fig. 14.2 Correct placement of narrow-tipped FOTI probe (0.75 mm) for posterior interproximal caries detection (left), carious enamel lesion on mesial surface of third molar (right, circled), contrast between composite restorative material and tooth tissue evident on second molar (right)

It is sometimes appropriate to use the FOTI tip on the lingual surface of lower incisors due to the reduced thickness of these teeth and observing the teeth directly. This method can also be employed for the upper teeth in some cases.

For posterior teeth, the FOTI tip should again be placed on the buccal cervical margin of each tooth—above the gingival margin but below the contact point. As before, the FOTI tip should be moved back and forth along the cervical margin whilst using a mouth mirror to observe the whole of the occlusal surface; particular attention should be paid to the pit and fissure patterns and marginal ridges (Fig. 14.2). In relation to pits and fissures, as with incisor palatal pits, look for the presence of shadows in the enamel in the immediate areas around the pits and fissures—a grey shadow tends to indicate enamel caries, whereas the presence of orange-brown or larger grey-blue shadows tends to suggest dentin caries—these shadows appear adjacent to the fissure pattern and dentin lesions tend to spread more widely than enamel lesions. Illumination of the tooth from the cervical aspect can also be helpful in some cases to improve contrast, depending on the site of the lesion.

The presence of stain in the depth of a fissure can confound the FOTI assessment, however, with increasing experience of using the FOTI technique, the clinician should be able to discern a stained fissure from a carious lesion. By moving both the probe and the viewing angle, the three-dimensional structure of a caries lesion can be observed and this can aid in discrimination of surface stain from underlying shadows. Stain and enamel caries are also readily discriminated by using the optical properties of the tooth. When the light is used to transilluminate the tooth, the grey shadow of carious enamel will tend to appear and disappear in intensity as the light is moved over the tooth surface. In contrast, a stained area will tend to remain consistent in intensity. The FOTI light can also be used to directly illuminate the tooth surface from 2 to 3 cm. In this case, tooth stain will tend to remain similar in appearance when transilluminated but enamel caries will now tend to appear white due to the backscattering properties of the tooth.

With regard to observation of marginal ridges during a FOTI examination, a clear difference between enamel and dentin translucency can be observed. Any shadows in enamel approaching, but not reaching, the EDJ should be discernible; with experience, one can begin to classify whether the enamel shadow is limited to the outer or inner half of the enamel layer. The EDJ is readily apparent, permitting easy identification of lesions extending into dentin. As discussed previously, these lesions tend to show up with orange-brown colour changes, especially if the tip is moved across the embrasure to the adjacent teeth increasing the range of light intensity passing through the tooth. This range can also be extended by moving the FOTI tip vertically to and from the cervical margin. The use of narrow FOTI tips (<1 mm) placed into the embrasure below the contact area of adjacent teeth will increase the relative intensity differences of the light scattering effects and allow two interproximal marginal ridges to be observed at the same time. Particular care is needed when using FOTI for the examination of teeth with large restorations, as these teeth are difficult to transilluminate and caries can often be missed. In addition, very large dentin lesions are often difficult to discern with FOTI due to lack of lesion boundary and contrast with sound enamel.

An additional FOTI technique involves placing the FOTI probe on the occlusal surface and observing the buccal and palatal aspects in turn using the dental mirror; this aids in examination of the approximal sites. As above, if the operator moves the tip of the light guide over the tooth surfaces to transilluminate different aspects of the tooth, differences between enamel and dentin become apparent, aiding in the judgement of lesion extent and proximity to pulp.

As with all clinical techniques, time is required to learn the skills and more importantly, become proficient in their use. As discussed in the introduction, linking FOTI to a direct visual evidence-based caries index adds invaluable diagnostic information to traditional visual assessment and encourages recording of FOTI findings in patient records.

14.2.2 DIFOTI Technique

Generally, DIFOTI systems will provide two attachments to permit anterior and posterior imaging. The anterior attachment shines light from either the buccal or lingual direction and captures the image using the CCD sensor on the opposite surface. In contrast, the posterior attachment shines light from both the buccal and lingual directions, capturing the image from the occlusal surface.

All teeth should be imaged in a methodical manner, taking care to capture images from a stable position with the light source(s) at right angles to the buccal and/or lingual surface. This allows better reproducibility of images for longitudinal monitoring and reduces the risk of an angulation change falsely altering the appearance of a lesion (i.e. false improvement or worsening).

The device-specific software will often automatically progress through the arch, taking approximately 10–15 min to capture a full mouth series [13]. Captured images should be reported in a similar manner to radiographic reporting, i.e. visually assessed with a description of any findings of interest—this is crucial to any longitudinal monitoring attempted using DIFOTI.

14.3 Additional Device-Specific Considerations

14.3.1 Microlux

The Microlux device (AdDent, Inc.) is a handheld, battery powered FOTI device (Fig. 14.3). The device offers a 2 and 3 mm light guide for posterior and anterior caries detection, respectively, to be used in the method described in Sect. 14.2.1. A fine-tipped 0.75 mm attachment is also available for use in posterior interproximal areas; intended to be placed into the gingival embrasure below the contact point, this tip may further increase the definition of any carious changes within posterior teeth [12]. Additionally, the device can be used with a variety of other tips, allowing the clinician to use the device for canal orifice detection, periodontal pocket depth assessment and oral cancer screening (Fig. 14.3).

14.3.2 DiaLUX

The DiaLUX probe (KaVo) is the most economical FOTI device considered in this chapter; this light probe fits onto pre-existing couplings on the dental chair (MultiFlex, KaVo). The device is used in the method described in Sect. 14.2.1,

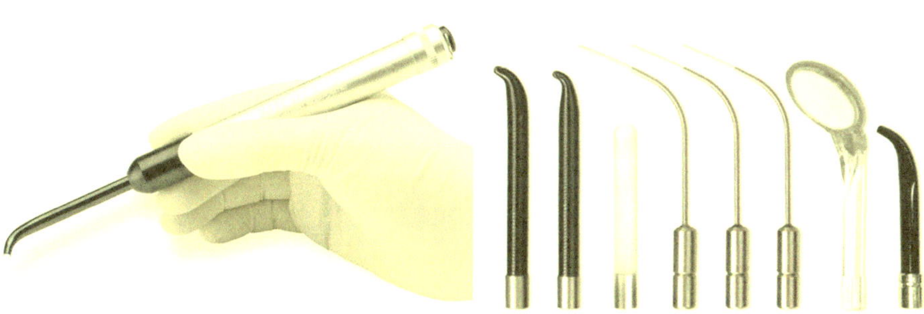

Fig. 14.3 Microlux device and range of available tips (Reproduced from AdDent 2017 [19])

however, whilst the DiaLUX is perhaps the simplest FOTI device available, its simplicity brings limitations; the device offers no additional tips to change the diameter of the probe or for use in other conditions. Other manufacturers may provide options to allow curing lights to be used for transillumination.

14.4 Concluding Remarks

To date, visual assessment supplemented with radiographic investigation remains the mainstay of caries examinations. Despite successful use in research for many years [5, 6], methods employing transillumination are rarely utilised in practice or taught in dental schools [7]. In recent years, the availability and affordability of digital dental devices have increased significantly; more than ever, clinicians are, rightly, excited by novel methods capable of supplementing their clinical practice. Whilst these technologies merit enthusiasm, this should not come at the expense of proven methods using the simplest of techniques [12]. Using only light, FOTI and DIFOTI are capable of improving caries detection for all lesions, on all teeth, and across all surfaces. When the additional uses for other conditions are considered, it would seem every clinician stands to improve his or her clinical practice through adoption of this method.

Summary table

Bitewing radiography	FOTI and DIFOTI			
Which surfaces/ sites is it useful for	Occlusal (pits and fissures)	Proximal/ (approximal)	Smooth surface (buccal and lingual)	Root caries
	Y	Y	Y	Y
What type of lesions is valuable for	Primary coronal	Secondary coronal	Primary root caries	Secondary root caries
	Y	Y	Y	Y
What type of dentition	Primary		Permanent	
	Y		Y	
Lesion severity	Enamel lesions		Dentinal lesions	
	Y		Y	
Sensitivity	4–94% [8, 9]			
Specificity	74–100% [8, 9]			
Perceived Ease Of Use (PEOU)[a]	1. (DI)FOTI is easy-to-use 2. Some experience is required to become skilful at using (DI)FOTI 3. Learning to operate (DI)FOTI is easy 4. (DI)FOTI is flexible to interact with 5. Interacting with (DI)FOTI is mostly clear and understandable, but can be confounded by other conditions (i.e. stain, enamel dysplasia, tooth fracture) 6. It is easy to interact with (DI)FOTI			

Advantages/ disadvantages	*Advantages* 1. Short learning curve 2. Non-invasive and non-irradiating 3. Suitable for all surfaces and lesion stages 4. Image storage for longitudinal monitoring and patient education (DIFOTI only) 5. Can be used for crown and root fracture detection and canal orifice location *Disadvantages* 1. Qualitative output requiring subjective interpretation 2. Experience needed to improve consistency of lesion detection and classification 3. Unsuitable for longitudinal monitoring (FOTI only)
Time	15–20 s per tooth surface
Cost	**DiaLUX** ≈£100–200 **Microlux** Device and one light guide (2 mm or 3 mm tip) ≈ £240 Additional light guide ≈ £115 Proximal caries attachment ≈ £100 (requires purchase of disposable tips) Disposable sleeves ≈ £35 per box of 250 **DIAGNOCam** ≈£4500 Reusable tips ≈£160 per tip

[a]Davis [20]

References

1. Hume W. Need for change in dental caries diagnosis. In: Stookey G, editor. Early detection of dental caries: proceedings of the 1st annual Indiana conference. Indianapolis: Indiana University School of Dentistry; 1996. p. 1–10.
2. Pine CM. Fibre-optic transillumination (FOTI) in caries diagnosis. In: Stookey G, editor. Early detection of dental caries: proceedings of the 1st annual Indiana conference. Indianapolis: Indiana University School of Dentistry; 1996. p. 51–65.
3. Gomez J. Detection and diagnosis of the early caries lesion. BMC Oral Health. 2015;15(Suppl 1):S3.
4. Pretty IA. Caries detection and diagnosis: novel technologies. J Dent. 2006;34(10):727–39.
5. Stephen KW, Russell JI, Creanor SL, Burchell CK. Comparison of fibre optic transillumination with clinical and radiographic caries diagnosis. Community Dent Oral Epidemiol. 1987;15(2):90–4.
6. Côrtes DF, Ellwood RP, Ekstrand KR. An in vitro comparison of a combined FOTI/visual examination of occlusal caries with other caries diagnostic methods and the effect of stain on their diagnostic performance. Caries Res. 2003;37:8–16.
7. Davies GM, Worthington HV, Clarkson JE, Thomas P, Davies RM. The use of fibre-optic transillumination in general dental practice. Br Dent J. 2001;191(3):145–7. Nature Publishing Group.
8. Gomez J, Tellez M, Pretty IA, Ellwood RP, Ismail AI. Non-cavitated carious lesions detection methods: a systematic review. Community Dent Oral Epidemiol. 2013;41(1):55–66.

9. Bader JD, Shugars DA, Bonito AJ. A systematic review of the performance of methods for identifying carious lesions. J Public Health Dent. 2002;62(4):201–13.
10. Pretty IA, Ellwood RP. The caries continuum: opportunities to detect, treat and monitor the re-mineralization of early caries lesions. J Dent. 2013;41(Suppl 2):S12–21.
11. Neuhaus KW, Ellwood RP, Lussi A, Pitts NB. Traditional lesion detection aids. In: Pitts N, editor. Detection, assessment, diagnosis and monitoring of caries. Basel: Karger; 2009. p. 42–51.
12. Strassler HE, Pitel ML. Using fiber-optic transillumination as a diagnostic aid in dental practice. Compend Contin Educ Dent. 2014;35(2):80–8.
13. Pretty IA, Maupomé G. A closer look at diagnosis in clinical dental practice: part 5. Emerging technologies. J Can Dent Assoc (Tor). 2004;70(8):540.
14. Schneiderman A, Elbaum M, Shultz T, Keem S, Greenebaum M, Driller J. Assessment of dental caries with Digital Imaging Fiber-Optic TransIllumination (DIFOTI): in vitro study. Caries Res. 1997;31(2):103–10. Karger Publishers.
15. Astvaldsdóttir A, Ahlund K, Holbrook WP, de Verdier B, Tranæus S. Approximal caries detection by DIFOTI: in vitro comparison of diagnostic accuracy/efficacy with film and digital radiography. Int J Dent. 2012;2012:326401. Hindawi Publishing Corporation.
16. Söchtig F, Hickel R, Kühnisch J. Caries detection and diagnostics with near-infrared light transillumination: clinical experiences. Quintessence Int (Berl). 2014;45(6):513–38.
17. Kühnisch J, Söchtig F, Pitchika V, Laubender R, Neuhaus KW, Lussi A, et al. In vivo validation of near-infrared light transillumination for interproximal dentin caries detection. Clin Oral Investig. 2016;20(4):821–9. Springer Berlin Heidelberg.
18. Liewehr F. An inexpensive device for transillumination. J Endod. 2001;27(2):130–1.
19. AdDent. Microlux device [Internet]. [cited 2 Aug 2017]. http://www.addent.com/microlux/.
20. Davis FD. Perceived usefulness, perceived ease of use, and user acceptance of information technology. MIS Q. 1989;13(3):319–40. https://doi.org/10.2307/249008.

Near-Infrared Light Transillumination 15

Jan Kühnisch

15.1 Introduction

Appropriate caries management requires a valid and reliable caries diagnosis with visual examination and additional diagnostic methods to reveal the caries burden [1–6]. Here, conventional (digital) bitewing radiography is frequently understood as the additional method of choice in daily clinical practice to detect and diagnose caries lesions on proximal and occlusal surfaces [7–9]. Obtaining satisfactory bitewing radiographs in children and teenagers is often problematic and sometimes impossible. Overlapping effects on X-rays or fixed orthodontic appliances may also hinder caries detection. Furthermore, the indication and repeatability of dental X-rays are considerably restricted because of the associated usage of ionizing radiation (for additional information on radiographs see Chaps. 11 and 12). Consequently, alternative diagnostic methods that do not rely on using dental X-rays may balance out the aforementioned disadvantages. Near-infrared light transillumination (NILT, DIAGNOcam, KaVo, Biberach, Germany/CariVu, DEXIS, Hatfield, PA, USA) was introduced on the European dental market as a novel X-ray-free imaging method for caries detection and diagnostics in posterior teeth in autumn 2012 [10]. This new method uses near-infrared light to visualize enamel and dentin caries lesions in molars and premolars. Technically, the intraoral camera (Fig. 15.1) emits near-infrared light with a wavelength of ~780 nm by two light emission windows, each arranged on the buccal and oral branches of the handpiece. The light is transmitted through the alveolar bone into the dental hard tissue. The image of the transilluminated tooth is captured with a CCD sensor over the occlusal surface (Fig. 15.2).

J. Kühnisch (✉)
Department of Conservative Dentistry and Periodontology, University Hospital, Ludwig-Maximilian-University of Munich, Munich, Germany
e-mail: jkuehn@dent.med.uni-muenchen.de

© Springer Nature Switzerland AG 2019

A. Ferreira Zandona, C. Longbottom (eds.), *Detection and Assessment of Dental Caries*, https://doi.org/10.1007/978-3-030-16967-1_15

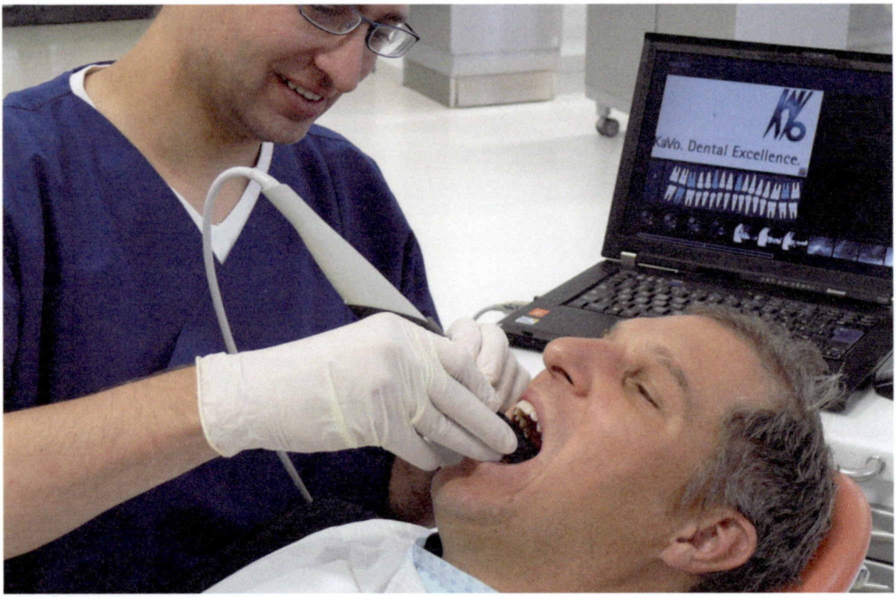

Fig. 15.1 The clinical set-up comprises of a camera system including a near-infrared light source, a USB connected intraoral camera and a computer equipped with specially developed capturing software

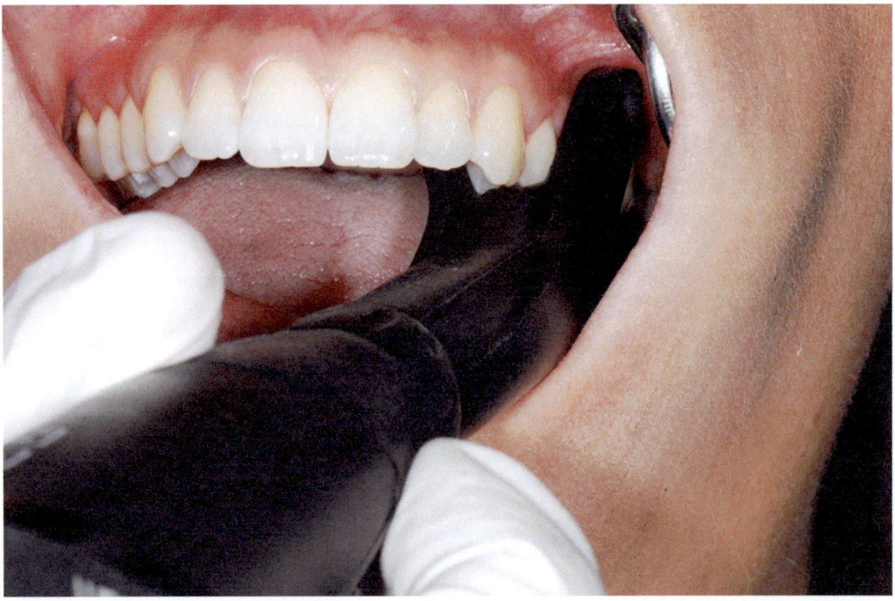

Fig. 15.2 Intraoral positioning of the NILT-based intraoral camera. The hand piece with the elastic arms has to be placed over the posterior teeth and alveolar margin

Caries lesions can be seen easily, as the optical properties of demineralized dental tissue differ distinctively from those of the surrounding sound hard tissue when longwave light is applied. The altered structure of demineralized enamel with larger numbers of pores and interprismatic water content causes an increase in light scattering and absorption in these tissues and therefore appears less transparent. Dentin caries lesions can be detected if the demineralization reaches the dentin–enamel junction (DEJ) or if, in addition, dentin appears less translucent. However, sound enamel is highly transparent in the near-infrared range [11–17].

15.2 Validation and Reproducibility Studies

Meanwhile, this novel diagnostic device was validated under in vivo conditions that aimed to estimate the diagnostic accuracy of the NILT camera for dentin caries detection on interproximal surfaces in comparison to the validated caries depth [18]. As a result, the registered sensitivity (99%) and Az values (0.992) indicated excellent accuracy, which was found to be comparable to digital bitewing radiography (SE: 96%; Az value: 0.984). It should be noted that it was not justifiable due to ethical reasons to validate any enamel caries lesions due to the availability of non-invasive, preventive dental treatment strategies at such sites. Importantly, none of the included sites were free of dentin caries or extended into the enamel only. This explains why no specificity values could be calculated. In another trial, 12 dentists evaluated the reproducibility based on 100 NILT and bitewing images. When considering all diagnostic ratings, the inter- and intra-examiner reliability showed good to excellent weighted Kappa values for NILT (Inter: wK = 0.86 for first round of examination/0.82 for second round of examination; Intra: wK = 0.84) and digital bitewing radiography (Inter: wK = 0.74/0.76; Intra: wK = 0.77). Based on these unpublished data, we concluded that NILT and bitewings showed a similar degree of diagnostic reliability. The findings from both studies strongly encourage the clinical usage of NILT for proximal caries detection.

15.3 Clinical Technique

Following the clinical principles in caries diagnostics, the use of additional methods, including NILT, must be justified on basis of the results from the visual examination, which should be understood as the first-choice method in dental practice due to its simplicity and lower cost. Here, the criteria of the International Caries Detection and Assessment System (ICDAS) (see Chap. 6) or the Universal Visual Scoring System for Caries Detection and Diagnosis (UniViSS) represent recommendable criteria [19–21]. In general, it should be recognized that first visual examination as well as photo-optical diagnostic caries detection and assessment methods require a professional tooth cleaning to eliminate potential confounders, e.g., calculus, plaque or staining (see Chap. 2). Second, teeth should be dried with compressed air before examination to remove any saliva and wetness. When considering possible indications for the prescription of additional diagnostic methods, clinically detectable (active) non-cavitated caries lesions on smooth, proximal or occlusal sites need to be counterchecked with respect to the potential of being more extensive than believed. Furthermore, the presence of non-cavitated caries lesions signals an increased caries risk, which indicates a detailed initial and periodical full-mouth evaluation.

The clinical usage of the NILT method follows some simple rules (Figs. 15.1 and 15.2). Practically, it has been recommended to switch off the light source of the dental unit while the images are being taken to prevent any light interference. In addition to cleanliness and dryness, the camera must be centered over an area of interest parallel to the occlusal plane and the dental arch. To focus the region of interest as precisely as possible, it is necessary to adjust the vertical positions—in other words, the focus-object distance. The optimal position of the intraoral camera could be verified using the live view mode on the computer screen. A full-mouth screening on posterior teeth can be performed by the dentist within 1 or 2 min. In addition, we observed a high level of acceptance of the NILT camera by patients, which may have resulted from the absence of ionizing radiation and the relatively pleasant examination. After each application, the removable tip must be sterilized. All the other surfaces of the device must be wiped with a cloth and an approved disinfectant for disinfection in accordance with the manufacturer's instructions.

Following the digital capture of relevant images, all findings must be analyzed and evaluated. Based on our clinical and scientific experience [10, 18] two sets of caries assessment criteria were used for caries detection and assessment on proximal and occlusal sites, respectively (Figs. 15.3 and 15.4). With respect to the clinical experience, it should be highlighted that the strength of the method must be seen in the early detection of enamel lesions on proximal sites, which are frequently not detectable on bitewing radiographs. Furthermore, it is possible to describe the extension of the lesion much more precisely in relation to the DEJ. It seems to be particularly important to evaluate the configuration of enamel lesions carefully to be able to draw conclusions about the dentin involvement. Early proximal caries lesions on the outer dentin cannot always be visualized, as the optical characteristics of such lesions differ only slightly from those of healthy dentin (Fig. 15.3). However, early dentin caries can be detected based on indirect markers. The leading indicator seems to be the involvement of the DEJ, which is frequently associated with the rectangular configuration of the demineralization in enamel. If the extent of the caries reached deeper parts in dentin, then the translucency of dentin might be reduced, leading to the visibility of the lesion as a dark shadow on NILT images (Fig. 15.3). The NILT method is also able to record occlusal caries lesions (Fig. 15.4). Significant markers of occlusal caries involve possible discoloration in pits and fissures and/or a reduced transillumination as a sign of undermined dentin.

Proximal surface	NILT image	Probable diagnostic / treatment needs
Sound surface No signs of demineralization in enamel	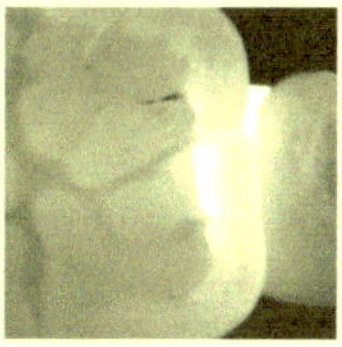	**No active dental care** - Daily self-management/biofilm removal - Monitoring
Enamel caries First visible signs of a demineralization in enamel	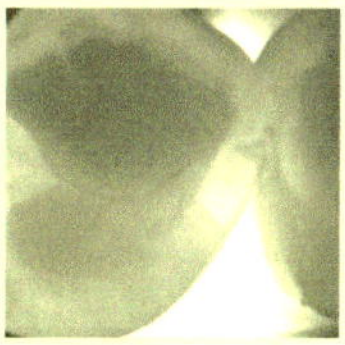	**Preventive dental care** - Daily self-management/biofilm removal - Regular diagnostic check-ups & professional fluoride application
Enamel caries Established demineralization in enamel	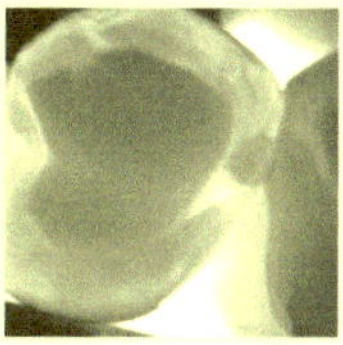	**Preventive or minimal invasive dental care** - Daily self-management/biofilm removal - Fluoridation or caries infiltration - Regular diagnostic check-ups & professional fluoride application
Enamel/dentin caries Established demineralization reaching the enamel-dentin junction	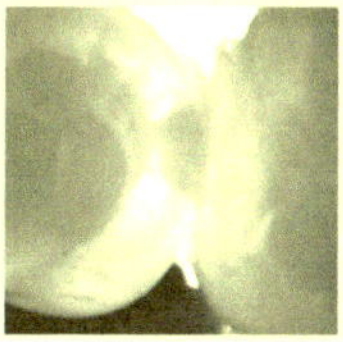	**Minimal invasive dental care** - Daily self-management/biofilm removal - Caries infiltration - Regular diagnostic check-ups & professional fluoridation
Dentin caries Established demineralization penetrating the enamel-dentin junction	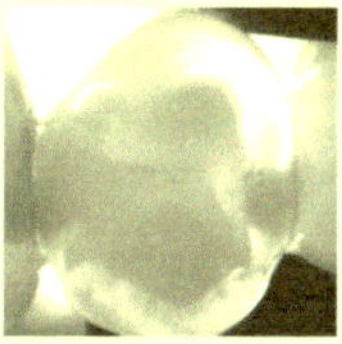	**Minimal invasive or operative dental care** - Daily self-management/biofilm removal - Bitewing radiography to determine lesion progression into dentin - Caries infiltration or restoration - Regular diagnostic check-ups & professional fluoridation
Dentin caries Established demineralization penetrating the enamel-dentin junction with presence of less translucent dentin or cavity	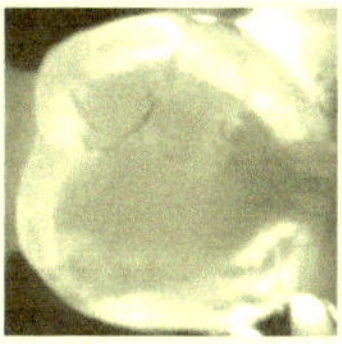	**Operative dental care** - Daily self-management/biofilm removal - Bitewing radiography to determine lesion progression into dentin - Restoration - Regular diagnostic check-ups & professional fluoridation

Fig. 15.3 Categorization of diagnostic findings and related treatment needs on proximal surfaces for near-infrared light transillumination (NILT)

The criteria shown in Figs. 15.3 and 15.4 should further help to link different lesion stages with probable treatment strategies (Table 15.1). If non-cavitated caries lesions were diagnosed, primarily preventative care should be recommended; these measures include optimal fluoride supplementation at home and during recall appointments, advice on tooth-friendly diets and guidance on optimal oral hygiene. In cases

Occlusal surfaces/Fissures	NILT image	Probable diagnostic/treatment needs
Sound surface No signs of demineralization	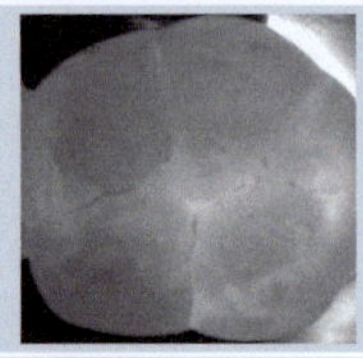	**No active dental care** - Daily self-management/biofilm removal - Monitoring
Enamel caries First or established demineralization restricted to enamel without any less translucent dentin	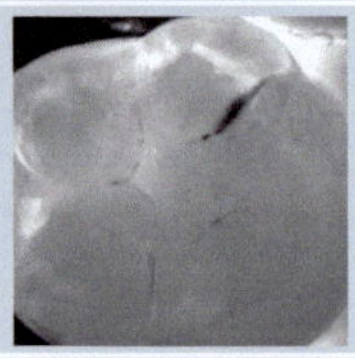	**Preventive dental care** - Daily self-management/biofilm removal - Fissure sealing or fluoridation - Regular diagnostic check-ups & professional fluoridation
Dentin caries Presence of less translucent dentin or cavity	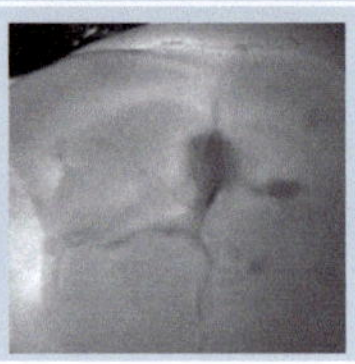	**Operative dental care** - Daily self-management/biofilm removal - Bitewing radiography to determine lesion progression into dentin - Restroration - Regular diagnostic check-ups & professional fluoridation

Fig. 15.4 Categorization of diagnostic findings and related treatment needs on occlusal surfaces for near-infrared light transillumination (NILT)

involving non-cavitated enamel caries lesions and those with minimal penetration of the DEJ into the outer dentin, the patient should be offered the option of resin infiltration. Clearly detectable dentin caries lesions must be treated operatively.

In addition, it is sometimes possible to detect caries lesions close to restoration margins (secondary caries). Otherwise, it is unable to diagnose residual caries left during caries excavation, which is located under the restoration. The same can be concluded for smooth surface caries, but in these clinical situations, diagnosis and assessment can be made easily by visual means. Interestingly, it was also feasible to diagnose cracks in several cases.

15.4 Concluding Remarks

Based on the given experiences, it can be concluded that novel NILT can complement visual examination as a second-choice method due to its diagnostic performance, especially for enamel caries detection, X-ray absence and clinical practicability. Bitewing radiographs should be prescribed in clinical situations where cavities or dentin caries lesions are diagnosed visually or by NILT. This diagnostic strategy will help to reduce possible risks of ionizing radiation, to prescribe diagnostic procedures on an individual basis and to meet all requirements to provide optimal preventive and operative dental care.

Table 15.1 Characterization of the near-infrared light transillumination (NILT) for caries detection and assessment

Bitewing radiography	Near-infrared light transillumination (NILT)			
Which surfaces/ sites is it useful for	Occlusal (pits and fissures)	Proximal/ (approximal)	Smooth surface (buccal and lingual)	Root caries
	Y	**Y**	**N**	**N**
What type of lesions is valuable for	Primary coronal	Secondary coronal	Primary root caries	Secondary root caries
	Y	**Y, with restrictions**	**N**	**N**
What type of dentition	Primary		Permanent	
	Y		**Y**	
Lesion severity	Enamel lesions		Dentinal lesions	
	Y		**Y**	
Sensitivity	99% for dentin caries detection on proximal surfaces under in vivo conditions [18]			
Specificity	No data available so far			
Perceived Ease Of Use (PEOU)	1. NILT is easy-to-use 2. It is easy to become skillful at using NILT 3. Learning to operate NILT is easy 4. NILT has to be applied exactly over the teeth—comparable to an intraoral camera 5. My interaction with NILT is clear and understandable 6. It is easy to interact with NILT			
Advantages/ disadvantages	*Advantages* 1. X-ray-free diagnostic method 2. Unlimited repeatability 3. Possible usage in uncooperative children and patients with special needs who normally dislike bitewing radiographs 4. Early detection of enamel caries 5. Detection of cracks *Disadvantages* 1. No possibility of imaging the caries extension in relation to the pulp			
Time	– Full-mouth screening: <1 min – Full-mouth screening and capturing of relevant images: approx. 2–3 min – Full-mouth screening and capturing of all images from all sites/ surfaces: approx. 5–8 min			
Cost	Catalog price US$ 6108/ € 5049			

References

1. Hopcraft MS, Morgan MV. Comparison of radiographic and clinical diagnosis of approximal and occlusal dental caries in a young adult population. Community Dent Oral Epidemiol. 2005;33:212–8.
2. Poorterman JH, Aartman IH, Kieft JA, Kalsbeek H. Value of bite-wing radiographs in a clinical epidemiological study and their effect on the DMFS index. Caries Res. 2000;34: 159–63.

3. Poorterman JH, Aartman IH, Kalsbeek H. Underestimation of the prevalence of approximal caries and inadequate restorations in a clinical epidemiological study. Community Dent Oral Epidemiol. 1999;27:331–7.
4. Mejàre I, Källest l C, Stenlund H. Incidence and progression of approximal caries from 11 to 22 years of age in Sweden: a prospective radiographic study. Caries Res. 1999;33:93–100.
5. Mejàre I, Källestål C, Stenlund H, Johansson H. Caries development from 11 to 22 years of age: a prospective radiographic study. Prevalence and distribution. Caries Res. 1998;32:10–6.
6. Kidd EA, Pitts NB. A reappraisal of the value of the bitewing radiograph in the diagnosis of posterior approximal caries. Br Dent J. 1990;169:195–200.
7. American Dental Association, Council on Scientific Affairs and U.S. Food and Drug Administration. Dental radiographic examinations: recommendations for patient selection and limiting radiation exposure. 2012. http://www.ada.org/en/member-center/oral-health-topics/x-rays. Accessed 15 May 2017.
8. European Commission. Radiation protection 136. European guidelines on radiation protection in dental radiology. The safe use of radiographs in dental practice. Luxembourg: Office for Official Publications of the European Communities; 2004.
9. Espelid I, Mejare I, Weerheijm K. EAPD guidelines for use of radiographs in children. Eur J Paediatr Dent. 2003;4:40–8.
10. Söchtig F, Hickel R, Kühnisch J. Caries detection and diagnostics with near-infrared light transillumination: clinical experiences. Quintessence Int. 2014;45:531–8.
11. Schneiderman A, Elbaum M, Shultz T, Keem S, Greenebaum M, Driller J. Assessment of dental caries with Digital Imaging Fiber-Optic Transillumination (DIFOTI): in vitro study. Caries Res. 1997;31:103–10.
12. Chung S, Fried D, Staninec M, Darling CL. Near infrared imaging of teeth at wavelengths between 1200 and 1600 nm. Proc SPIE Int Soc Photo Opt Eng. 2011;7884:78840X.
13. Staninec M, Lee C, Darling CL, Fried D. In vivo near-IR imaging of approximal dental decay at 1.310 nm. Lasers Surg Med. 2010;42:292–8.
14. Jones GC, Jones RS, Fried D. Transillumination of interproximal caries lesions with 830-nm light. Proc SPIE 5313, Lasers in Dentistry X. 2004;17.
15. Jones R, Huynh G, Jones G, Fried D. Near-infrared transillumination at 1310-nm for the imaging of early dental decay. Opt Express. 2003;11:2259–65.
16. Fried D, Glena RE, Featherstone JD, Seka W. Nature of light scattering in dental enamel and dentin at visible and near-infrared wavelengths. Appl Opt. 1995;34:1278–85.
17. Hall A, Girkin JM. A review of potential new diagnostic modalities for caries lesions. J Dent Res. 2004;83(Spec Issue No C):C89–94.
18. Kühnisch J, Söchtig F, Pitchika V, Laubender R, Neuhaus KW, Lussi A, Hickel R. In vivo validation of near-infrared light transillumination for interproximal dentin caries detection. Clin Oral Investig. 2016;20:821–9.
19. Pitts NB. Detection, assessment, diagnosis and monitoring of caries. Monographs in oral science, vol. 21. Basel: Karger; 2009.
20. Kühnisch J, Bücher K, Henschel V, Albrecht A, Garcia-Godoy F, Mansmann U, Hickel R, Heinrich-Weltzien R. Diagnostic performance of the universal visual scoring system (UniViSS) on occlusal surfaces. Clin Oral Investig. 2011;15:215–23.
21. Kühnisch J, Goddon I, Berger S, Senkel H, Bücher K, Oehme T, Hickel R, Heinrich-Weltzien R. Development, methodology and potential of the new universal visual scoring system (UniViSS) for caries detection and diagnosis. Int J Environ Res Public Health. 2009;6:2500–9.

Quantitative Light-Induced Fluorescence 16

Baek-Il Kim

16.1 Introduction

Quantitative light-induced fluorescence (QLF) is a representative optical technology for early detection and quantification of dental caries as the first introduced technology in clinical dentistry.

It has been developed continuously over the past 30 years and is now available for application in dental fields according to the main purpose of use. The QLF technology can measure both the mineral content as a fluorescence loss and bacterial activity as a red fluorescence simultaneously. The fluorescence changes detected by QLF can be visualized as an image, which enables to nondestructively quantify the physical characteristics of caries lesions and monitor its changes as numerical values. Based on these properties, this method enables to give evidence for providing preventive care. In this chapter, an overview of the QLF technology is provided regarding the principle of QLF, its history, and its clinical technique for detecting dental plaque and various types of dental caries.

16.2 Background

16.2.1 Principles and History of QLF

Teeth are hard tissues composed of multiple layers comprising various mineral contents. Dental caries is a disease in which the mineral content of teeth is chemically dissolved by acids produced by oral microorganisms as final metabolites in these hard tissues. The first subtle changes occur in the surface layer of the enamel, which

B.-II. Kim (✉)
Department of Preventive Dentistry and Public Oral Health, Yonsei University College of Dentistry, Seoul, Republic of Korea
e-mail: drkbi@yuhs.ac

© Springer Nature Switzerland AG 2019

A. Ferreira Zandona, C. Longbottom (eds.), *Detection and Assessment of Dental Caries*, https://doi.org/10.1007/978-3-030-16967-1_16

are followed by the formation of a cavity that breaks the continuity of the surface layer. In conventional dentistry these changes are detected using visual, tactile, and radiological examinations (as discussed in Chaps. 3, 5–7, 11, and 12), but these methods show low sensitivities of 20–30% in detecting minute changes in early caries. There have been many attempts to overcome the limitations associated with the detecting microscale changes in teeth based on applying various technologies such as light (see Chaps. 14 and 15), electric conductivity, and ultrasonic waves (see Chap. 21) [1]. The various caries detection technologies that have been developed to date are mainly based on two measurement principles: (1) measuring changes in the mineral content of teeth, comprising techniques for measuring the electrical resistance of teeth and optical instruments using light scattering phenomena such as the DIFOTI device (see Chap. 14), and (2) assessing bacterial activity, which includes the DIAGNOdent device (see Chap. 17) that detects metabolites of bacteria such as porphyrin. The quantitative light-induced fluorescence (QLF) technology can measure both the mineral content and also the bacterial activity simultaneously. Most of the light-based devices developed so far evaluate the subtle changes in tooth structure using light at a specific wavelength. The theoretical basis of QLF was provided by Bjelkhagen and Sundstrom et al. reporting the ability to clearly distinguish between an initial caries lesion and sound teeth by assessing fluorescence loss under irradiation with blue laser light with a wavelength of 488 nm [2].

The principles underlying the use of QLF to optically detect early caries lesions are as follows: visible blue light irradiating the teeth and reaching the dentinoenamel junction (DEJ) will induce fluorescence that acts like a lamp inside the tooth after passing through the enamel, and this fluorescence is amplified by fluorophores within the DEJ. This mechanism results in light scattering inside a white spot being 5–10 times higher than that in normal enamel when using QLF. The lesion appears darker than sound enamel tissue due to light scattering of the generated fluorescence, which allows such lesions to be seen by the naked eye [3]. The fluorescence loss detected by QLF can be visualized as an image, and from such images it is possible to nondestructively quantify the physical characteristics of caries lesions as numerical values in image analysis, which is a unique strength of QLF. One of the key quantitative parameters from a QLF system is delta F (ΔF), which represents the lesion depth and is calculated by comparing the fluorescence properties between a caries lesion and sound tooth. Previous studies have found that ΔF is strongly correlated with lesion depths as obtained using transverse microradiography (TMR) ($r = 0.88$), which is widely used as the gold standard for measuring lesion depth in vitro [4]. In addition, dedicated software (QA2) yields other parameters such as lesion size (area in mm^2) and lesion volume (ΔQ in $mm^2\%$). Furthermore, the intensity of red fluorescence that reflects bacterial activity can be calculated by delta R (ΔR, in %).

16.2.2 QLF Devices

The Inspektor Pro, which was introduced in 2004, is a first-generation QLF device that includes an intraoral camera attached to a special filter (Table 16.1). This device can provide two functions: (1) detecting changes in mineral contents using fluorescence differences between initial caries lesions and sound enamel, and (2) detecting the bacterial

Table 16.1 Characteristics of various QLF devices

	Inspektor™	QLF-D Biluminator™	Qraycam™	Qraypen™	Qrayview™	Qscan™
Generation	1st	2nd	3rd			
Release date	2004	2012	2014	2015	2012	2014
Light source	Halogen lamp	Dual color LEDs	Dual color LEDs	Dual color LEDs	Dual peak LEDs (405 and 460 nm) and LCUs (light curing units)	Single color LEDs
Filters	Single long high pass yellow filter (>520 nm)	Inspektor filter	Integrated glass Inspektor filter	Integrated glass Inspektor filter	A goggle with integrated Inspektor filter	Integrated Inspektor filter
Type of device	Intra-oral camera	DSLR (digital single lens reflex) camera	Handy camcorder	Intra-oral camera	Light pen and filter goggle	Handy homecare device
Range of capturing	Individual tooth (individual element surfaces)	From partial to whole oral cavity	From partial to whole oral cavity	From individual tooth to whole oral cavity	–	–
Zoom and focus	Fixed focus	Manual focus	Manual zoom and focus	Auto-adjust focus	Not available	Not available
Portability	Poor	Fair	Good	Good	Excellent	Excellent
Main purpose	Research	Research	Clinical practice	Clinical practice	Clinical practice	Education and home-use
Upgraded version (release date)	–	–	–		Qrayview Dual™ (2017)	Qscan Plus™ (2017)
Product image	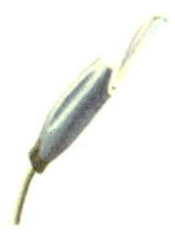	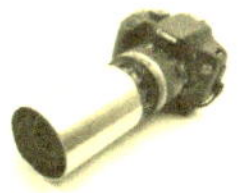	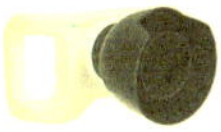	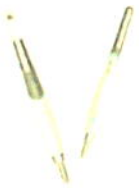	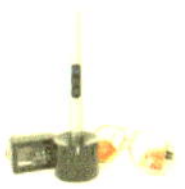	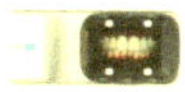

activity from the porphyrin reaction of oral bacteria. In detail, blue visible light with a wavelength of 405 nm induces fluorescence within the tooth structure. The emitted fluorescence is filtered by a single high-pass filter, and the resulting images captured by a micro-CCD camera in the Inspektor Pro are used to produce a QLF image.

A second-generation QLF device was introduced in 2012 and later upgraded to the digital Biluminator 2+ QLF device (QLF-D), which consisted of a special light source (Biluminator) and filters mounted on a DSLR (digital single lens reflex) camera with a 60-mm macro lens (Table 16.1). This advanced device was able to analyze the entire oral cavity extraorally. Compared with the first-generation QLF device with an Inspektor filter, the filter set of QLF-D comprised a high-pass filter (>480 nm) and a pink-color filter. The Inspektor filter enhanced the red fluorescence caused by bacterial metabolites and allowed it to be detected more clearly than with the first-generation device.

After the release of QLF-D, third-generation QLF, Qray devices were developed in 2012, whose design provides superior clinical capabilities. Qray devices can be divided into those containing a built-in camera (i.e., Qraycam and Qraypen) and those without a camera function that are only for real-time visual inspections (i.e., Qrayview and Qscan, Table 16.1). The consumer-friendly Qscan device was developed to provide patients and consumers with an easy-to-use device for self-checking their dental plaque at home without the use of disclosing agents. This device was regarded as a useful tool for providing oral health education to the general public.

A recent study found no difference in the ΔF values (representing the mineral content in teeth) measured using the different generations of QLF devices. However, the level of red fluorescence reflecting bacterial activity was significantly higher in the second- and third-generation QLF devices than in the first-generation device, which is due to the more recent devices focusing on the red fluorescence. It is considered that dental practitioners can use these devices to simultaneously improve both the reliability of image interpretations and their communication with patients.

16.3 Clinical Techniques

16.3.1 Dental Plaque

Dental plaque is a biofilm that is the main cause of dental caries, and it consists of bacteria colonies that have not been removed from the tooth surface. The biofilm attached to the tooth surface gradually enlarges due to bacterial growth, resulting in more complex types of bacteria colonies being present simultaneously, with the number of pathogenic bacteria also increasing [5]. During the growth phase of the dental biofilm, secondary colonizer bacteria produce a unique bacterial metabolite called porphyrin. These porphyrin-containing biofilms manifest as red fluorescence, and the fluorescence intensity is significantly correlated with various variables related to dental caries [6]. The red fluorescent biofilm detected using QLF is a mature plaque existing on the tooth surface that has been present for at least 3 days [7], and it is very similar to the mature, thick plaque that is stained blue by standard two-tone disclosure solution [8, 9]. A previous study showed a significant correlation between visual evaluation indices (the Turesky modified Quigley-Hein plaque index and the Silness & Löe plaque index) and the QLF index, confirming the possibility of quantitative plaque assessment using the red fluorescence index as calculated from QLF images [10].

It is vital for orthodontic patients to manage their oral hygiene when they are wearing complicated orthodontic appliances. Miller et al. reported that a repeated oral hygiene training program that included showing QLF images to orthodontic patients at 6-week intervals significantly improved their oral hygiene management ability (Fig. 16.1) [11]. It is expected that plaque assessments using QLF technology is an effective alternative to conventional plaque staining method because it can considerably reduce both patient discomfort and the time required for visual observations based on a staining process.

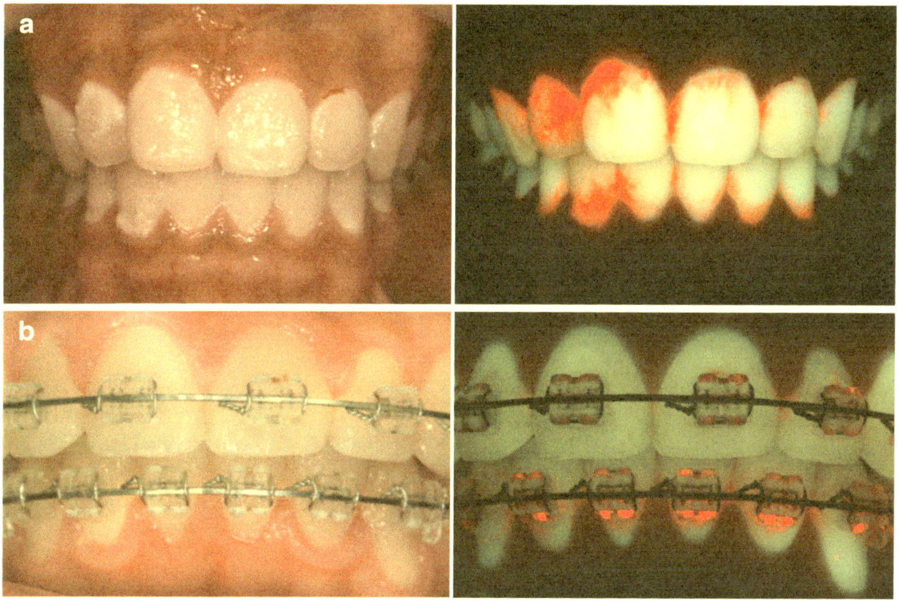

Fig. 16.1 QLF images (white-light and fluorescence images) of normal (**a**) and orthodontic (**b**) patients obtained using the Qraycam device

16.3.2 Occlusal Caries

Occlusal tooth surfaces having irregular structures such as pits and fissures are vulnerable to dental caries due to the niches where biofilm can accumualte undisturbed, which results in an eighfold higher risk of caries on occlusal surfaces compared to smooth surfaces. In the case of initial occlusal caries, the dentist must mainly rely on visual examinations because it is difficult to detect caries lesions using radiography (see Chaps. 11 and 12). The criteria of the International Caries Detection and Assessment System (ICDAS) (see Chap. 6) are commonly used for visual examinations aimed at distinguishing caries lesions. However, ICDAS exhibits a poor performance for teeth categorized as code 1 or 2. This limitation could be overcome by combining QLF with visual inspection to increase the sensitivity and specificity of diagnoses (Fig. 16.2) [12].

QLF uses quantitative parameters such as ΔF and ΔQ to describe small changes in the mineral content of the occlusal surface, and these values can be used to support decision-making regarding treatments for occlusal caries. Alammari et al. found that ΔF and ΔQ at baseline (i.e., before restorative treatment) differed significantly between groups treated with sealant and resin, and suggested that quantitative QLF values could be utilized when making decisions regarding occlusal restorative treatment [13].

It is relatively easy to detect the red fluorescence emitted from a biofilm when using second- and third-generation QLF devices. If an occlusal surface still exhibits red fluorescence after performing oral prophylaxis, it can be concluded that biofilm remains on

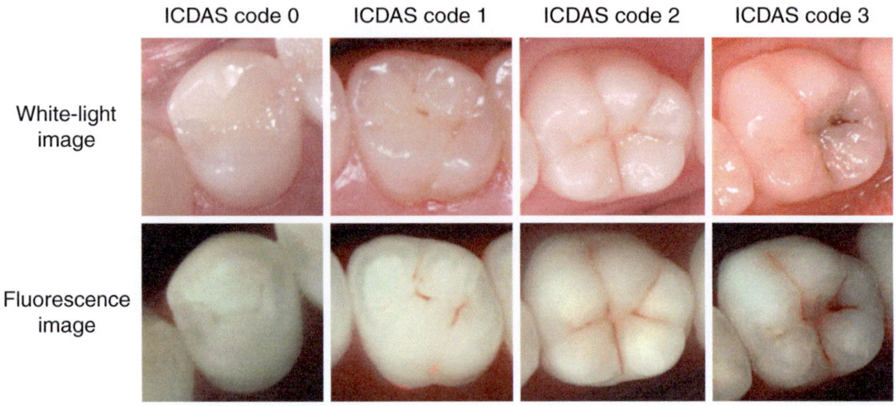

Fig. 16.2 QLF images (white-light and fluorescence images) of occlusal caries lesions according with different ICDAS codes obtained using the QLF-D device

the tooth and hence that caries progression is possible. In the case of stains in pits and fissures on occlusal surfaces, noncariogenic discoloration can be caused by staining by materials such as coffee, foods, and cigarettes, which will appear dark black in QLF-D. On the other hand, cariogenic discoloration involving bacteria appears as red fluorescence around stains, which can facilitate clinical decision-making.

16.3.3 Proximal Caries

Bitewing radiography (see Chaps. 11 and 12) has traditionally been used as the gold standard for detecting proximal caries. However, bitewing radiography shows maximum sensitivities of 50% and 40% for proximal and early proximal caries, respectively [1]. In addition, the need to develop nonradiographic imaging techniques has increased recently due to reports of risks associated with frequent radiography exposure [14]. QLF technology can be used to evaluate both mineral content and bacterial activity in the detection of proximal caries [15]. Pretty et al. reported that a first-generation QLF device could longitudinally monitor early caries lesion on the proximal surface of a deciduous tooth by using the ΔF parameter, which reflects changes in mineral contents [16]. Ko et al. reported that QLF-D could detect proximal caries lesions on the enamel and dentin surfaces with sensitivities of 71% and 64%, respectively, and specificities of 84% and 88% (Fig. 16.3) [17].

The clinical application of second- and third-generation QLF devices can identify the presence of proximal caries lesions based on red fluorescence, since this is an indirect indicator of bacterial activity. If an extraoral camera-type second- or third-generation QLF device is used with an occlusal mirror, it is possible to obtain occlusal fluorescent images of the entire arch. This makes it possible to rapidly screen the entire mouth and thereby dramatically reduce the image-taking time compared to using an intraoral camera.

A new QLF scoring scheme using ΔF and ΔR calculated from the images captured by a second-generation QLF device showed a moderate correlation ($r = 0.537$,

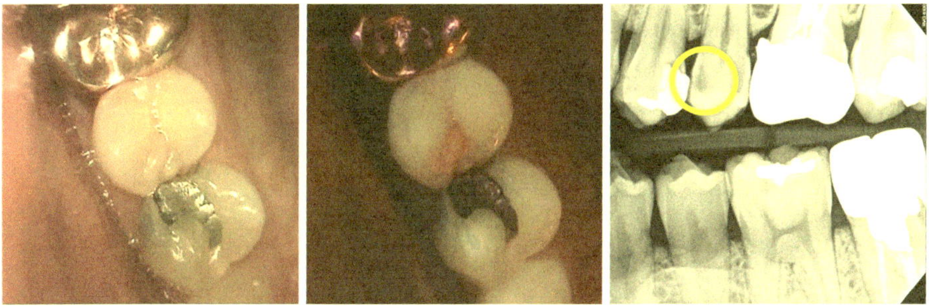

Fig. 16.3 QLF images (white-light and fluorescence images) of proximal caries obtained using the Qraypen device, and a bitewing X-ray

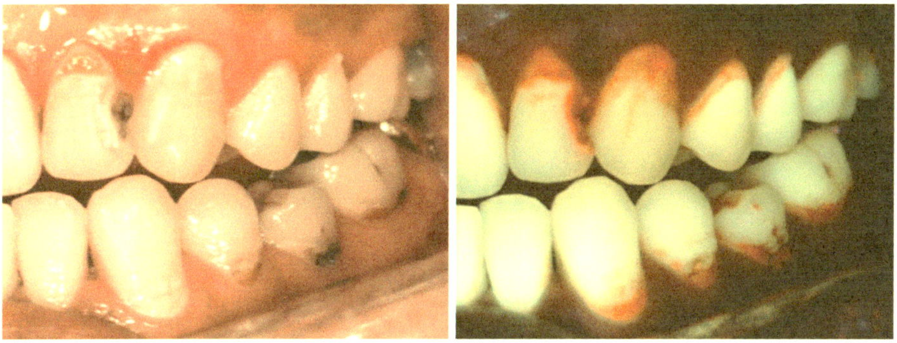

Fig. 16.4 QLF images (white-light and fluorescence images) of smooth-surface caries obtained using the Qraycam device

$P < 0.001$) and a high area under the receiver operating characteristics (AUROC) curve of over 0.8 compared to the radiographic score [18]. If a lesion is present below the contact point of the proximal surface, it is difficult to observe the changes in fluorescence when the tooth is irradiated by light on the occlusal surface. This makes it necessary to observe not only the occlusal surface but also the buccal and lingual surfaces when attempting to detect proximal caries using QLF devices [17].

16.3.4 Smooth-Surface Caries

Smooth-surface caries can exist around dental plaque that has accumulated in the gingival margin of the buccal and lingual surfaces. Because a smooth surface is easy to observe directly by the naked eye, visual inspections have been mainly used for detecting these kinds of lesions. A 4-year follow-up study found that AUROC was higher for a first-generation QLF device (0.82–0.87) than for ICDAS (0.65–0.80) [19]. A new index developed by combining QLF technology with ICDAS, called QLF-I, showed higher reliability than when using ICDAS alone, with kappa indexes of 0.79 and 0.70, respectively. In particular, this method was better for detecting white spots at stages according to ICDAS codes 1 and 2 (Fig. 16.4) [12].

It has been difficult to predict the level of remineralization obtained after applying fluoride treatment. However, evaluating the lesion severity with the Δ*F* parameter using QLF before fluoride treatment makes it possible to predict the severity of a lesion recovered by the topical application of fluoride. Kim and Kim reported that at least 50% of lesions were recovered when applying fluoride treatment to lesions with a Δ*F* of –14.6 or less [20].

QLF shows various red fluorescence intensities for different smooth-surface lesions. The difference in the level of red intensity could be a useful indicator of the severity of caries activity. Felix et al. reported a strong relationship between the red-to-orange fluorescence intensity of a lesion and the level of caries progression when evaluating the red fluorescence intensity of caries lesions with Δ*R*, followed by a first-generation QLF device for 4 years in children [14]. Because the second- and third-generation QLF devices were equipped with a dual filter that can capture red fluorescence with a higher sensitivity, the caries activity can be seen more clearly compared to when using first-generation QLF devices [21]. A recent study using a second-generation QLF device found that the level of red fluorescence was much higher for active lesions than for inactive lesions as classified by the Nyvad criteria (for the Nyvad criteria see Chap. 5) [22]. When detecting smooth-surface caries using QLF, the residual mature plaque on the surface might act as a confounding factor when assessing the red fluorescence of a lesion, which makes it necessary to remove any remaining plaque on the tooth surface by performing a tooth-cleaning procedure before such evaluations.

16.3.5 Root Caries

Root caries are caused by dental biofilm covering the exposed root surface. The prevalence of root caries has been increasing rapidly due to the increasing elderly retaining teeth longer. Although root caries occur in dentin containing a lower mineral content than enamel, they can be easily detected by utilizing QLF. A previous in vitro study investigating the detection of root caries found that the QLF (as quantified by Δ*Q*) was strongly correlated with TMR findings after demineralization ($r = 0.89$) and remineralization ($r = 0.84$) [23]. An in vivo study using a first-generation QLF device showed that the Δ*Q* value for noncavitated root caries lesions increased significantly after applying a fluoride varnish repeatedly over a 4-week period [24].

Figure 16.5 shows the sound root surfaces of maxillary anterior teeth with a bright color and the root caries lesions of mandibular anterior teeth with strong red fluorescence. Plaque or calculus remaining on the root surface might be a confounding factor when evaluating root caries lesions using QLF technology. It is therefore recommended to perform scaling and root planning to remove any plaque and calculus remaining on the root surface prior to evaluating root caries lesions.

16.3.6 Secondary Caries

Secondary caries can form from microleakages along the tooth–restoration interface. It is important to understand differences in the optical properties of various types of restorations when evaluating secondary caries using QLF, because the optical responses when applying this technology vary with the type of restoration. Metal

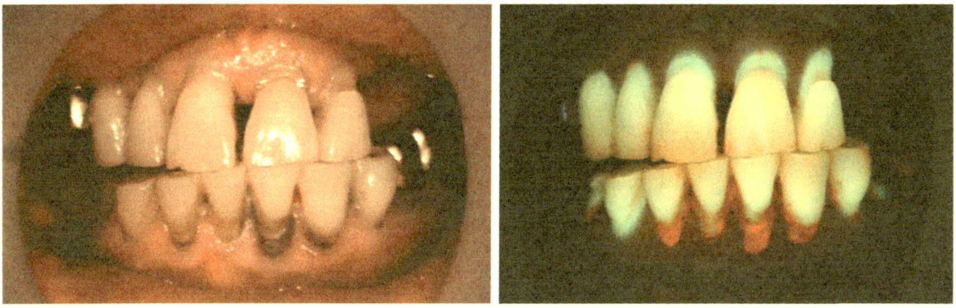

Fig. 16.5 QLF images (white-light and fluorescence images) showing sound root surfaces of maxillary anterior teeth and root caries lesions of mandibular anterior teeth obtained using the Qraycam device

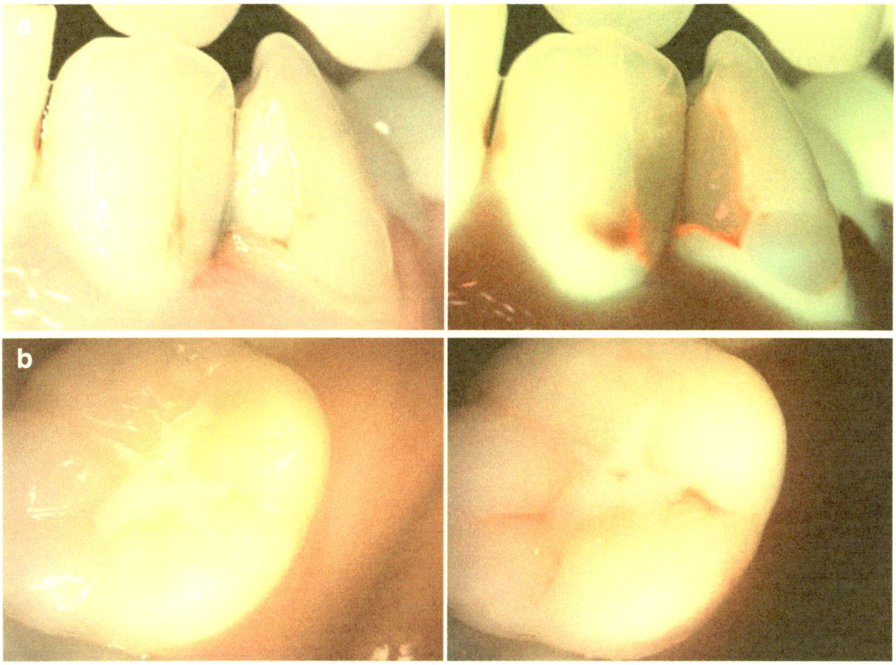

Fig. 16.6 QLF images (white-light and fluorescence images) of secondary caries around resin restorations (**a**) and marginal leakage around sealant restorations (**b**) obtained using QLF-D

restorations such as those involving gold and amalgam appear as black shadows since visible light does not penetrate metal restorations and they cannot produce fluorescent light. Meanwhile, the fluorescence characteristics of various composite resin restorations may be classified into bright and dark, with this difference originating from the different chemical compositions of the resins [25]. Figure 16.6 shows a difference in fluorescence values between two resins from two different sites: one is a cervical site and the other is a proximal site of a mandibular canine.

A previous study investigating secondary caries adjacent to amalgam restorations using several optical devices and visual inspection methods found that QLF technology had the highest sensitivity in detecting secondary caries lesions [26]. A recent study found that QLF technology showed a higher sensitivity in detecting secondary caries around resin components and amalgam than ICDAS and other techniques [27]. Second- and third-generation QLF devices show greater sensitively in detecting red fluorescence, making this easier to detect at the margins of a restoration, which is where secondary caries form the most frequently. In particular, secondary caries around composite resin restorations are much easier to detect based on red fluorescence from marginal leakage due to differences in the fluorescence intensity between sound enamel and composite resin. The physical weakness of filler-free resin sealant makes it important to detect initial leakages and defects of the sealant when attempting to prevent secondary caries. Fontana et al. reported that QLF technology can be used to confirm the occurrence of sealant failure and can be useful for decisions regarding sealant repair [28]. Therefore, second- and third-generation QLF devices can be a useful tool for determining whether or not restorations need to be repaired based on evaluating increases and decreases in red fluorescence around them.

When evaluating secondary caries using QLF for in the clinical setting, it is necessary to perform oral prophylaxis for removing dental plaque around restorations prior to examinations. Variations in the characteristics of the fluorescence such as its color and intensity with the type of restoration materials also need to be considered.

Other devices are available for caries detection based on fluorescence. CamX Spectra Caries Detection Aid (Air Techniques) uses light at the 405 nm wavelength. The software used automatically analyze the images displaying a numerical indicator between 0 and 5 indicating the extent of the lesion, 0 being sound tooth structure and 5 deep dentin caries. SOPROLIFE Caries Detector and Intraoral camera (ACTEON) uses light at 450-nm wavelength and magnification of up to 50×. The software used to collect the images does not analyze the images.

16.4 Concluding Remarks

QLF technology was introduced in 1981 as the first optical evaluation technique in the field of dentistry (after X-rays) for nondestructively evaluating the fluorescence changes in early caries lesions using blue visible light and filters. It has been developed continuously over the past 30 years, and is now available for application in clinical dentistry. The third-generation QLF devices focus on the red fluorescence that reflects bacterial activity, which improves the convenience of image interpretation and ease of communication with patients in the clinical situation. The future implementation of QLF technology on smartphones could enable everyone to check their oral condition in real time and share the results with dental professionals, thereby greatly facilitating their ability to continuously monitor the oral health status of their patients.

Summary table

Bitewing radiography				
Which surfaces/sites is it useful for	Occlusal (pits and fissures)	Proximal (approximal)	Smooth surface (buccal and lingual)	Root caries and which of the four surfaces?
	Y	**Y**	**Y**	**Y**

What type of lesions is valuable for	Primary coronal **Y**	Secondary coronal **Y**	Primary root caries **Y**	Secondary root caries **Y**
What type of dentition	Primary **Y**		Permanent **Y**	
Lesion severity	Enamel lesions **Y**		Dentinal lesions **Y**	
Sensitivity	Literature reported range in 64–94% (minimum-maximum value, it depends on the sites, type of lesion, and lesion severity)			
Specificity	Literature reported range in 84–100% (minimum-maximum value, it depends on the sites, type of lesion, and lesion severity)			
Perceived Ease Of Use (PEOU)[a]	1. "QLF" is easy-to-use 2. It is easy to become skillful at using "QLF" 3. Learning to operate "QLF" is easy 4. "QLF" is flexible to interact with 5. My interaction with "QLF" is clear and understandable 6. It is easy to interact with "QLF"			
Advantages/ disadvantages	*Advantages* 1. Easy-to-use, portable, easy to communicate with patients, time-consuming, quantitative analysis (possible to assess lesion severity and monitor its changes) *Disadvantages* 1. Sensitive to the ambient light, difficult to reposition of intraoral camera type devices for the next image taking			
Time	For all tooth surfaces – 1–2 min (for visual examination and image taking) – Within 5 min (for quantitative analysis using dedicated software)			
Cost	Qscan Plus™: USD 90 Qrayview Dual™: USD 900 Qraypen™: USD 2000 Qraycam Pro™: USD 5000			

[a]Davis (1989)

References

1. Pretty IA. Caries detection and diagnosis: novel technologies. J Dent. 2006;34(10):727–39.
2. Bjelkhagen H, Sundstrom F, Angmar-Mansson B, Ryden H. Early detection of enamel caries by the luminescence excited by visible laser light. Swed Dent J. 1982;6(1):1–7.
3. van der Veen MH, de Josselin de Jong E. Application of quantitative light-induced fluorescence for assessing early caries lesions. Monogr Oral Sci. 2000;17:144–62.
4. Shi XQ, Tranaeus S, Angmar-Mansson B. Comparison of QLF and DIAGNOdent for quantification of smooth surface caries. Caries Res. 2001;35(1):21–6.
5. Kim YS, Kang SM, Lee ES, Lee JH, Kim BR, Kim BI. Ecological changes in oral microcosm biofilm during maturation. J Biomed Opt. 2016;21(10):101409.
6. Lee ES, Kang SM, Ko HY, Kwon HK, Kim BI. Association between the cariogenicity of a dental microcosm biofilm and its red fluorescence detected by Quantitative Light-induced Fluorescence-Digital (QLF-D). J Dent. 2013;41(12):1264–70.
7. Kim YS, Lee ES, Kwon HK, Kim BI. Monitoring the maturation process of a dental microcosm biofilm using the Quantitative Light-induced Fluorescence-Digital (QLF-D). J Dent. 2014;42(6):691–6.
8. Han SY, Kim BR, Ko HY, Kwon HK, Kim BI. Assessing the use of Quantitative Light-induced Fluorescence-Digital as a clinical plaque assessment. Photodiagn Photodyn Ther. 2016;13:34–9.

9. Volgenant CMC, Fernandez YMM, Rosema NAM, van der Weijden FA, Ten Cate JM, van der Veen MH. Comparison of red autofluorescing plaque and disclosed plaque—a cross-sectional study. Clin Oral Investig. 2016;20(9):2551–8.
10. Han SY, Kim BR, Ko HY, Kwon HK, Kim BI. Validity and reliability of autofluorescence-based quantification method of dental plaque. Photodiagn Photodyn Ther. 2015;12(4): 587–91.
11. Miller CC, Burnside G, Higham SM, Flannigan NL. Quantitative Light-induced Fluorescence-Digital as an oral hygiene evaluation tool to assess plaque accumulation and enamel demineralization in orthodontics. Angle Orthod. 2016;86(6):991–7.
12. Ferreira Zandona A, Santiago E, Eckert G, Fontana M, Ando M, Zero DT. Use of ICDAS combined with quantitative light-induced fluorescence as a caries detection method. Caries Res. 2010;44(3):317–22.
13. Alammari MR, Smith PW, de Josselin de Jong E, Higham SM. Quantitative light-induced fluorescence (QLF): a tool for early occlusal dental caries detection and supporting decision making in vivo. J Dent. 2013;41(2):127–32.
14. Felix Gomez G, Eckert GJ, Ferreira Zandona A. Orange/red fluorescence of active caries by retrospective quantitative light-induced fluorescence image analysis. Caries Res. 2016;50(3):295–302.
15. Claus EB, Calvocoressi L, Bondy ML, Schildkraut JM, Wiemels JL, Wrensch M. Dental x-rays and risk of meningioma. Cancer. 2012;118(18):4530–7.
16. Pretty IA, Edgar WM, Higham SM. Detection of in vitro demineralization of primary teeth using quantitative light-induced fluorescence (QLF). Int J Paediatr Dent. 2002;12(3):158–67.
17. Ko HY, Kang SM, Kim HE, Kwon HK, Kim BI. Validation of quantitative light-induced fluorescence-digital (QLF-D) for the detection of approximal caries in vitro. J Dent. 2015;43(5):568–75.
18. Kim ES, Lee ES, Kang SM, Jung EH, de Josselin de Jong E, Jung HI, Kim BI. A new screening method to detect proximal dental caries using fluorescence imaging. Photodiagnosis Photodyn Ther. 2017;20:257–62.
19. Ferreira Zandona A, Ando M, Gomez GF, Garcia-Corretjer M, Eckert GJ, Santiago E, et al. Longitudinal analyses of early lesions by fluorescence: an observational study. J Dent Res. 2013;92(Suppl 7):84s–9s.
20. Kim HE, Kwon HK, Kim BI. Recovery percentage of remineralization according to severity of early caries. Am J Dent. 2013;26(3):132–6.
21. Kim HE, Kim BI. Analysis of orange/red fluorescence for bacterial activity in initial carious lesions may provide accurate lesion activity assessment for caries progression. J Evid Based Dent Pract. 2017;17(2):125–8.
22. Kim BR, Kang SM, Kwon HK, Kim BI. In vitro assessment of quantitative light-induced red fluorescence related to activity of caries lesions [abstract]. Caries Res. 2017;51(4):344.
23. Pretty IA, Ingram GS, Agalamanyi EA, Edgar WM, Higham SM. The use of fluorescein-enhanced quantitative light-induced fluorescence to monitor de- and re-mineralization of in vitro root caries. J Oral Rehabil. 2003;30(12):1151–6.
24. Durmusoglu O, Tagtekin DA, Yanikoglu F. Clinical evaluation of demineralization and remineralization of intact root surface lesions in the clinic by a quantitative light-induced fluorescence system. Lasers Med Sci. 2012;27(2):397–402.
25. Kim BR, Kang SM, Kim GM, Kim BI. Differences in the intensity of light-induced fluorescence emitted by resin composites. Photodiagn Photodyn Ther. 2016;13:114–9.
26. Ando M, Gonzalez-Cabezas C, Isaacs RL, Eckert GJ, Stookey GK. Evaluation of several techniques for the detection of secondary caries adjacent to amalgam restorations. Caries Res. 2004;38(4):350–6.
27. Diniz MB, Eckert GJ, Gonzalez-Cabezas C, Cordeiro Rde C, Ferreira-Zandona AG. Caries detection around restorations using ICDAS and optical devices. J Esthet Restor Dent. 2016;28(2):110–21.
28. Fontana M, Platt JA, Eckert GJ, Gonzalez-Cabezas C, Yoder K, Zero DT, et al. Monitoring of sound and carious surfaces under sealants over 44 months. J Dent Res. 2014;93(11):1070–5.

DIAGNOdent

17

Klaus W. Neuhaus and Adrian Lussi

17.1 Introduction

In the 1990s it was found that caries emits fluorescence when activated with red light at the wavelength of about 650 nm.

The DIAGNOdent device was consequently developed in the late 1990s for assessment of occlusal sites. In the early 2000s a pen-type DIAGNOdent device was developed for approximal sites as well. Both devices operate at a wavelength of 655 nm. The light is emitted from a specific laser diode, which induces fluorescence of bacterial porphyrins. The intensity of caries fluorescence is correlated with the intensity of bacterial contamination, i.e., with lesion depth. DIAGNOdent has been intended to act as a second opinion device in case of questionable occlusal and proximal surfaces, or when radiography is not applicable. DIAGNOdent was conceptualized as a hand-held device that is easy-to-use in daily dental practice. Because DIAGNOdent is sensitive also for initial caries lesions it was intended to be used as a device for caries monitoring as well. The device is applicable on both deciduous and permanent teeth. Next to numerous laboratory trials that all demonstrate a high reliability of DIAGNOdent [1–3], nowadays there is a

K. W. Neuhaus (✉)
Clinic of Periodontology, Endodontology and Cariology, University Center for Dental Medicine Basel, University of Basel, Basel, Switzerland

Herzogenbuchsee, Switzerland
e-mail: klaus.neuhaus@unibas.ch

A. Lussi
Department of Preventive, Restorative and Preventive Dentistry, School of Dental Medicine, University of Bern, Bern, Switzerland
e-mail: adrian.lussi@zmk.unibe.ch

© Springer Nature Switzerland AG 2019

A. Ferreira Zandona, C. Longbottom (eds.), *Detection and Assessment of Dental Caries*, https://doi.org/10.1007/978-3-030-16967-1_17

sufficient body of evidence gained from clinical trials that supports the device's use in primary care dentistry [4–6].

17.2 Clinical Technique

The device needs to be applied on cleaned teeth. Make sure that your prophy paste or prophy powder is completely rinsed off to avoid wrong measurements. Remnants of several prophylaxis pastes, but also calculus give a false positive fluorescence signal. The assessment of occlusal and approximal sites needs different tips. It should be noted that each tip needs to be calibrated separately against a ceramic standard before clinical use. The display on the pen device is the same as the display on the external viewer. Your assistant should focus on the external display.

17.2.1 Measurement of Occlusal Sites

Insert the round-ended occlusal tip. Because every tooth has an auto-fluorescence, the device should be calibrated against a healthy aspect of the tooth before assessing the occlusal surface. The healthy aspect should be localized on the occlusal third of the buccal side. Slight air-drying of the surface is recommended. If no calibration is performed, you can subtract 2 digits from your readings. But be aware, that sometimes the auto-fluorescence of teeth can be up to 5. Then, start measuring the suspected occlusal aspect by bringing the sapphire tip into pressure-less contact with the tooth surface. It is then indispensable to make a circular movement of your wrist in order to tilt the tip on the same spot on the tooth surface. Remember that caries is a three-dimensional process that can spread in different directions beneath the fissure. The reflection intensity of fluorescence signal is a digital value between 0 and 99. A peak-holder function remembers the highest fluorescence value. The device gives an acoustic signal, but more importantly, take down notes of the peak value. Before measuring another spot, you might want to set back the peak value to zero by pressing the ring once. A new calibration is not needed after the first measurement in the same patient.

17.2.2 Measurement of Approximal Sites

Insert the sharp-edged approximal tip with the red and yellow point at the base (Figs. 17.1 and 17.2). The light-beam is directed towards the red point. Perform a calibration on a healthy aspect on the buccal upper third as described above. Then insert the tip from the vestibular aspect beneath the contact area, red point directed towards the tooth whose adjacent surface is to be measured. Reset to zero, then re-insert the tip from the lingual aspect in the same interdental space. Be aware of the red dot and slightly turn the tip if necessary. Take down the higher peak value of the two measurements.

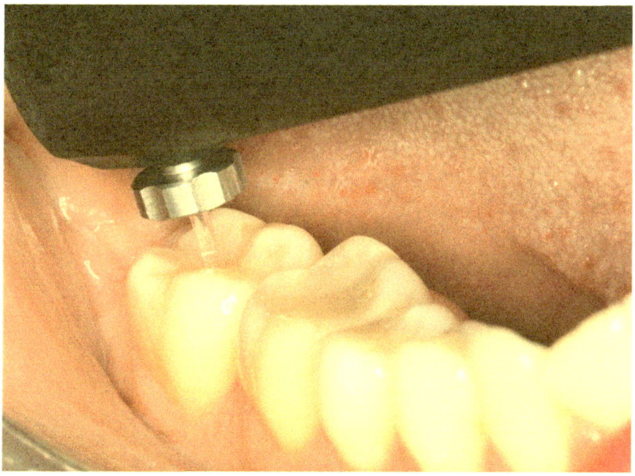

Fig. 17.1 DIAGNOdent pen used for occlusal caries detection (cylindric tip)

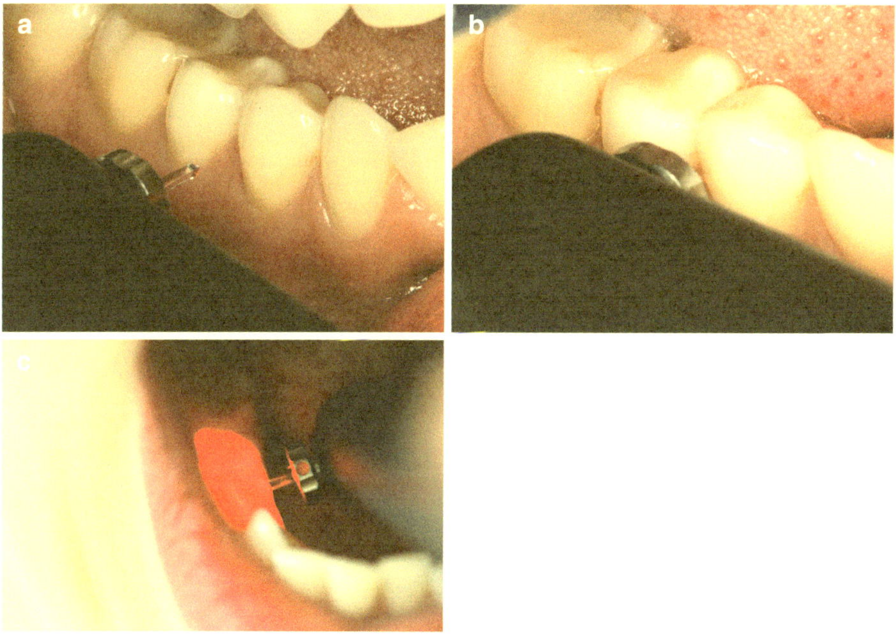

Fig. 17.2 (**a**) For caries detection of a single approximal surface with DIAGNOdent pen. (**b**) The wedge-shaped tip has to be inserted in the approximal space from both the vestibular (**c**) and the oral aspect. The red dot marks the direction of the laser beam

For secondary caries detection, there is evidence that DIAGNOdent is not helpful. It was described that in composite restorations the composite material itself gives false positive readings [7], and in amalgam restorations tiny amounts of calculus also lead to false positive signals [8]. For other materials, no studies have been carried out. The findings regarding the diagnostic performance for root caries are discouraging [9]. For root caries diagnostics, there is no clinical study at hand, and the scarce in vitro evidence found that the correlations between DIAGNOdent readings and clinical features or histology are weak.

It is also noteworthy that the cut-off levels for the occlusal and approximal measurements are different.

Cut-off levels in vivo (and in vitro)

Device	DIAGNOdent	DIAGNOdent pen	DIAGNOdent pen
Aspect	Occlusal	Occlusal	Approximal
Sound	0–13 (0–4)	0–12 (0–6)	0–7 (0–6)
Enamel caries	14–20 (5–10)	13–25 (6–17)	8–16 (7–15)
Dentin caries	>20 (>10)	>25 (>17)	>16 (>15)

[4, 5, 8–11]

Summary table

Bitewing radiography	Laser fluorescence			
Which surfaces/sites is it useful for	Occlusal (pits and fissures)	Proximal/ (approximal)	Smooth surface (buccal and lingual)	Root caries and which of the four surfaces?
	Y	**Y**	**Y**	**N**
What type of lesions is valuable for	Primary coronal	Secondary coronal	Primary root caries	Secondary root caries
	Y	**N**	**N**	**N**
What type of dentition	Primary		Permanent	
	Y		**Y**	
Lesion severity	Enamel lesions		Dentinal lesions	
	Y		**Y**	
Sensitivity	Enamel caries: 0.68–0.96 Dentin caries: 0.67–0.81			
Specificity	Enamel caries: 0.6–0.85 Dentin Caries: 0.79–0.87			
Perceived Ease Of Use (PEOU) [12]	2 It is easy to become skillful at using "DIAGNOdent"			
Advantages/ disadvantages	*Advantages* 1. Caries detection without ionizing radiation 2. Caries monitoring possible 3. Might enhance treatment decision 4. Sufficient clinical validation			
	Disadvantages 1. Punctual measurement (no images) 2. No detection of cavitation 3. Approximal tip too thick to assess tight contact areas 4. Approximal tip not flexible, likely to break upon bending			
Time	Occlusal: 10–40 s Approximal: 20 s from buccal and oral aspect Plus calibration time before the first measurement: 15 s			
Cost	Ca $3′500			

17.2.3 Midwest Caries I.D.

An attempt was made to replace the red laser diode by a red LED; the device was marketed as Midwest Caries I.D. (Dentsply, Tulsa, USA). The device was found to have sufficient accuracy for occlusal dentin caries [13], but not for occlusal enamel caries [10, 13] nor for approximal caries [11].

17.3 Concluding Remarks

DIAGNOdent device is based on inducing fluorescence of bacterial porphyrins. DIAGNOdent has been intended to act as a second opinion device. Use of the device requires clean teeth and calibration prior to using it on a sound surface. The device can be used on occlusal surfaces and proximal surfaces, but it is not reliable for detection of caries around restorations or root caries. It is also noteworthy that the cut-off levels for the occlusal and approximal measurements are different.

References

1. Lussi A, Hack A, Hug I, Heckenberger H, Megert B, Stich H. Detection of approximal caries with a new laser fluorescence device. Caries Res. 2006;40:97–103.
2. Lussi A, Hellwig E. Performance of a new laser fluorescence device for the detection of occlusal caries in vitro. J Dent. 2006;34:467–71.
3. Lussi A, Imwinkelried S, Pitts N, Longbottom C, Reich E. Performance and reproducibility of a laser fluorescence system for detection of occlusal caries in vitro. Caries Res. 1999;33:261–6.
4. Huth KC, Lussi A, Gygax M, Thum M, Crispin A, Paschos E, Hickel R, Neuhaus KW. In vivo performance of a laser fluorescence device for the approximal detection of caries in permanent molars. J Dent. 2010;38:1019–26.
5. Huth KC, Neuhaus KW, Gygax M, Bücher K, Crispin A, Paschos E, Hickel R, Lussi A. Clinical performance of a new laser fluorescence device for detection of occlusal caries lesions at permanent molars. J Dent. 2008;36(12):1033–40.
6. Lussi A, Megert B, Longbottom C, Reich E, Francescut P. Clinical performance of a laser fluorescence device for detection of occlusal caries lesions. Eur J Oral Sci. 2001;109:14–9.
7. Rodrigues JA, Neuhaus KW, Hug I, Stich H, Seemann R, Lussi A. In vitro detection of secondary caries associated with composite restorations on approximal surfaces using laser fluorescence. Oper Dent. 2010;35:564–71.
8. Neuhaus KW, Rodrigues JA, Seemann R, Lussi A. Detection of proximal secondary caries at cervical class II-amalgam restoration margins in vitro. J Dent. 2012;40:493–9.
9. Karlsson L, Johansson E, Tranaeus S. Validity and reliability of laser-induced fluorescence measurements on carious root surfaces in vitro. Caries Res. 2009;43:397–404.
10. Diniz MB, Eckert GJ, Gonzalez-Cabezas C, Cordeiro R d, Ferreira Zandona AG. Caries detection around restorations. J Esthet Restor Dent. 2016;28:110–21. https://doi.org/10.1111/jerd.12183.
11. Neuhaus KW, Ciucchi P, Rodrigues JA, Hug I, Emerich M, Lussi A. Diagnostic performance of a new red light LED device for approximal caries detection. Lasers Med Sci. 2015;30:1443–7.
12. Davis FD. Perceived usefulness, perceived ease of use, and user acceptance of information technology. MIS Quarterly. 1989;13(3):319–40. Published by: Management Information Systems Research Center, University of Minnesota. https://doi.org/10.2307/249008.
13. Rodrigues JA, Hug I, Neuhaus KW, Lussi A. Light-emitting diode and laser fluorescence-based devices in detecting occlusal caries. J Biomed Opt. 2011;16:107003.

Photothermal Radiometry and Modulated Luminescence: The Canary System

18

Bennett T. Amaechi

18.1 Introduction

The Canary System, developed and distributed by Quantum Dental Technologies, has a very different approach to caries detection. It is a nonionizing caries detection procedure to aid detecting, quantifying, monitoring, and recording changes in structure of tooth tissues. The Canary System investigates the status of the tooth crystal structure by using Photothermal Radiometry and Luminescence (PTR-LUM) technology. The Canary System pulses low-energy laser light on the tooth surface, and the laser light, upon interaction with the crystalline structure of tooth tissue, is converted to heat (Photothermal Radiometry or PTR) and light (luminescence or LUM), which are emitted from the tooth surface when the laser is modulated [1, 2]. The device then collects the emitted infrared radiation (heat) and luminescence that provide information about the health of the tooth tissue. The Canary System measures four signals:

1. The strength or amplitude of the converted heat or PTR signal
2. The time delay or phase of the converted heat or PTR to reach the surface
3. The strength or amplitude of the emitted luminescence (LUM)
4. The time delay or phase of the emitted luminescence (LUM)

A Canary Number is created from an algorithm combining these four signals and is directly linked to the status of the tooth crystal structure [3].

These harmless pulses of laser light allow one to examine up to 5 mm below the tooth surface. Demineralization (caries lesions) modifies the thermal properties (PTR) and glow (LUM) from the healthy teeth, which changes how fast and how

B. T. Amaechi (✉)
Department of Comprehensive Dentistry, University of Texas Health Science Center at San Antonio, San Antonio, TX, USA
e-mail: amaechi@uthscsa.edu

© Springer Nature Switzerland AG 2019

A. Ferreira Zandona, C. Longbottom (eds.), *Detection and Assessment of Dental Caries*, https://doi.org/10.1007/978-3-030-16967-1_18

much light and heat can travel. As a suspected lesion grows, there is a corresponding change in the signal (the Canary Number) because the heat is confined to the region with crystalline disintegration (dental caries) and PTR increases and LUM decreases. As remineralization progresses and enamel prisms begin to reform their structure, the thermal and luminescence properties begin to revert back in the direction of healthy teeth. The system detects very small changes in temperature. The temperature rise in the tooth is less than 1–2 °C (1.8–3.6 °F), much less than that generated by a conventional dental curing light [4], and it is undetectable by patients and has no effect on vital tissues. There is no alteration of any of the tissues and no safety issues such as those associated with dental X-rays. The Canary System can be used on both primary and permanent teeth.

The Canary System software can be installed on dental practice workstations throughout the dental office. It captures both signal and images of the tooth surface being examined. The images are displayed on computer monitors for immediate chairside review with the patient. Images are presented on an Odontogram, incorporating Canary Numbers and color codes for the examined teeth, along with the dentist's treatment recommendation. Lower numbers indicate the need for Canary remineralization therapy, depending on the caries risk assessment. Higher Canary color-coded numbers indicate the probability of advanced disease, and the need for restorative management. The Canary System creates an opportunity for dialogue and co-diagnosis, two strong motivators for a new long-term, recurring patient relationship. With the Detail Scan, odontograms also are added to patients' files so treatment progress can be monitored over time. The data is saved on the computer and merged into detailed user-friendly reports, including information on risk factors and their impact on developing caries lesions.

Research has shown that PTR-LUM technology used in the Canary System can detect occlusal pit and fissure caries [5–7], smooth surface caries [6, 8], acid erosion lesions [9], root caries [10], proximal caries lesions [10–13], progression and remineralization of early caries lesions [14–16], caries underneath opaque sealants [17], caries around orthodontic brackets [18], and caries around and underneath restorations [19]. A clinical trial and in vitro studies confirmed the effectiveness of The Canary System to detect proximal caries [10–13, 20]. Two multicenter clinical trials have confirmed the safety of The Canary System, along with its accuracy in detecting early caries lesion (white or brown spots) on both wet and dry tooth surfaces and the ability to detect lesions on tooth surfaces with moderate stain [3, 19].

Thus, as an aid to the conventional visual assessment of the teeth, PTR-LUM can be used to perform the following functions as a second step in the lesion detection and monitoring process: (1) investigate suspect sites for "hidden caries" in pits/fissures, proximal surfaces, around and underneath restorations, beneath clear and opaque sealants, and clear resin infiltrants; (2) obtain the estimate of the severity of the caries lesion in terms of depth and breadth, as Canary Number, to facilitate treatment decision; (3) measure and record the initial quantitative value of the demineralization, as Canary Number, to enable (4) quantitative monitoring of the changes in lesion activities (progress or remineralization) over time during nonoperative lesion management; (5) detect and measure cracks and erosion of teeth; and (6) use an integrated intra-oral camera to capture the image of the examined surface/lesion for future reference. The Canary System, currently available through Quantum Dental Technologies, Canada, can be used on adults and children.

18.2 Clinical Technique

The Canary System is comprised of a console with handpiece, software (that is loaded directly on to computer workstations or laptops), and various accessories: plastic sleeve, plastic tip, and calibration block and safety goggles. The system is ready for scanning following calibration, using the provided calibration block, to make sure that the laser is operating properly and at full power. You will be prompted to calibrate the System during the initial setup routine and every 23 h.

The Canary System has options of "Quick Scan" or "Detail Scan". Quick Scan allows the user to examine teeth without saving any images or information. The information is displayed on the computer screen, and it is up to the user to record this information (if desired) in the patient's clinical record. If you want to save information to a patient record, the "Detail Scan" should be used instead. Before scanning, the handpiece should be covered with the disposable plastic sleeve, which provides a barrier to prevent cross-contamination between patients and a plastic tip attached over the plastic sleeve to create the proper focal distance for the laser from handpiece to tooth. Teeth undergoing examination must be devoid of food, relatively clear of pools of saliva or water, and must be free of all surface residues (plaque, calculus, and heavy stain) that might influence the Canary Number. It is recommended that patients brush their teeth prior to a scanning procedure in order to remove food debris. However, two clinical trials showed that the presence of moisture and moderate plaque and stain does not confound the PTR-LUM assessment of caries on any tooth surface [3].

The examination should begin by using the tracking beam to identify areas to be scanned. When the desired region on the tooth is selected, position the cone of the plastic tip in direct contact with the surface to be measured. One must maintain direct contact with the tooth without movement for the duration of the 5 s measurement. The handpiece should be held directly perpendicular (at right angle, 90°) and parallel from both right/left and up/down perspectives to the tooth surface being measured, using the aiming laser beam to ensure correct positioning. Angulation of the laser beam influences the reproducibility of the system. Laser beam travels on a straight course and scans the tooth tissues along its path; thus change of angulation of the laser beam in subsequent measurement means scanning different tissues, resulting in the examining different areas of crystal structure. Considering that "Right angle (90°)" is the most easily reproducible angulation, it is advised that repeated measurements should be performed on the same spot and at the same beam angulation. Other factors that may influence the Canary Number are the thickness of the overlying enamel, the angulation of the laser beam, thickness of the caries, and surrounding healthy dentin. Lesions that occur on smooth surfaces will have differing behaviors to lesions that occur proximally or in the deep pits and fissures of teeth. Detection performance for deep enamel or dentin caries may be stronger than that for shallow initial lesions.

Following positioning and stabilization of the plastic tip on the tooth surface, the Canary scanning is initiated by selecting the "Start or Scan" button. The Canary System is based on the concept of "point scanning," and it is up to the user's discretion to determine how many areas will be scanned per tooth surface. During the scanning procedure, the handpiece pulses laser light on the tooth surface for approximately 5 s, and the device collects the emitted infrared radiation (heat) and luminescence upon interaction with the crystalline structure of enamel and dentin. The emitted luminescence and heat provide accurate information about the health of the tooth crystal structure. The information is interpreted by the computer software, and each scan is assigned a "Canary Number" on a graduated scale (Fig. 18.1), where lower numbers suggest healthy enamel and higher numbers suggest a greater suspicion of more advanced tooth decay. The Canary Number is displayed on the computer screen and a voice also provides the Canary Number in either French or English (depending upon the language selected). On completion of the scanning of a tooth, a *Scan–Summary* screen will display a summary of all the scanned teeth and their corresponding Canary Numbers. The data can be saved on the cloud.

18.3 Interpreting the Canary Number

The Canary Scale (Fig. 18.1) is a relative scale that reflects the state of tooth mineralization, a measure of the integrity of the surface being scanned. This is a graduated scale where lower numbers suggest healthy enamel and higher numbers suggest the presence of caries and cracks. It is not recommended that treatment decisions be based exclusively on the Canary Numbers. The Canary Numbers should be used as a guide and interpreted by trained professionals using sound clinical judgment in order to develop an appropriate treatment approach. The Canary Scale can be used to assist in treatment planning and monitoring treatment effectiveness. It is often not possible to link the Canary Number to visual

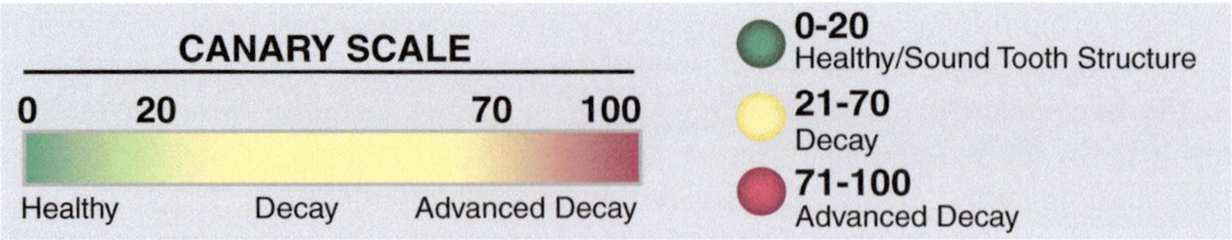

Fig. 18.1 The Canary Scale

examination or radiographs since each of these technologies has limitations in the ability to detect/diagnose early lesions beneath the enamel or root surface (depending on the location).

18.4 Examination of Proximal Surfaces and Visible Margins of Restorations

To assess for caries around restorations (Fig. 18.2), the tip of the handpiece should be positioned approximately 0.50 mm away from the visible margin of the restoration. Allowances have to be made if it appears that the restoration walls are not parallel and are in the path of the laser beam. This is particularly important when examining older amalgam restorations. To identify suspicious proximal caries (Fig. 18.3), scan should be performed from the buccal and lingual embrasure surfaces of the proximal surface in question [10, 13]. Practitioners should use their discretion to determine the appropriate number of scans. One can also scan the occlusal surface of a contact region, but the overlying enamel may dampen the signal and thus decrease the Canary Number. Other tooth surfaces such as occlusal (Figs. 18.4 and 18.5), buccal, and lingual can be examined using the clinical technique described in Sect. 18.2.

Case Study: Caries Beneath an Amalgam

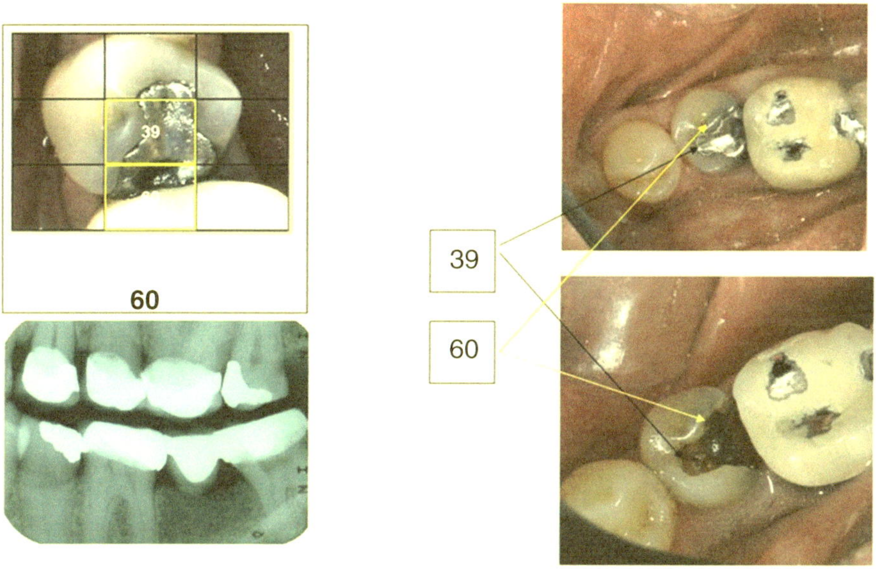

Fig. 18.2 Is it caries or amalgam discoloration? The Canary System was able to confirm shadowing underneath enamel adjacent to an amalgam restoration to be active caries undermining the enamel and dentin

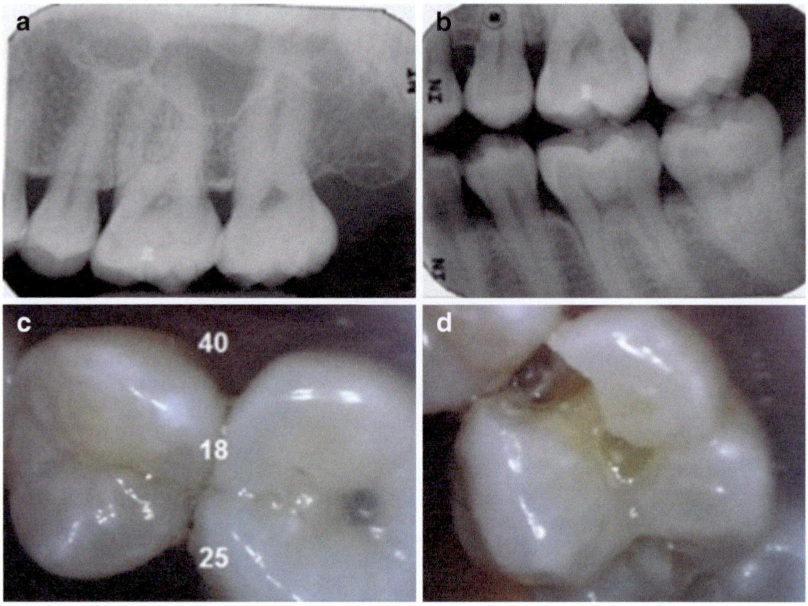

Fig. 18.3 Interproximal caries: (**a**) No evidence of radiographic decay on mesial of the upper left molar first molar; (**b**) Canary Scan was indicated due to gray shadow beneath the mesial marginal ridge of the maxillary first molar; (**c**) Canary Scan of interproximal contact from the mesiobuccal contact indicated CN 40 and from mesiolingual contact indicated CN 25, scan of mesial marginal ridge from the occlusal was not significant; (**d**) Extent of decay visible during preparation extending to the gingival seat and more toward the buccal aspect of the tooth

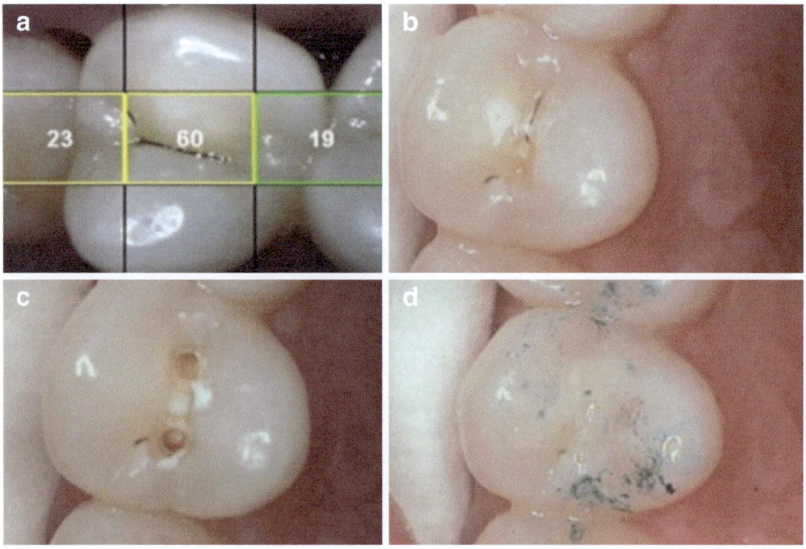

Fig. 18.4 Premolar pit and fissure caries: (**a**) Clinical stain is evident in pits and fissures, typically this would be considered simply a stain; (**b**) Canary exam revealed CN 60 indicating caries beneath the surface; (**c**) Initial excavation followed by deeper further extension to expose deeper caries after further preparation; (**d**) Final restoration after checking the bite

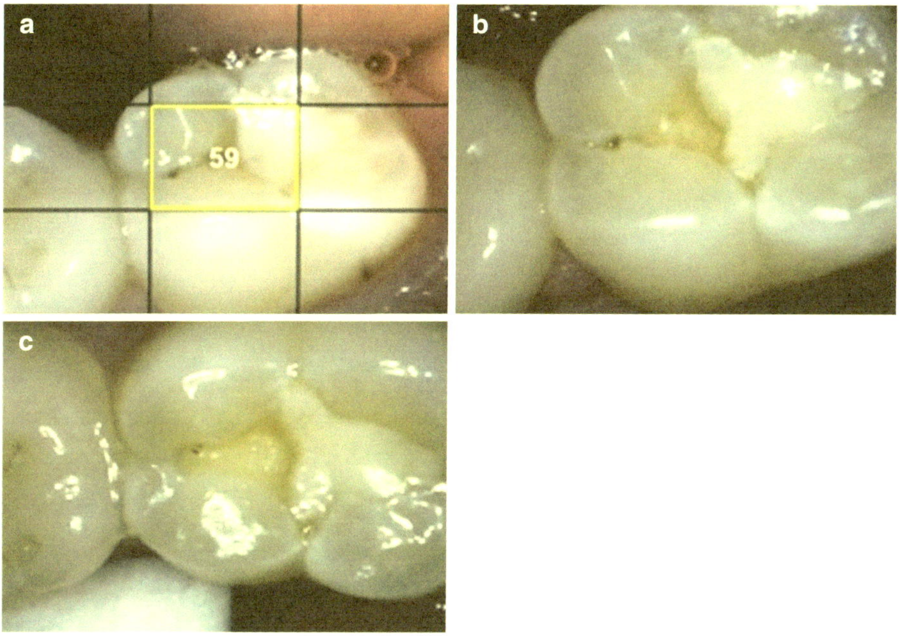

Fig. 18.5 Molar pit and fissure caries: (**a**) Clinical observation of stained pits and grooves in a coalescence fissure adjacent to an existing composite; (**b**) Canary Scan revealed CN 59 in the central groove; (**c**) Excavation of early caries extending just into the dentin

Summary table

Bitewing radiography	Photothermal Radiometry/Luminescence (PTR-LUM). Laser-based technology that can detect and measure the integrity of the crystal structure of the tooth including enamel, dentin, and cementum. It is able to detect lesions up to 5 mm below the tooth surface including around the intact margins of restorations			
Which surfaces/sites is it useful for	Occlusal (pits and fissures)	Proximal/(approximal)	Smooth surface (buccal and lingual)	Root caries and which of the four surfaces?
	Y	**Y**	**Y**	**Y on all surfaces**
What type of lesions is it valuable for	Primary coronal	Secondary coronal	Primary root caries	Secondary root caries
	Y	**Y**	**Y**	**Y**
What type of dentition	Primary		Permanent	
	Y		**Y**	
Lesion severity	Enamel lesions		Dentinal lesions	
	Y		**Y**	
Sensitivity	Literature reported range in 97% [15, 16]			
Specificity	Literature reported range in 97% [15, 16]			

Additional clinical situations	1. Can detect secondary caries around the intact margins of composites, amalgams, and all ceramic crowns 2. Can detect caries beneath clear and opaque sealants 3. Can detect caries around the margins of orthodontic brackets 4. Can detect and monitor caries beneath clear resin infiltrants such as ICON (DMG) 5. Can detect and monitor changes in teeth treated with CURODONT repair (P11-4) 6. Able to use the ADA code D0600 for examination with The Canary System 7. Able to use the new Canadian Dental Association code for caries detection
Perceived Ease Of Use (PEOU)	1. Canary Software bridges with practice management software, so that it can be easily moved around a dental office—simply plug and use 2. Canary Software can be loaded on to computers in the dental office, creating a very portable system 3. Voice provides Canary Number at the end of each scan which engages the patient 4. Intra-oral camera and Canary controlled by two buttons on the handpiece 5. Data stored on the cloud meeting all privacy regulations in North America 6. Training videos and manuals available on Canary Cloud for ongoing training 7. Virtual in-office training allowing the dental team to learn how to use the system at their convenience
Advantages/ disadvantages	*Advantages*
	1. Quantifiable measurements that can track remineralization 2. Integrated intra-oral camera 3. Cloud-based technology for storage and analysis of data 4. Able to create graphs and reporting letters on status and changes in lesions 5. Patients can access their reports on the Canary Cloud 6. High inter- and intra-operator repeatability 7. Portable between operatories
	Disadvantages
	1. Bridged but not fully integrated with Practice Management Software
Time	5 s per scan
Cost	US$10,000–disposables $1.75 per patient

18.5 Concluding Remarks

The Canary System is a non-ionizing caries detection procedure. The Canary Numbers should be used as a guide and interpreted by trained professionals using sound clinical judgment in order to develop an appropriate treatment approach. It is often not possible to link The Canary Number to visual examination or radiographs since each of these technologies have limitations in the ability to detect/diagnose early lesions beneath the enamel or root surface (depending on the location).

References

1. Jeon RJ, Han C, Mandelis A, Sanchez V, Abrams SH. Non-intrusive, non-contacting frequency-domain photothermal radiometry and luminescence depth profilometry of carious and artificial sub-surface lesions in human teeth. J Biomed Opt. 2004;9(4):804–19.
2. Jeon RJ, Sivagurunathan K, Garcia J, Matvienko A, Mandelis A, Abrams S. Dental diagnostic clinical instrument ("Canary") development using photothermal radiometry and modulated luminescence. J Phys Conf Ser. 2010;214:012023.
3. Silvertown JD, Abrams SH, Sivagurunathana KS, Kennedy J, Jeon J, Mandelis A, Hellen A, Hellen W, Elman G, Ehrlich R, Chouljian R, Finer Y, Amaechi BT. Multi-centre clinical evaluation of photothermal radiometry and luminescence correlated with international benchmarks for caries detection. Open Dent J. 2017;11:636–47.
4. Guiraldo RD, Consani S, de Souza AS. Influence of light energy density on heat generation during photoactivation of dental composites with different dentin and composite thickness. J Appl Oral Sci. 2009;17(4):289–93.
5. Jeon RJ, Han C, Mandelis A, Sanchez V, Abrams SH. Dental depth profilometric diagnosis of pit & fissure caries using frequency-domain infrared photothermal radiometry and modulated laser luminescence. In: Stookey G, editor. Early detection of caries III: proceedings of the sixth Indiana conference. Indianapolis: Indiana University Press; 2003. p. 49–67.
6. Jeon RJ, Han C, Mandelis A, Sanchez V, Abrams SH. Diagnosis of pit and fissure caries using frequency-domain infrared photothermal radiometry and modulated laser luminescence. Caries Res. 2004;38:497–513.
7. Jeon RJ, Mandelis A, Abrams SH. Dental depth profilometric diagnosis of pit and fissure caries using frequency-domain infrared photothermal radiometry and modulated luminescence. In: Oraevsky AA, Wang LV, editors. Photons plus ultrasound: imaging and sensing, vol. 5320. Bellingham, WA: SPIE; 2004. p. 29–39.
8. Jeon RJ, Mandelis A, Abrams SH. Depth profilometric case studies in caries diagnostics of human teeth using modulated laser radiometry and luminescence. Rev Sci Instr. 2003;74:380–3.
9. Jeon RJ, Phan TDT, Wu A, Kulkarni G, Abrams SH, Mandelis A. Photothermal radiometric quantitative detection of the different degrees of demineralization of dental enamel by acid etching. J Phys IV France. 2005;125:721–5.
10. Jan J, Wan Bakar WZ, Mathews SM, Okoye LO, Ehler BR, Louden C, Amaechi BT. Proximal caries lesion detection using the Canary Caries Detection System: an in vitro study. J Investig Clin Dent. 2016;7(4):383–90. https://doi.org/10.1111/jicd.12163. Epub 2015 May 27.
11. Jeon RJ, Matvienko A, Mandelis A, Abrams SH, Amaechi BT, Kulkarni G. Detection of interproximal demineralized lesions on human teeth in vitro using frequency-domain infrared photothermal radiometry and modulated luminescence. J Biomed Opt. 2007;12(3):034028.
12. Jeon RJ, Matvienko A, Mandelis A, Abrams SH, Amaechi BT, Kulkarni G. Interproximal dental caries detection using photothermal radiometry and modulated luminescence. Eur Phys J Spec Top. 2008;153:467–9.
13. Uzamere EO, Jan J, Wan Bakar WZ, Mathews SM, Amaechi BT. Clinical trial of the canary system for proximal caries detection. J Dent Res. 2015;94(Spec. Iss A.): 0346. www.iadr.org.
14. Matvienko A, Mandelis A, Hellen A, Jeon RJ, Abrams SH, Amaechi BT. Quantitative analysis of incipient mineral loss in hard tissues, vol. 7166. Bellingham WA: SPIE; 2009; p. 1–12, 29–39.
15. Hellen A, Mandelis A, Finer Y. Photothermal radiometry and modulated luminescence examination of demineralized and remineralized lesions. J Phys Conf Ser. 2010;214(1):012024.
16. Silvertown JD, Wong BP, Sivagurunathan KS, Abrams SH, Kirkham J, Amaechi BT. Remineralization of natural early caries lesions in vitro by P_{11} -4 monitored with

photothermal radiometry and luminescence. J Investig Clin Dent. 2017;8(4):e12257. https://doi.org/10.1111/jicd.12257. Epub 2017 Jan 4.
17. Silvertown JD, Wong BP, Abrams SH, Sivagurunathan KS, Mathews SM, Amaechi BT. Comparison of The Canary System and DIAGNOdent for the in vitro detection of caries under opaque dental sealants. J Investig Clin Dent. 2017;8(4):e12239. https://doi.org/10.1111/jicd.12239. Epub 2016 Sep 26.
18. Dorfman JM. Cement composition effects on enamel demineralization adjacent to orthodontic brackets: an in vitro study using the canary system [Dissertation/Thesis]. ProQuest Dissertations & Theses Global. (1951782587): Temple University; 2017.
19. Abrams TE, Abrams SH, Sivagurunathan K, Silvertown JD, Hellen WMP, Elman GI, Amaechi BT. In vitro detection of caries around amalgam restorations using four different modalities. Open Dent J. 2017;11:609–20.
20. Jeon RJ, Hellen A, Matvienko A, Mandelis A, Abrams SH, Amaechi BT. In vitro detection and quantification of enamel and root caries using infrared photothermal radiometry and modulated luminescence. J Biomed Opt. 2008;13(3):034025. https://doi.org/10.1117/1.2942374.

Part IV

Caries Diagnostic Methods in the Making

Near-Infrared Reflectance Imaging of Caries Lesions

19

Daniel Fried

19.1 Introduction

Even though near-IR (NIR) imaging devices for caries detection have only been introduced recently, several in vitro and in vivo studies carried out over the past 20 years have demonstrated the unique advantages of imaging caries in this wavelength region. Multiple imaging geometries have proven to be valuable including NIR proximal and occlusal transillumination and NIR reflectance [1]. Light scattering in dental enamel decreases with increasing wavelength, and enamel is most transparent near λ = 1300 nm [2, 3]. At that wavelength, NIR light can penetrate a factor of 30 times further through the tooth enamel than is possible in the visible range without scattering for markedly better performance. A plot of the attenuation of light in enamel and water is shown in Fig. 19.1 as a function of wavelength from 400 to 2000 nm [2–4]. Light scattering increases by 2–3 orders of magnitude with demineralization at λ = 1300 nm, indicating that high contrast in transillumination between sound and carious tissues is found near λ = 1300 nm as well [5].

19.2 NIR Proximal and Occlusal Transillumination

The first NIR proximal transillumination images of natural lesions were acquired at 1310 nm [6]. The contrast of simulated lesions in sections of enamel from 2 to 7 mm thickness was compared for visible, 830 and 1310 nm wavelengths [7]. The contrast was higher at 830 nm than the visible, but the contrast was highest at 1310 nm, and only at 1310 nm, were the lesions visible through 6–7 mm of enamel [7].

D. Fried (✉)
Division of Biomaterials and Bioengineering, Department of Preventive and Restorative Dental Sciences, University of California, San Francisco, San Francisco, CA, USA
e-mail: daniel.fried@ucsf.edu

© Springer Nature Switzerland AG 2019

A. Ferreira Zandona, C. Longbottom (eds.), *Detection and Assessment of Dental Caries*, https://doi.org/10.1007/978-3-030-16967-1_19

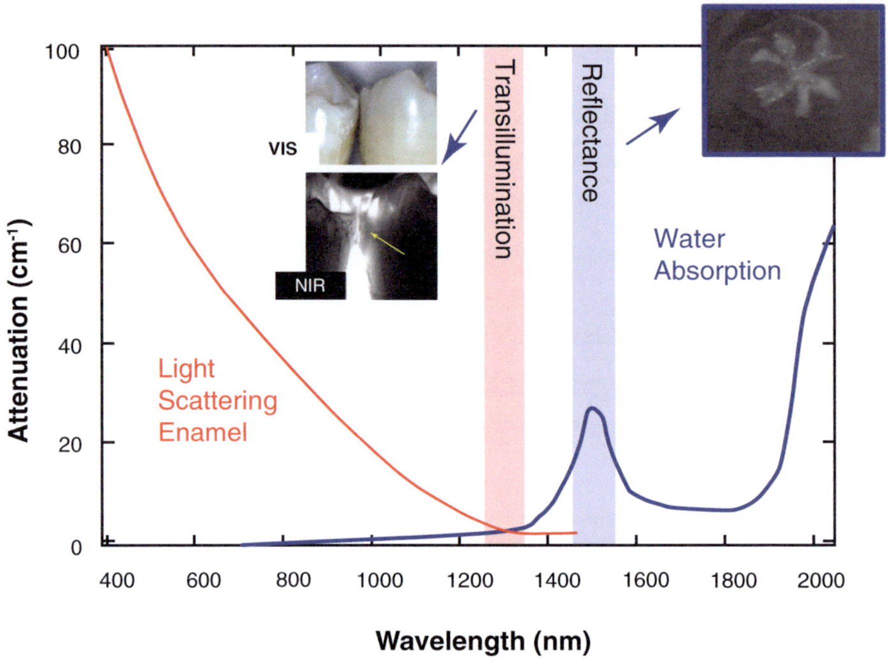

Fig. 19.1 The attenuation coefficient for dental enamel (red) and the absorption coefficient of water (black) in the visible and NIR [2–4]. Best wavelengths for transillumination (1300 nm) and best wavelengths for reflectance (1450 and 1940 nm) and example images are shown for each modality

Due to the high transparency of enamel in the NIR, lesions can be imaged from the occlusal surface after shining light at and below the gum line, which we call occlusal transillumination [8, 9]. Both approximal lesions [6, 7, 9] and occlusal lesions [8–13] can be viewed with high contrast.

The known chromophores responsible for stains on teeth do not absorb light at longer wavelengths since there is not sufficient energy for electronic excitation [8, 14]. Almaz et al. demonstrated that it is necessary to use NIR wavelengths greater than 1150 nm to avoid significant interference from stains when measuring lesion contrast in reflectance and transillumination modalities [15]. Therefore, stains can be easily differentiated from actual demineralization in the NIR range, which is not possible at visible wavelengths or at NIR wavelengths less than 1100 nm as demonstrated in Fig. 19.2. Chung et al. [16] showed that absorption due to stains contributed more to the lesion contrast than increased scattering due to demineralization at visible wavelengths. Since it is impractical to remove stains from the deep grooves and fissures on tooth occlusal surfaces, lack of interference from stains at longer NIR wavelengths is a significant advantage.

In the first NIR clinical study in 2009, it was demonstrated that approximal lesions that appeared on radiographs could be detected with NIR proximal and occlusal transillumination with similar sensitivity [9]. Figure 19.3 shows

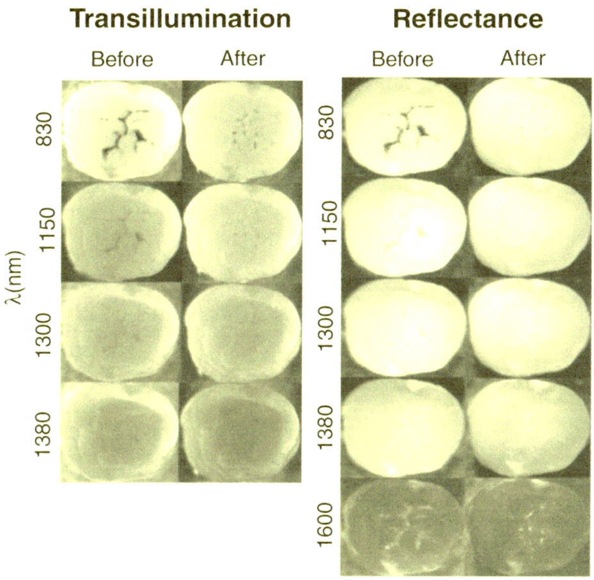

Fig. 19.2 NIR transillumination and reflectance images before and after stain removal with various bandpass (BP) and longpass (LP) filters at BP830, BP1150, BP1300, BP1380, and LP1500

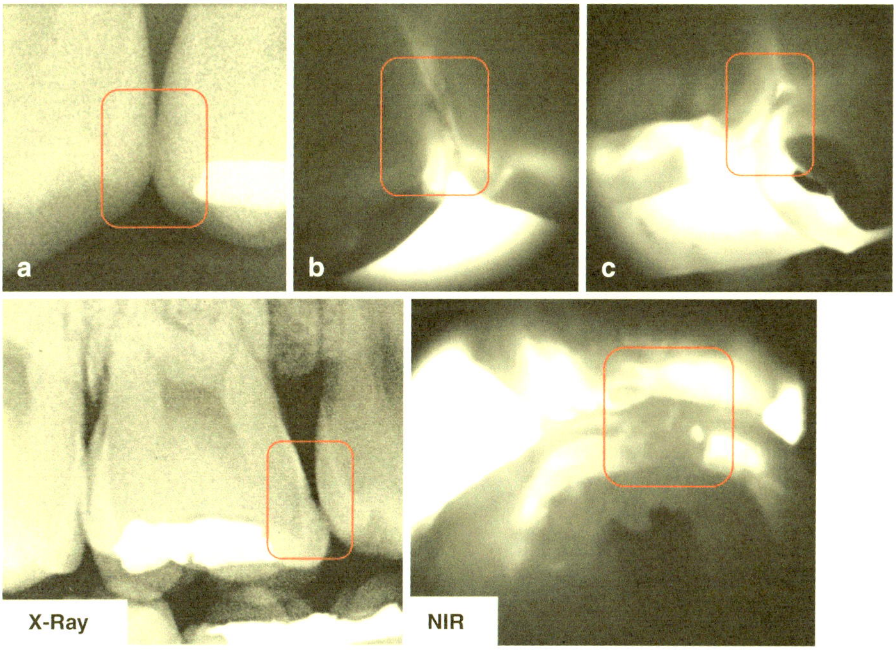

Fig. 19.3 Radiograph (**a**) and in vivo proximal transillumination images at 1300 nm, buccal (**b**) and lingual (**c**) views of the contact point. Radiograph (X-ray) and in vivo occlusal transillumination image (NIR) at 1300 nm of a tooth from the first NIR clinical study

radiographs and proximal and occlusal transillumination images acquired at 1310 nm from that study. Even though the sensitivity of radiographs is not very high [17–21], most studies indicate that the specificity of radiographs is above 90%, which made it a suitable standard for comparison for the first test of this new imaging technology. In addition to demonstrating that the sensitivity of NIR transillumination was as high as radiography, multiple imaging geometries were employed to aid in diagnosis, and it was shown that occlusal imaging geometry in which light is applied at and below the cementum–enamel junction (CEJ) is extremely valuable for detecting approximal lesions [9]. In the second study completed in 2011, teeth with non-cavitated occlusal caries lesions that were not radiopositive were examined in test subjects using NIR occlusal transillumination at 1300 nm prior to restoration [22]. That study demonstrated that occlusal caries lesions can be imaged with high contrast in vivo and that NIR occlusal transillumination is an excellent screening tool for occlusal lesions. In addition, secondary caries lesions can be detected as well. Figure 19.4 shows NIR proximal and transillumination images of secondary caries acquired in vivo.

In the most recent clinical study [1], NIR proximal and occlusal transillumination and NIR reflectance were used to screen premolar teeth scheduled for extraction. The teeth were collected and sectioned and examined with polarized light microscopy and transverse microradiography which served as the gold standard. In addition, extraoral radiographs were taken of teeth and the diagnostic performance of NIR imaging was compared with radiography. The sensitivity of the combined NIR imaging probes was significantly higher ($P < 0.05$) than radiographs for both occlusal and approximal lesions in vivo. It was anticipated that NIR methods would be more sensitive than radiographs since the radiographic sensitivity for occlusal lesions is extremely poor; however, the sensitivity was also much higher for approximal lesions than radiography, 0.53 vs. 0.23. In addition, the sensitivity of each individual NIR probe was either individually equal to or higher than radiography.

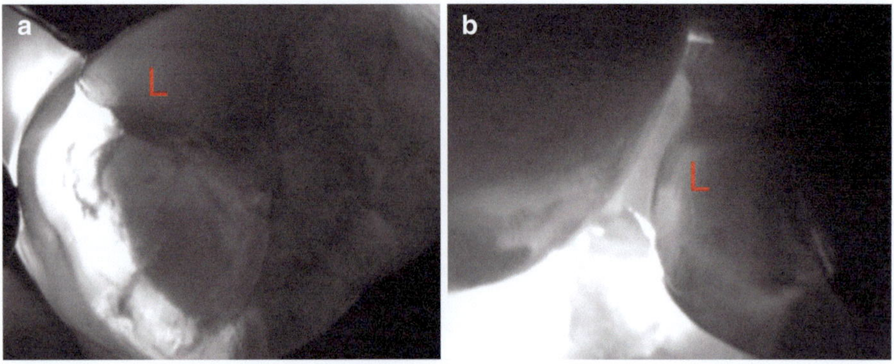

Fig. 19.4 In vivo NIR images of a tooth with secondary caries around a composite restoration, occlusal (**a**) and proximal (**b**) transillumination at 1300 nm

The first commercially available NIR imaging device called the Diagnocam from Kavo (Biberach, Germany) uses an occlusal transillumination probe with 780 nm light [23, 24]. The shorter wavelength allows the use of less expensive silicon-based detectors. However, a previous in vitro study indicated that transillumination imaging at 830 nm with a low-cost silicon CCD sensor optimized for the NIR was capable of higher performance than visible systems, but the contrast was significantly lower than that at 1300 nm and simulated lesions could not be imaged through the full enamel thickness [7]. It is also important to point out that stains still interfere at 780 nm [15]. (For additional information on NIR, see Chap. 15).

19.3 NIR Reflectance Imaging

Early enamel white spot lesions can be discriminated from sound enamel by visual observation or by visible light diffuse reflectance imaging [25, 26]. Very early lesions can be detected visually; however, color in addition to the intensity of the reflected light plays a large role in detecting those changes, and such changes are difficult to quantify; moreover, the color of sound tooth structure varies markedly. Specular reflectance is also a problem since enamel has a high refractive index. However, the visibility of scattering structures on highly reflective surfaces such as teeth can be enhanced by use of crossed polarizers to remove the glare from the surface [27, 28]. The contrast between sound and demineralized enamel can be further enhanced by depolarization of the scattered light in the area of demineralized enamel [10, 29]. A more difficult problem to overcome is visible light absorption due to stains. In a recent imaging study of natural lesions in the occlusal surfaces of extracted teeth, the image contrast was actually negative as opposed to being positive in visible reflectance measurements indicating that absorption due to stains contributed more than increased scattering due to demineralization to the reflectivity in the visible range [16]. This renders the method useless in areas that are subject to heavy staining, namely the areas where most lesions are likely to develop. In fact, visible light reflectance was proposed two decades ago for use in monitoring early demineralization on tooth surfaces but has proven to be unsuccessful due to the problems indicated above [26].

The contrast between sound and demineralized enamel is greatest in the NIR due to the minimal scattering of sound enamel, and this can be exploited for reflectance imaging of early demineralization [5]. The first NIR reflectance study was carried out by Wu et al. [30], and they found that the contrast of early demineralization was significantly higher at 1310 nm than in the visible range. Zakian acquired hyperspectral reflectance images of occlusal caries lesions and demonstrated that multi-wavelength images could be used to aid diagnosis [14]. The highest contrast is achieved at longer NIR wavelengths coincident with higher water absorption [31]. Water in the underlying dentin and surrounding sound enamel absorbs the deeply penetrating light and reduces the reflectivity in sound areas, and this in turn results in higher contrast between sound and demineralized enamel. The highest contrast is at 1450 nm where there is a water absorption band (Fig. 19.1). A study by Chung et al. [16] of natural occlusal lesions indicated that other NIR wavelengths where water absorbs provided significantly higher contrast than at 1310 nm and the visible range.

Monte Carlo simulations suggest that the optimal spectral region for the highest lesion contrast depends on the lesion depth and severity and that shorter wavelengths are likely to yield higher contrast for shallow lesions while longer wavelengths should yield higher contrast for deeper lesions [32]. An imaging method that shows a concomitant increase in lesion contrast with increasing lesion severity is more useful since the lesion severity can more easily be estimated from the images. NIR reflectance at wavelengths coincident with higher water absorption produced the greatest range of lesion contrast values, and the contrast increased linearly with increasing lesion depth and severity [33].

In the first clinical study employing NIR reflectance [1], images of premolar teeth were taken prior to extraction at wavelengths from 1500 to 1700 nm. The performance of NIR reflectance was higher than the other NIR transillumination probes, and approximal lesions located well below the tooth surface could be seen with high contrast. Figure 19.5 shows in vivo reflectance images acquired during that study. Recently, a commercial NIR reflectance system operating at 850 nm was introduced, Vistacam iX Proxi from Durr Dental (Bietigheim-Bissingen, Germany) [34].

NIR imaging is best suited for screening for caries lesions, while optical coherence tomography (see Chap. 20) is well suited for aiding in diagnosis. Both methods exploit the high transparency of enamel and utilize similar wavelengths. Figure 19.6 shows visible, NIR occlusal transillumination, NIR reflectance, and cross-polarization optical coherence tomography (CP-OCT) images of a tooth that was diagnosed with both occlusal and proximal lesions while NIR methods show that there is only a lesion on the proximal surface. These images demonstrate the clinical potential of these new NIR imaging technologies for the management of caries.

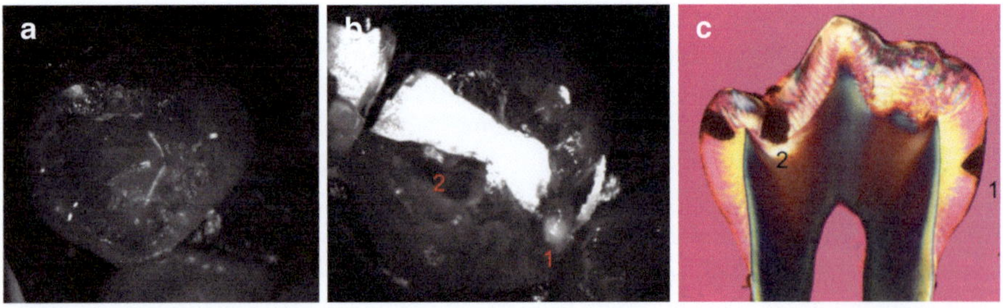

Fig. 19.5 NIR in vivo reflectance images of two teeth at 1500–1700 nm (**a** and **b**) along with a polarized light micrograph (**c**) of a section cut from the tooth shown in (**b**) from the first clinical study utilizing NIR reflectance

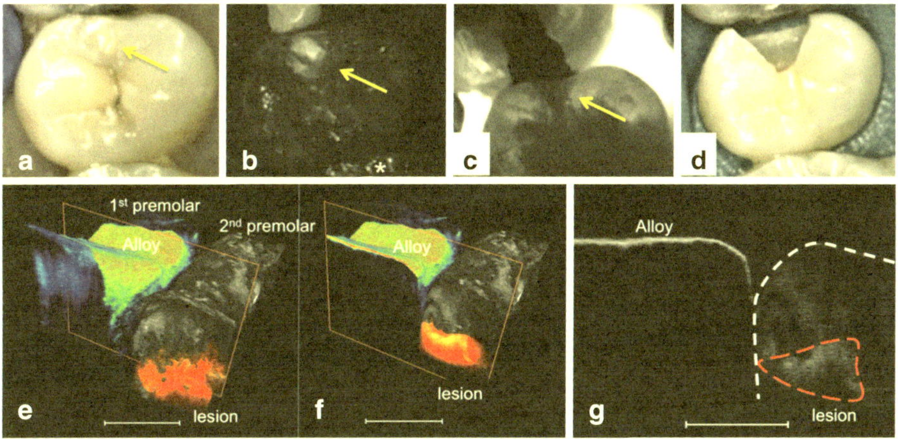

Fig. 19.6 Images of a tooth with a suspected occlusal lesion in the central fissure (stained fissure) and an interproximal lesion indicated at the position of the yellow arrow in the visible light reflectance image (**a**) of the tooth are shown. Near-IR reflectance (**b**) and near-IR occlusal transillumination images (**c**). Visible image of the preparation (**d**) are also shown. A rendered CP-OCT 3D image (**e**) shows the amalgam (alloy) filling on the adjoining first premolar in green and the lesion in red. The length of the bar in images (**e**–**g**) is 300 μm. In (**f**), the same 3D CP-OCT image is shown with the image truncated at the position of the extracted b-scan shown in (**f**) to better show the lesion. In the extracted b-scan (**g**), the surface of the second premolar and the subsurface lesion are shown by the white and red dashed lines, respectively

Summary table

Near-IR imaging				
Which surfaces/sites is it useful for	Occlusal (pits and fissures)	Proximal/ (approximal)	Smooth surface (buccal and lingual)	Root caries
	Y	**Y**	**Y**	**Y**
What type of lesions is valuable for	Primary coronal	Secondary coronal	Primary root caries	Secondary root caries
	Y	**Y**	–	–
What type of dentition	Primary		Permanent	
	Y		**Y**	
Lesion severity	Enamel lesions		Dentinal lesions	
	Y		**Y**	
Sensitivity	Literature reported 0.53 proximal and 0.49 occlusal [1]			
Specificity	Literature reported 0.86 proximal and 0.70 occlusal [1]			
Perceived Ease Of Use (PEOU)	Easy to use and interpret			
Advantages/ disadvantages	*Advantages* 1. No interference from stains *Disadvantages* 1. Expensive			
Time	Real-time video rates			
Cost	Not yet available commercially			

19.4 Concluding Remarks

Enamel is highly transparent in the NIR allowing approximal and occlusal lesions to be viewed with high contrast. At longer NIR wavelengths there is a lack of interference from stains frequently found on occlusal surfaces. NIR transillumination is at least as sensitive as radiography for detection of occlusal and proximal caries. NIR imaging is best suited for screening for caries lesions.

References

1. Simon JC, Lucas SA, Lee RC, Staninec M, Tom H, Chan KH, et al. Near-IR transillumination and reflectance imaging at 1300-nm and 1500–1700-nm for in vivo caries detection. Lasers Surg Med. 2016;48(6):828–36.
2. Fried D, Glena RE, Featherstone JD, Seka W. Nature of light scattering in dental enamel and dentin at visible and near-infrared wavelengths. Appl Opt. 1995;34(7):1278–85.
3. Jones RS, Fried D, editors. Attenuation of 1310-nm and 1550-nm laser light through sound dental enamel. Lasers in dentistry VIII Proc SPIE, vol. 4610. San Jose; 2002. p. 187–90.
4. Hale GM, Querry MR. Optical constants of water in the 200-nm to 200-μm wavelength region. Appl Opt. 1973;12:555–63.
5. Darling CL, Huynh GD, Fried D. Light scattering properties of natural and artificially demineralized dental enamel at 1310-nm. J Biomed Opt. 2006;11(3):34023.
6. Jones RS, Huynh GD, Jones GC, Fried D. Near-IR transillumination at 1310-nm for the imaging of early dental caries. Opt Express. 2003;11(18):2259–65.
7. Jones G, Jones RS, Fried D, editors. Transillumination of interproximal caries lesions with 830-nm light. Lasers in dentistry X SPIE, vol. 5313. San Jose; 2004. p. 17–22.
8. Buhler C, Ngaotheppitak P, Fried D. Imaging of occlusal dental caries (decay) with near-IR light at 1310-nm. Opt Express. 2005;13(2):573–82.
9. Staninec M, Lee C, Darling CL, Fried D. In vivo near-IR imaging of approximal dental decay at 1,310 nm. Lasers Surg Med. 2010;42(4):292–8.
10. Fried D, Featherstone JDB, Darling CL, Jones RS, Ngaotheppitak P, Buehler CM. Early caries imaging and monitoring with near-IR light. Dent Clin North Am. 2005;49(4):771–94.
11. Hirasuna K, Fried D, Darling CL. Near-IR imaging of developmental defects in dental enamel. J Biomed Opt. 2008;13(4):044011.
12. Lee C, Lee D, Darling CL, Fried D. Nondestructive assessment of the severity of occlusal caries lesions with near-infrared imaging at 1310 nm. J Biomed Opt. 2010;15(4):047011.
13. Karlsson L, Maia AMA, Kyotoku BBC, Tranaeus S, Gomes ASL, Margulis W. Near-infrared transillumination of teeth: measurement of a system performance. J Biomed Opt. 2010;15(3):036001–8.
14. Zakian C, Pretty I, Ellwood R. Near-infrared hyperspectral imaging of teeth for dental caries detection. J Biomed Opt. 2009;14(6):064047.
15. Almaz EC, Simon JC, Fried D, Darling CL, editors. Influence of stains on lesion contrast in the pits and fissures of tooth occlusal surfaces from 800–1600-nm. Lasers in dentistry XXII Proc SPIE, vol. 96920X; 2016. p. 1–6.
16. Chung S, Fried D, Staninec M, Darling CL. Multispectral near-IR reflectance and transillumination imaging of teeth. Biomed Opt Express. 2011;2(10):2804–14.
17. Peers A, Hill FJ, Mitropoulos CM, Holloway PJ. Validity and reproducibility of clinical examination, fibre-optic transillumination, and bite-wing radiology for the diagnosis of small approximal carious lesions. Caries Res. 1993;27:307–11.
18. Pine CM, ten Bosch JJ. Dynamics of and diagnostic methods for detecting small carious lesions. Caries Res. 1996;30(6):381–8.

19. Purdell-Lewis DJ, Pot T. A comparison of radiographic and fibre-optic diagnoses of approximal caries lesions. J Dent. 1974;2(4):143–8.
20. Vaarkamp J, ten Bosch JJ, Verdonschot EH, Bronkhoorst EM. The real performance of bitewing radiography and fiber-optic transillumination in approximal caries diagnosis. J Dent Res. 2000;79(10):1747–51.
21. Stephen KW, Russell JI, Creanor SL, Burchell CK. Comparison of fibre optic transillumination with clinical and radiographic caries diagnosis. Community Dent Oral Epidemiol. 1987;15(2):90–4.
22. Staninec M, Douglas SM, Darling CL, Chan K, Kang H, Lee RC, et al. Nondestructive clinical assessment of occlusal caries lesions using near-IR imaging methods. Lasers Surg Med. 2011;43(10):951–9.
23. Kuhnisch J, Sochtig F, Pitchika V, Laubender R, Neuhaus KW, Lussi A, et al. In vivo validation of near-infrared light transillumination for interproximal dentin caries detection. Clin Oral Investig. 2015;20(4):821–9.
24. Sochtig F, Hickel R, Kuhnisch J. Caries detection and diagnostics with near-infrared light transillumination: clinical experiences. Quintessence Int. 2014;45(6):531–8.
25. Angmar-Mansson B, ten Bosch JJ. Optical methods for the detection and quantification of caries. Adv Dent Res. 1987;1(1):14–20.
26. ten Bosch JJ, van der Mei HC, Borsboom PCF. Optical monitor of in vitro caries. Caries Res. 1984;18:540–7.
27. Benson PE, Ali Shah A, Robert Willmot D. Polarized versus nonpolarized digital images for the measurement of demineralization surrounding orthodontic brackets. Angle Orthod. 2008;78(2):288–93.
28. Everett MJ, Colston BW, Sathyam US, Silva LBD, Fried D, Featherstone JDB, editors. Noninvasive diagnosis of early caries with polarization sensitive optical coherence tomography (PS-OCT). Lasers in dentistry V SPIE, vol. 3593. San Jose; 1999. p. 177–83.
29. Fried D, Xie J, Shafi S, Featherstone JDB, Breunig T, Lee CQ. Early detection of dental caries and lesion progression with polarization sensitive optical coherence tomography. J Biomed Opt. 2002;7(4):618–27.
30. Wu J, Fried D. High contrast near-infrared polarized reflectance images of demineralization on tooth buccal and occlusal surfaces at lambda = 1310-nm. Lasers Surg Med. 2009;41(3):208–13.
31. Fried WA, Chan KH, Fried D, Darling CL. High contrast reflectance imaging of simulated lesions on tooth occlusal surfaces at near-IR wavelengths. Lasers Surg Med. 2013;45(8):533–41.
32. Zhang L, Nelson LY, Seibel EJ. Spectrally enhanced imaging of occlusal surfaces and artificial shallow enamel erosions with a scanning fiber endoscope. J Biomed Opt. 2012;17(7):076019.
33. Simon JC, Chan KH, Darling CL, Fried D. Multispectral near-IR reflectance imaging of simulated early occlusal lesions: variation of lesion contrast with lesion depth and severity. Lasers Surg Med. 2014;46(3):203–15.
34. Jablonski-Momeni A, Jablonski B, Lippe N. Clinical performance of the near-infrared imaging system VistaCam iX Proxi for detection of approximal enamel lesions. BDJ Open. 2017;3:17012.

Optical Coherence Tomography for Imaging Dental Caries

20

Daniel Fried

20.1 Introduction

Optical coherence tomography (OCT) is a noninvasive technique for creating cross-sectional images of internal biological structure [1]. The intensity of the reflected/backscattered light is measured as a function of its axial position in the tissue. OCT can be used to measure the reflectivity within dental hard tissues to a depth of up to 3–5 mm in enamel and 1–2 mm in dentin with an axial (depth) resolution exceeding 10 μm. The first images of the soft and hard tissue structures of the oral cavity were acquired by Colston et al. [2]. Feldchtein et al. [3] presented the first images of dental caries in vivo.

Figure 20.1 shows a 3D OCT tomographic image of a 6 × 6 mm^2 area of a tooth occlusal surface with demineralization in the fissure. The b-scan image shows position and depth and the magnitude of the reflectivity or backscattered light at each pixel is displayed in a grayscale false color image with white indicating high reflectivity and black low reflectivity. Two a-scans of reflectivity vs. depth are shown in sound lesion areas. The reflectivity from the area of demineralization is orders of magnitude larger than the sound reflectivity.

20.2 Use of OCT for Quantitative Measurements of Lesion Severity

Since OCT provides measurements of the optical reflectivity with depth, the most obvious method for quantifying the severity of demineralization in OCT images is to integrate the reflectivity over the lesion depth. However, the strong reflection at the tooth surface is typically several orders of magnitude higher than the reflectivity/

D. Fried (✉)
Division of Biomaterials and Bioengineering, Department of Preventive and Restorative Dental Sciences, University of California, San Francisco, San Francisco, CA, USA
e-mail: Daniel.Fried@ucsf.edu

© Springer Nature Switzerland AG 2019

A. Ferreira Zandona, C. Longbottom (eds.), *Detection and Assessment of Dental Caries*, https://doi.org/10.1007/978-3-030-16967-1_20

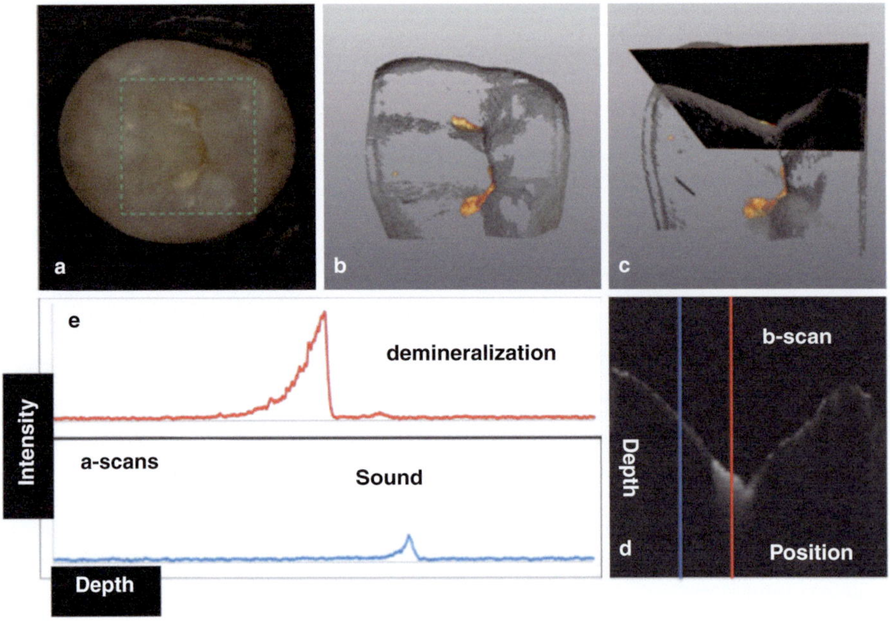

Fig. 20.1 A visible image of an extracted tooth (**a**) with demineralization in the fissure, a 5 × 5 mm box was cut to mark the ROI. (**b** and **c**) Show the acquired CP-OCT 3D scans segmented to show areas of demineralization (red/yellow). A 2D slice extracted from the image at the position indicated in (**c**) is shown in (**d**), this is called a b-scan. The b-scan is displayed in grayscale with higher reflectivity in white which corresponds to demineralization. Two lineouts of depth vs. intensity, called a-scans, were extracted (red and blue lines) at sound and lesion (demineralization) areas and are shown in (**e**)

scattering from the lesion. Therefore it is problematic with a conventional OCT system to use this value as a measure of lesion severity. Because of this problem, the first attempts to use OCT to monitor demineralization utilized the loss of optical penetration as a measure of lesion severity [4]. Even though the loss of optical penetration can be invaluable for identifying lesions in OCT images, there are major problems with using the loss of light penetration to quantify the extent of demineralization. One must arbitrarily choose a distance from the surface to serve as a cutoff point, based on an arbitrary intensity loss. More recently, other researchers with conventional OCT systems have used attenuation coefficients to quantify lesion severity [5, 6]. Both approaches have problems since increased demineralization can lead to either an increase in attenuation of the reflectivity with depth or an increase due to the complex optical behavior. The strong surface reflection in OCT images can be reduced and the contrast between sound and demineralized tissues enhanced by use of polarization.

Baumgartner et al. [7] presented the first polarization resolved images of dental caries. Later polarization sensitive OCT (PS-OCT) measurements demonstrated the advantage of using the cross-polarization OCT (CP-OCT) image to quantify lesion severity [8]. If the incident light is linearly polarized, surface reflections do not scramble the polarization so the surface reflection does not appear strongly in the CP-OCT image. The strong scattering in demineralized lesion areas scrambles incident linearly polarized light, and the reflectivity in the CP image can be directly integrated to provide a measure of the lesion severity [8].

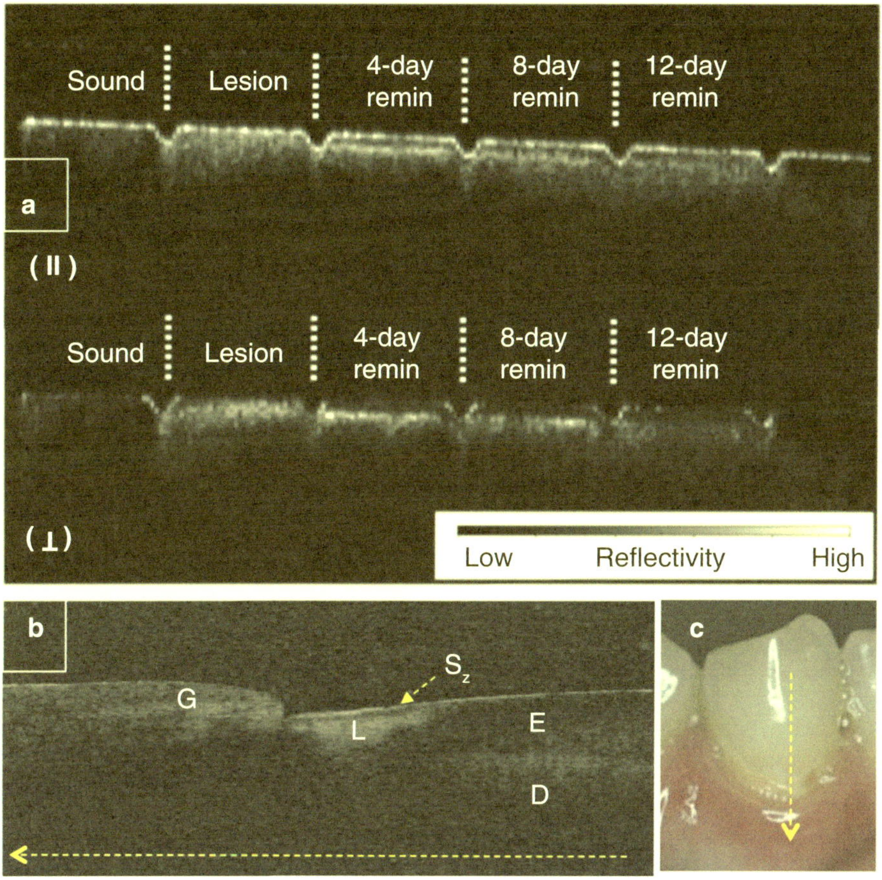

Fig. 20.2 (**a**) PS-OCT b-scan images of a bovine enamel block showing the sound (protected) regions located on the extreme left and right side of the sample, the lesion area (0 days exposed to remin. soln), and the areas exposed for increasing periods of time to the remineralization solution, 4, 8, and 12 days. The (‖) image represents the light reflected in the original polarization while the (⊥) image is the orthogonal polarization or cross-polarization image which was used for analysis in these studies. The incisions are ~100-μm deep and separated by 1.4 mm from [16]. (**b**) An in vivo CP-OCT b-scan and a visible image (**c**) of a cervical enamel lesion that appears arrested. There was no change in the lesion structure after treatment with fluoride varnish after 30 weeks. The lesion is clearly visible and it has a well-defined surface zone (S_Z) that is visible. The dentinal enamel junction (DEJ) and the gingival (*G*) are visible in the image and the position of the scans are indicated on the photograph of the tooth from [22]

The advantages of using PS-OCT to monitor demineralization has been demonstrated in several studies utilizing various lesion models and natural lesions [8–14]. The ability of PS-OCT to monitor remineralization and the formation of a distinct transparent surface zone [15, 16] has also been demonstrated. Figure 20.2 shows PS-OCT co-polarization (‖) and cross-polarization (⊥) images of a bovine enamel sample with six windows showing lesion areas that have been exposed to a remineralization solution. The most obvious change was the formation of a distinct transparent outer surface layer ~50-μm thick. Note the large difference in intensity between the surface in the (‖) and (⊥) images.

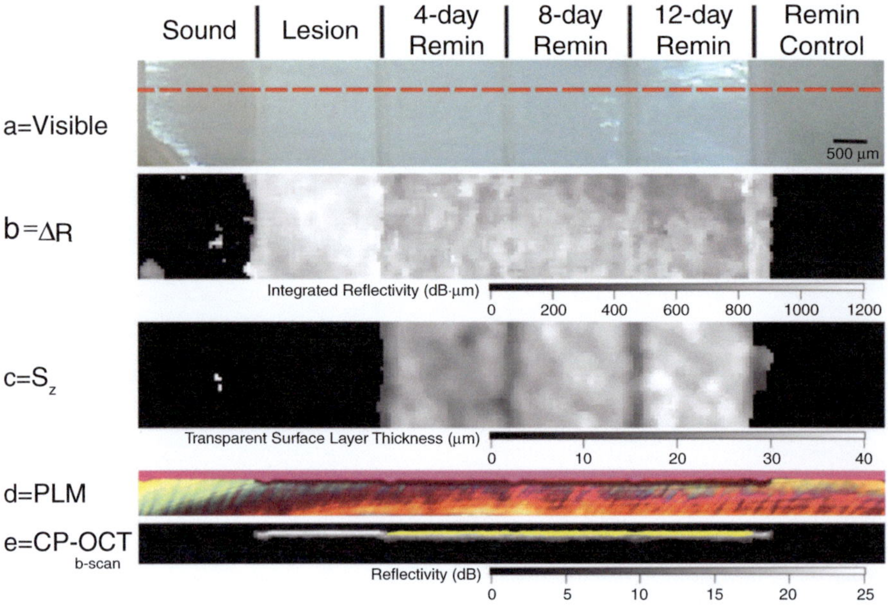

Fig. 20.3 A visible, CP-OCT and cross-sectional PLM images of a bovine enamel sample with six windows. Initial lesions were produced after 24 h demineralization on the central four windows and then the right four windows were exposed to a remineralization solution. The red dotted line in the visible light reflectance image (**a**) represents the position of the section shown in (**d**) and (**e**). Two-dimensional CP-OCT surface projection images of the same sample are shown including (**b**) integrated reflectivity and (**c**) the transparent surface layer thickness. PLM (**d**) and processed CP-OCT B-scan (**e**) images show an increase in transparent surface layer thickness over the periods of exposure to the remineralizing solution. The transparent surface layer is highlighted in yellow (**e**) from [14]

Automated methods have been developed for converting 3D CP-OCT images to 2D projection images of the lesion depth and the integrated reflectivity over the lesion depth which we call ΔR, a convenient unit analogous to the integrated mineral loss, ΔZ the standard unit used to represent lesion severity assessed using transverse microradiography and μCT [13, 17–19]. Automated methods can be used to generate 2D projection maps of the lesion depth (L_d), integrated reflectivity with lesion depth (ΔR), and the thickness of the transparent surface zone (S_z) from 3D images [13, 14]. Figure 20.3 shows a bovine enamel slab (10 mm × 2 mm × 2 mm) with lesion areas that have been exposed to remineralization [14]. The 3D CP-OCT image was converted to 2D projection images of ΔR and S_z. A polarized light micrograph of a histological section is also shown for comparison.

In the first clinical study using OCT to monitor demineralization, the development of demineralization on tooth occlusal and smooth surfaces was monitored using the handheld PS-OCT probe shown in Fig. 20.4 that acquires individual b-scans [20]. PS-OCT was able to non-destructively measure significant increases in demineralization on both the buccal and occlusal surfaces after 30 days [20]. In a subsequent

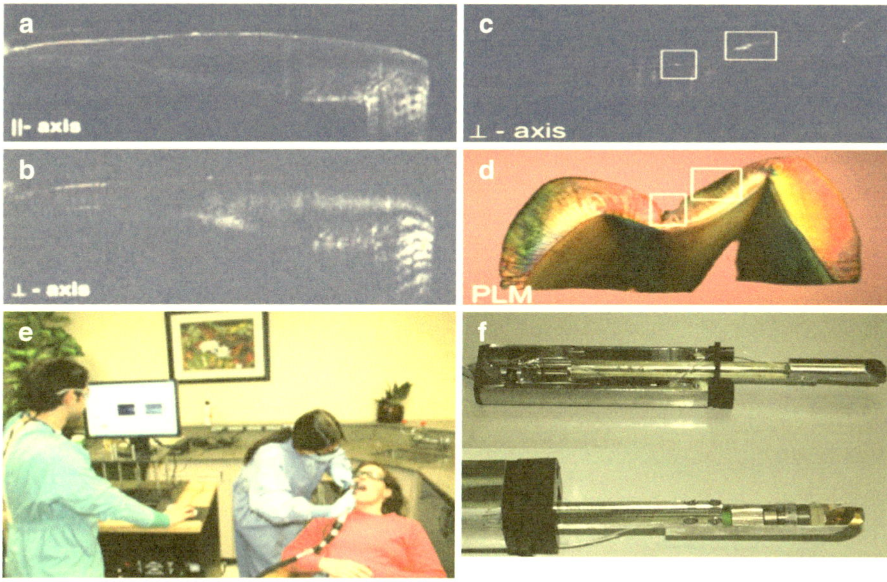

Fig. 20.4 Co-polarization (**a**) and cross-polarization (**b**) OCT b-scans of a sound area of a tooth from the first clinical study monitoring demineralization in vivo showing clear resolution of the dentinal enamel junction from the crown to the root. The CP-OCT image of the occlusal surface of another tooth (**c**) shows demineralization that was confirmed using polarized light microscopy (**d**) after tooth extraction. The PS-OCT system is shown in use (**e**) along with images of the custom fabricated scanning probe (**f**) from [20]

study, a high-speed swept-source CP-OCT system with an integrated MEMS scanner from Santec (Komaki Aichi, Japan) was used to acquire 3D volumetric images of the area at the base of orthodontic brackets over a period of 12 months after placement (Fig. 20.5). Even though an increase in demineralization was not visibly apparent in images taken before and after 12 months, CP-OCT was successful in monitoring a small but significant ($p < 0.05$) increase in the mean lesion depth (L_d) and integrated reflectivity (ΔR) with time over the area cervical to the brackets further validating the utility of CP-OCT for monitoring early demineralization [21].

In a clinical study recently completed, existing smooth surface enamel was monitored using CP-OCT over a period of 30 weeks before and after application of a fluoride varnish [22]. Each lesion was imaged before application of the varnish and at 6-week intervals. It was interesting to observe that a transparent surface zone was visible in CP-OCT images for all but one of the enamel lesions, 62/63. A CP-OCT image of one of the arrested lesions with the transparent surface zone clearly visible is shown in Fig. 20.2. Only a small fraction of the lesion manifested changes after treatment indicating that most were likely arrested; however, the study demonstrated that changes in the internal microstructure of caries lesions can be monitored over time during preventative intervention. This ability offers many intriguing possibilities for caries research and future clinical use.

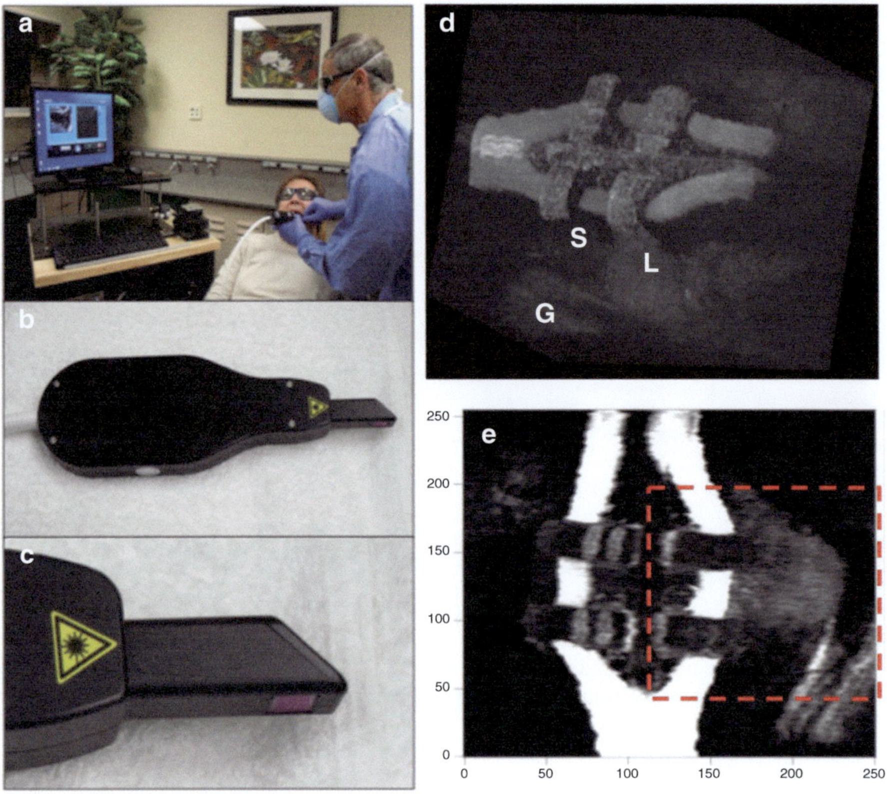

Fig. 20.5 Images from the first clinical study monitoring demineralization with a high-speed 3D CP-OCT system. The Santec system is shown in (**a**) along with the handpiece with integrated interferometer and MEMS scanner in (**b** and **c**). (**d**) Surface rendering of 6 × 6 × 7 mm 3D CP-OCT image around bracket; *G* gingiva, *S* sound, and *L* lesion. (**e**) Collapsed 2D image of ΔR (rotated by 90°) showing the area monitored over time in red box from [21]

20.3 Use of OCT for the Diagnosis of Questionable Occlusal Caries (QOC) Lesions

Most clinicians are interested in knowing how deep the occlusal lesions have actually penetrated into the tooth so that they can decide whether a restoration is necessary. Even though the optical penetration of near-IR light can easily exceed 7 mm through sound enamel to image lesions on proximal surfaces with high contrast, the large increase in light scattering due to demineralization [23] typically limits optical penetration in highly scattering lesions (also dentin and bone) to 1–2 mm, thus cutting off the OCT signal before it reaches the dentinal enamel junction (DEJ). However, most occlusal lesions rapidly spread laterally under the enamel upon contacting the more soluble dentin. OCT can be used to determine if occlusal lesions have penetrated to the underlying dentin [24] by detecting the lateral spread across the DEJ. In a clinical study, 12 out of 14 of the lesions examined in vivo using OCT that were scheduled for restoration exhibited increased reflectivity below the DEJ

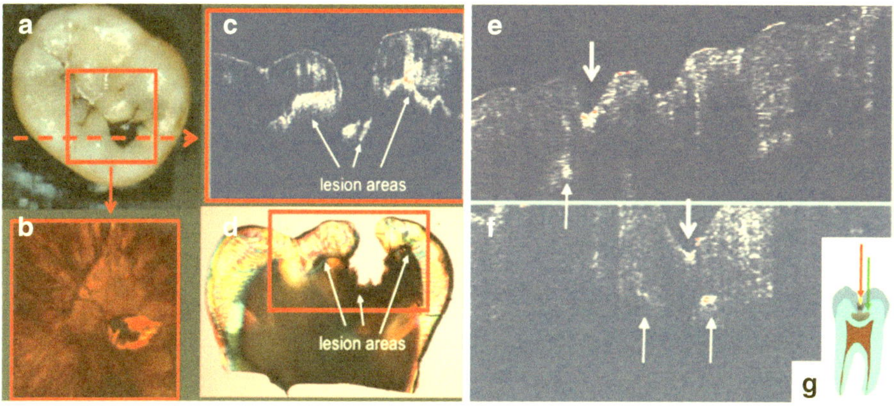

Fig. 20.6 A tooth with a cavitated occlusal lesion that has spread laterally in the underlying dentin (**a**). A surface rendering of the 3D OCT scan (**b**) and an OCT b-scan across the lesion with a PLM image of the matching section (**d**). (**e** and **f**) Two in vivo OCT b-scans of occlusal lesions showing the higher reflectivity at the DEJ peripheral to each fissure shown by the upward pointing arrows. Downward pointing arrows demarcate the center of the fissure and lesion. Intensity scale for **c**, **e**, **f** is red > white > blue. Diagram in (**g**) shows that lesion in fissure blocks optical penetration (red arrow) while light can penetrate to the underlying lesion through the sound enamel (green arrow)

indicating that the lesions had spread to the dentin. Sample images from that study are shown in Fig. 20.6. Since none of the lesions showed up on a radiograph, this is a remarkable improvement over existing technology [24].

The visibility of QOC lesions can be significantly increased by the use of optical clearing agents and image analysis methods [25]. Optical clearing agents have routinely been used in biological microscopy and have found recent application in clinical imaging including OCT [26, 27]. In a recent study, extracted teeth with QOC were imaged with optical coherence tomography (OCT) with and without the addition of a transparent vinyl polysiloxane impression material (VPS) currently used in vivo. VPS enhances the visibility of occlusal lesions that have penetrated to the underlying dentin and also enhance the visibility of the dentinal enamel junction (DEJ) [25].

20.4 Use of OCT for the Diagnosis of Root Caries

Even though the penetration depth of near-IR light is more limited in dentin than for enamel, one can still acquire images of early root caries and demineralization in dentin [28]. PS-OCT studies have successfully measured demineralization in simulated caries models in dentin and on root surfaces (cementum) [29–31]. PS-OCT can effectively be used to discriminate demineralized dentin from sound dentin and cementum [29]. PS-OCT has also been used to measure remineralization on dentin surfaces and to detect the formation of a highly mineralized layer on the lesion surface after exposure to a remineralization solution [31]. Cementum has lower reflectivity than dentin in OCT images making it possible to easily discriminate the remaining cementum thickness [29, 31]. Shrinkage in lesion areas particularly for dentin is also of interest. Shrinkage occurs in dentin due to the high collagen content when the lesion area loses water. More severe lesions manifest greater shrinkage and lesions exposed to remineralization with an intact highly mineralized surface zone have reduced shrinkage [31]. Inspection of the lesions exposed to remineralization indicates that there is markedly less shrinkage. There was a correlation between the lesion severity (ΔZ) and the degree of shrinkage measured using PS-OCT [31].

20.5 Use of OCT for the Diagnosis of Secondary and Residual Caries

OCT has also been used to look at different restorative materials and identify pit and fissure sealants [3, 32].

The penetration depth of PS-OCT through composite has been shown to be sufficient to detect and track early demineralization or secondary caries on the occlusal surface under a sealant or restoration in vitro. The penetration depth was not influenced by the composition of the filler. The reflectivity, however, is markedly increased when an optical pacifier such as titanium dioxide is added [9]. The advantage of having polarization sensitivity to quantify lesion severity is even more apparent for imaging secondary caries under sealants or composite restorations. Most composites/sealants have sufficient transparency in the near-IR to allow imaging through the composite to resolve early demineralization under sealants and restorations. Polarization sensitivity may also help in identifying particular sealants since they apparently depolarize light at different rates. Jones et al. [9] showed that one particular sealant had minimal reflectivity in the orthogonal polarization image, i.e., does not depolarize the incident light and has minimal birefringence. The fact that there is minimal reflectivity from overlying composite also greatly facilitates direct integration of the reflectivity from the demineralized area. These images demonstrate that polarization sensitivity is advantageous for differentiating demineralized enamel under composite sealants and restorations for imaging secondary caries lesions. Other studies have investigated the use of OCT for the detection of demineralization beneath sealants and composites in addition to primary lesions [33–35].

Summary table

Optical coherence tomography				
Which surfaces/sites is it useful for	Occlusal (pits and fissures)`	Proximal/ (approximal)	Smooth surface (buccal and lingual)	Root caries
	Y	**Y**	**Y**	**Y**
What type of lesions is valuable for	Primary coronal	Secondary coronal	Primary root caries	Secondary root caries
	Y	**Y**	**Y**	**Y**
What type of dentition	Primary		Permanent	
	Y		**Y**	
Lesion severity	Enamel lesions		Dentinal lesions	
	Y		**Y**	
Sensitivity	Not appropriate			
Specificity	Not appropriate			
Perceived Ease Of Use (PEOU)[a]	OCT images are similar to ultrasound images			

Optical coherence tomography	
Advantages/ disadvantages	*Advantages* 1. Capable of acquiring high resolution image of lesion structure *Disadvantages* 1. Assessment of lesion penetration into dentin is done by detecting the lateral spread across the DEJ since the OTC signal is cutoof before it reaches the DEJ due to the high scattering in the demineralized enamel
Time	3D image acquisition in 1 s
Cost	Not yet available commercially

[a]Davis (1989)

20.6 Concluding Remarks

Optical coherence tomography (OCT) is a noninvasive technique for creating cross-sectional images of internal biological structure. PS-OCT is able to access lesion severity. It non-destructively measures changes in the internal microstructure of caries lesions monitoring both demineralization and remineralization. Studies have demonstrated its utility in occlusal, smooth, proximal surfaces as well as for root caries and caries around restorations.

References

1. Bouma BE, Tearney GJ. Handbook of optical coherence tomography. New York: Marcel Dekker; 2002.
2. Colston B, Everett M, Da Silva L, Otis L, Stroeve P, Nathel H. Imaging of hard and soft tissue structure in the oral cavity by optical coherence tomography. Appl Opt. 1998;37(19):3582–5.
3. Feldchtein FI, Gelikonov GV, Gelikonov VM, Iksanov RR, Kuranov RV, Sergeev AM, et al. In vivo OCT imaging of hard and soft tissue of the oral cavity. Opt Express. 1998;3(3):239–51.
4. Amaechi BT, Higham SM, Podoleanu AG, Rodgers JA, Jackson DA. Use of optical coherence tomography for assessment of dental caries. J Oral Rehabil. 2001;28(12):1092–3.
5. Sowa MG, Popescu DP, Friesen JR, Hewko MD, Choo-Smith LP. A comparison of methods using optical coherence tomography to detect demineralized regions in teeth. J Biophotonics. 2011;4(11–12):814–23.
6. Espigares J, Sadr A, Hamba H, Shimada Y, Otsuki M, Tagami J, et al. Assessment of natural enamel lesions with optical coherence tomography in comparison with microfocus x-ray computed tomography. J Med Imaging. 2015;2(1):014001.
7. Baumgartner A, Dicht S, Hitzenberger CK, Sattmann H, Robi B, Moritz A, et al. Polarization-sensitive optical coherence tomography of dental structures. Caries Res. 2000;34:59–69.
8. Fried D, Xie J, Shafi S, Featherstone JDB, Breunig T, Lee CQ. Early detection of dental caries and lesion progression with polarization sensitive optical coherence tomography. J Biomed Opt. 2002;7(4):618–27.
9. Jones RS, Staninec M, Fried D. Imaging artificial caries under composite sealants and restorations. J Biomed Opt. 2004;9(6):1297–304.
10. Jones RS, Darling CL, Featherstone JD, Fried D. Imaging artificial caries on the occlusal surfaces with polarization-sensitive optical coherence tomography. Caries Res. 2006;40(2):81–9.
11. Chong SL, Darling CL, Fried D. Nondestructive measurement of the inhibition of demineralization on smooth surfaces using polarization-sensitive optical coherence tomography. Lasers Surg Med. 2007;39(5):422–7.
12. Hirasuna K, Fried D, Darling CL. Near-IR imaging of developmental defects in dental enamel. J Biomed Opt. 2008;13(4):044011.

13. Chan KH, Chan AC, Fried WA, Simon JC, Darling CL, Fried D. Use of 2D images of depth and integrated reflectivity to represent the severity of demineralization in cross-polarization optical coherence tomography. J Biophotonics. 2015;8(1–2):36–45.
14. Lee RC, Kang H, Darling CL, Fried D. Automated assessment of the remineralization of artificial enamel lesions with polarization-sensitive optical coherence tomography. Biomed Opt Express. 2014;5(9):2950–62.
15. Jones RS, Fried D. Remineralization of enamel caries can decrease optical reflectivity. J Dent Res. 2006;85(9):804–8.
16. Kang H, Darling CL, Fried D. Nondestructive monitoring of the repair of enamel artificial lesions by an acidic remineralization model using polarization-sensitive optical coherence tomography. Dent Mater. 2012;28(5):488–94.
17. Ngaotheppitak P, Darling CL, Fried D. Measurement of the severity of natural smooth surface (interproximal) caries lesions with polarization sensitive optical coherence tomography. Lasers Surg Med. 2005;37(1):78–88.
18. Le MH, Darling CL, Fried D. Automated analysis of lesion depth and integrated reflectivity in PS-OCT scans of tooth demineralization. Lasers Surg Med. 2010;42(1):62–8.
19. Kang H, Jiao JJ, Chulsung L, Le MH, Darling CL, Fried DL. Nondestructive assessment of early tooth demineralization using cross-polarization optical coherence tomography. IEEE J Sel Top Quantum Electron. 2010;16(4):870–6.
20. Louie T, Lee C, Hsu D, Hirasuna K, Manesh S, Staninec M, et al. Clinical assessment of early tooth demineralization using polarization sensitive optical coherence tomography. Lasers Surg Med. 2010;42:738–45.
21. Nee A, Chan K, Kang H, Staninec M, Darling CL, Fried D. Longitudinal monitoring of demineralization peripheral to orthodontic brackets using cross polarization optical coherence tomography. J Dent. 2014;42(5):547–55.
22. Chan KH, Tom H, Lee RC, Kang H, Simon JC, Staninec M, et al. Clinical monitoring of smooth surface enamel lesions using CP-OCT during nonsurgical intervention. Lasers Surg Med. 2016;48(10):915–23.
23. Darling CL, Huynh GD, Fried D. Light scattering properties of natural and artificially demineralized dental enamel at 1310-nm. J Biomed Opt. 2006;11(3):34023.
24. Staninec M, Douglas SM, Darling CL, Chan K, Kang H, Lee RC, et al. Nondestructive clinical assessment of occlusal caries lesions using near-IR imaging methods. Lasers Surg Med. 2011;43(10):951–9.
25. Kang H, Darling CL, Fried D. Use of an optical clearing agent to enhance the visibility of subsurface structures and lesions from tooth occlusal surfaces. J Biomed Opt. 2016;21(8):081206.
26. Tuchin VV. Optical clearing of tissues and blood. Bellingham, WA: SPIE; 2006.
27. Jones RS, Fried D, editors. The effect of high index liquids on PS-OCT imaging of dental caries. Lasers in dentistry XI. San, Jose, CA: SPIE; 2005.
28. Amaechi BT, Podoleanu AG, Komarov G, Higham SM, Jackson DA. Quantification of root caries using optical coherence tomography and microradiography: a correlational study. Oral Health Prev Dent. 2004;2(4):377–82.
29. Lee C, Darling C, Fried D. Polarization sensitive optical coherence tomographic imaging of artificial demineralization on exposed surfaces of tooth roots. Dent Mater. 2009;25(6):721–8.
30. Manesh SK, Darling CL, Fried D. Nondestructive assessment of dentin demineralization using polarization-sensitive optical coherence tomography after exposure to fluoride and laser irradiation. J Biomed Mater Res B Appl Biomater. 2009;90(2):802–12.
31. Manesh SK, Darling CL, Fried D. Polarization-sensitive optical coherence tomography for the nondestructive assessment of the remineralization of dentin. J Biomed Opt. 2009;14(4):044002.
32. Otis LL, Al-Sadhan RI, Meiers J, Redford-Badwal D. Identification of occlusal sealants using optical coherence tomography. J Clin Dent. 2000;14(1):7–10.
33. Lenton P, Rudney J, Chen R, Fok A, Aparicio C, Jones RS. Imaging in vivo secondary caries and ex vivo dental biofilms using cross-polarization optical coherence tomography. Dent Mater. 2012;28(7):792–800.
34. Holtzman JS, Osann K, Pharar J, Lee K, Ahn YC, Tucker T, et al. Ability of optical coherence tomography to detect caries beneath commonly used dental sealants. Lasers Surg Med. 2010;42(8):752–9.
35. Tom H, Simon JC, Chan KH, Darling CL, Fried D. Near-infrared imaging of demineralization under sealants. J Biomed Opt. 2014;19(7):77003.

Use of Ultrasound for Caries Detection

21

Funda Çalışkan Yanıkoğlu and Dilek Tağtekin

21.1 Introduction

Sound is the propagation of mechanical energy through gases, liquids, and solids. Sound propagates well through most elastic or near-elastic solids and liquids, particularly those with low viscosities at ultrasonic frequencies above 20 kHz [1]. Human ear can perceive sound in the range of 50–18,000 cycles per second. Ultrasound means high-frequency sound waves in the range of 2–16 million cycles per second [1–3]. Human cannot hear ultrasound. In nature, bats and dolphins navigate by sonar capability.

As in general principle, the scanner used for ultrasonography generates electrical impulses that are converted into high-frequency sound waves by a transducer, electrical energy into ultrasonic energy [2]. Abrupt change in medium begins a series of vibrations that produce the sound waves transmitted into the test material or tissue being examined. Because of its acoustic impedance, a tissue has an internal echo pattern that is characteristic. Those echo patterns delineate different tissues, which may also be correlated with pathologic changes in a tissue. Any surface irregularities may cause diffusion and scattering. Sonic waves that are reflected back (echoes) toward the transducer cause a change in the thickness of the piezoelectric crystal, which in turn produces an electrical signal processed, and ultimately displayed on the monitor. The echoes will be reflected back with the existence of any discontinuity, and the presence of the defect will appear with low amplitude (Fig. 21.1) [2, 3].

F. Ç. Yanıkoğlu (✉)
Department of Operative Dentistry, Faculty of Dentistry, Marmara University, Istanbul, Turkey
e-mail: funday@tnn.net

D. Tağtekin
Faculty of Dentistry, Marmara University, Istanbul, Turkey

© Springer Nature Switzerland AG 2019

A. Ferreira Zandona, C. Longbottom (eds.), *Detection and Assessment of Dental Caries*, https://doi.org/10.1007/978-3-030-16967-1_21

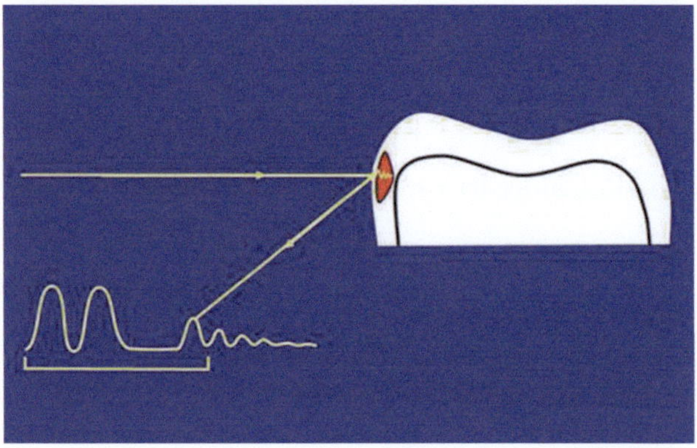

Fig. 21.1 The reflected echoes form the lesion and its amplitude seen on the screen indicating presence of difference and its predictable depth

Ultrasonic system (USG) could be adjusted according to the velocity of the material to be tested or just the thickness measurements of the test material can be performed [4, 5].

Ultrasound is extensively used on soft tissues such as measuring thickness of masticatory mucosa, besides hard tissue, bone for evaluation of intactness [6, 7].

21.2 In Dentistry

In daily clinical practice, USG has been implemented in periodontology in order to remove calculus, in endodontics for irrigation of root canals and for cleaning debris from the dental instruments [8]. It has been suggested as a method to measure the thickness of the masticatory mucosa [6] which may prove to be useful for determining the extent of soft tissue displacement under dentures by the forces of occlusion. It has been used as detection of dentino–enamel junction, dentino–pulp interface, and sonic velocities of enamel and dentin tissues of human, bovine, and dog teeth [2, 7, 9].

21.3 For Caries Detection

Specific acoustic impedance of mineral content of the body of enamel lesion has been introduced that the high-frequency pulse-echo ultrasound waves (18 MHz) can distinguish an intact and demineralized enamel surface [10–14]. Some studies detect the potential of USG in enamel demineralization and initial enamel caries [15–20, 23–30]. Briefly, studies (Table 21.1) have showed that USG provides promising and reliable results in detecting dental caries [16, 17, 24, 26], depth of lesion and wear [21, 22, 25], showing similar results to a gold standard measurement (microscopy and QLF) [13]), with high sensitivity and specificity [18].

Table 21.1 Studies on efficacy of ultrasound systems in diagnosis of initial caries lesions *(Marmara University, Faculty of Dentistry, Department of Restorative Dentistry)*

Authors and study design	Specimens	Methods	Outcomes
Yanikoglu et al. (1999) [20] In vitro	20 teeth with natural white spot lesions 890 μm in depth	USG, histological evaluation (microscope)	USG is qualitatively and quantitatively compatible with histological values on measuring natural white spot lesion with 890 μm
Caliskan Yanikoglu et al. (1999) [29] In vitro	1.5 × 2 × 1.5 mm of enamel specimens (*n* = 8), 60–70 μm	USG, Vickers hardness	USG may detect 60–70 μm demineralization and its remineralization (0, 300, 1500, 3000 ppm F)
Çalışkan Yanıkoglu et al. (2000) [18] In vitro	50 extracted human molars with natural white spot and no cavitation	USG, histological evaluation (microscope)	Sensitivity 88%; specificity 86% USG is able to detect subsurface structural changes
Bozkurt et al. (2002) [19] In vivo	710 μm enamel lesion; four patients, eight teeth	USG; light microscope	USG is able to detect lesions on buccal surface of enamel, even differentiate differences in lesion depth at mesial, distal, and central areas of buccal enamel
Tagtekin et al. (2008) [23] In vitro	42 permanent white/brown lesion	USG; DIAGNOdent; confocal laser scanning microscopy (CLSM)	Sensitivity 86%; specificity 84%; USG is able to detect enamel and dentine caries lesion
Bilgin et al. (2012) [30] In vitro	50 μm artificial enamel lesion	USG; microhardness	USG is able to detect 50 μm lesion and its remineralization by NaF toothpaste, herbal ginger and honey mixture, and rosemary oil
Bozkurt et al. (2013) [24] In vitro	64 enamel specimen	USG; QLF; confocal laser scanning microscopy (CLSM)	CLSM could detect lesions (20 μm), USG and QLF could not detect lesions in that depth
Avci et al. (2017) [26] In vitro	ICDAS I, II, III, IV, 200 teeth with natural caries lesion	USG; FluoreCam, light microscope	USG is consistent with ICDAS clinical evaluation on detecting lesion differences numerically
Yanikoglu et al. (2017) [27] In vitro	70 μm root caries lesion	USG; QLF; DIAGNOdent; CLSM	USG is able to detect lesions with 70 μm enamel caries lesion
Turkmen et al. (2018) [28] In vitro	53, 80, 140 μm of artificial enamel caries lesion	USG; microhardness; FluoreCam, light microscope	USG is able to detect lesions with 53, 80, 140 μm of enamel caries lesion

21.4 Clinical Technique

1. Adjustment of the ultrasonic instrument according to the procedure of desired process, such as velocity or depth measurements (Fig. 21.1).
2. Cleaning of tooth surface and air drying for 5 s.
3. Application of the coupling agent to tooth surface (Glycerin, medium gel).
4. Calibration of the probe using aluminum blocks and enamel/dentin specimens with standardized thickness and known velocity (Figs. 21.2 and 21.3).
5. Measurement of the sound enamel/dentin surface using the calibrated probe. Record the value when the first irregularity in amplitude is observed (repeat ×3 giving 5 s pause before measurements; calculate the mean value).

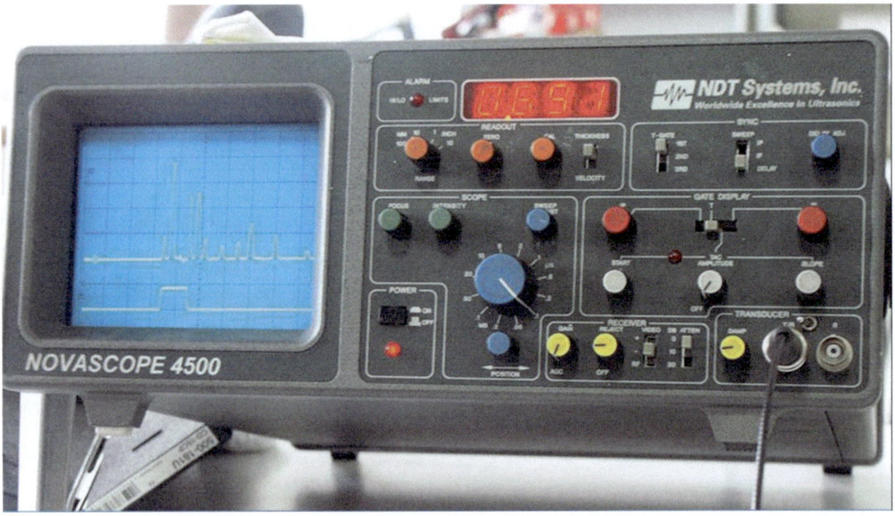

Fig. 21.2 Ultrasonic system (NDT, Novascope 4500)

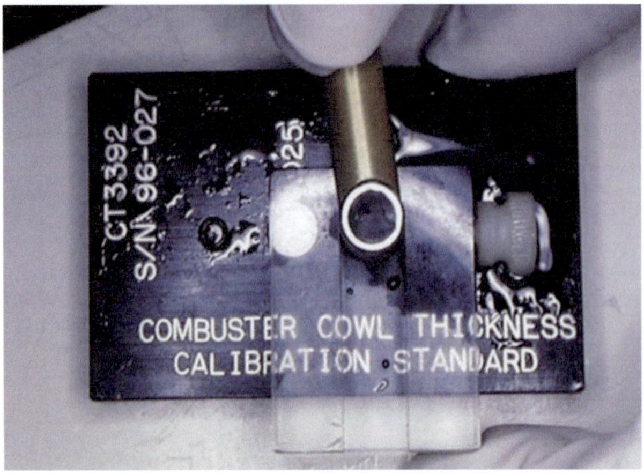

Fig. 21.3 Aluminum calibration block

6. Measurement of the carious enamel/dentin surface using the calibrated probe. Record the value when the first irregularity in amplitude is observed (repeat ×3 giving 5 s pause before measurements; calculate the mean value) (Figs. 21.4, 21.5, and 21.6).

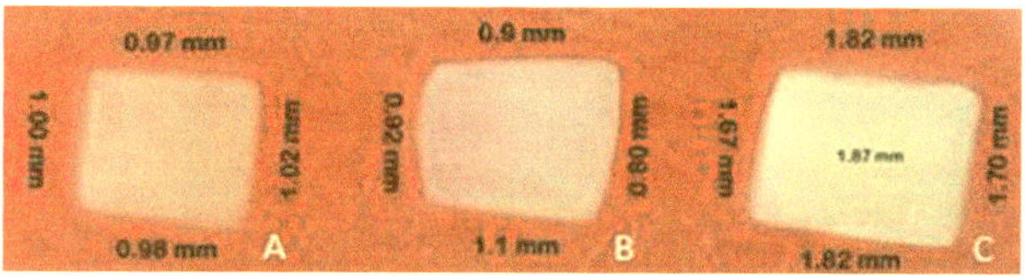

Fig. 21.4 Enamel calibration blocks (**a**, **b**); Enamel–dentin calibration block (**c**)

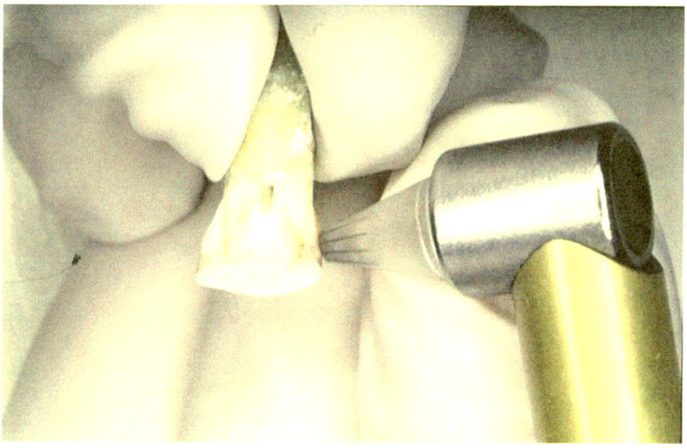

Fig. 21.5 Measurement by ultrasonic transducer

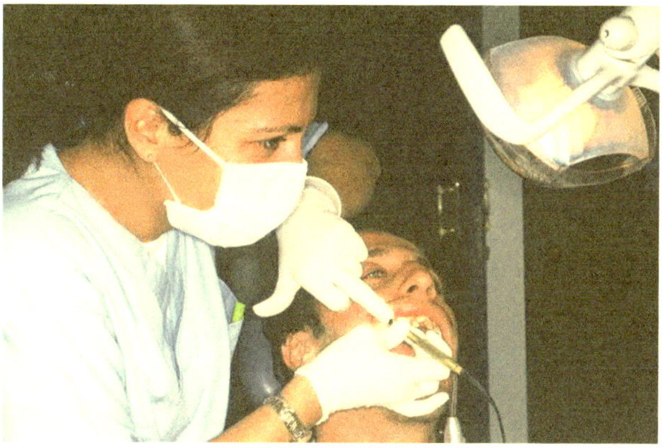

Fig. 21.6 Clinical application of the ultrasonic system by the operator

Summary table

Bitewing radiography	**Ultrasound**			
Which surfaces/ sites is it useful for	Occlusal (pits and fissures)	Proximal/ (approximal)	Smooth surface (buccal and lingual)	Root caries and which of the four surfaces?
	Unknown	**Unknown**	**Y**	**Y**

What type of lesions is valuable for	Primary coronal	Secondary coronal	Primary root caries	Secondary root caries
	Y	**Unknown**	**Y**	**Unknown**
What type of dentition	Primary		Permanent	
	Unknown		**Y**	
Lesion severity	Enamel lesions		Dentinal lesions	
	Y		**Y**	
Sensitivity	Literature reported range in **88%**			
Specificity	Literature reported range in **86%**			
Perceived Ease Of Use (PEOU)[a]	1. "**Ultrasonic device**" is easy to use 2. It is easy to become skillful at using "**Ultrasonic device**" 3. Learning to operate "**Ultrasonic device**" is easy 4. "**Ultrasonic device**" is flexible to interact with (resemble to handpiece) 5. My interaction with "**Ultrasonic device**" is clear and understandable 6. It is easy to interact with "**Ultrasonic device**"			
Advantages/ disadvantages	*Advantages*			
	1. Noninvasive 2. Quantitative 3. Repeatable and reproducible 4. Painless 5. Harmless 6. Easy to apply 7. Predicted depth of lesion 8. Differentiates structural differences over the time 9. Distinguish lesion depth differences 10. Distinguish tooth wear 11. Designed for benchtop use (Fig. 21.1)			
	Disadvantages			
	1. Lesion activity cannot be detected 2. Lesion size cannot be detected 3. It necessitates specific training 4. It works on smooth surfaces 5. It needs a coupling agent (glycerin)			
Time	**15–60 s**			
Cost	**$3500**			

[a]Davis (1989)

21.5 Concluding Remarks

Ultrasonic system can distinguish an intact and demineralized enamel surface due to specific acoustic impedance caused by changes in the mineral content. Some studies have demonstrated the potential use of USG for detection of initial enamel caries lesions, assessing lesion depth and wear with high sensitivity and specificity.

Acknowledgements We would like to thank **Dt. Zeynep Ceren Pehlivan** for her help in preparation of this manuscript and NDT Service of Turkish Airlines and valuable employees helping us with the system.

References

1. Curry TS, Dowdey JE, Murry RC. Christensen's physics of diagnostic radiology. 4th ed. Philadelphia: Lea & Febiger; 1990.
2. Barber FE, Lees S, Lobene RR. Ultrasonic pulse-echo measurements in teeth. Arch Oral Biol. 1969;14:745–60.
3. Cheeke N, David J. Fundamentals and applications of ultrasonic waves. 2nd ed. Boca Raton: Taylor & Francis; 2012.
4. Krautkramer J, Krautkramer H. Ultrasonic testing of materials. 2nd ed. New York: Springer; 1977.
5. Gratt BM. Imaging principles and techniques. In: Goaz PW, White SC, editors. Oral biology: principles and interpretation. St. Louis: Mosby; 1994. p. 286–90.
6. Kydd WL, Daly CH, Wheeler JB. The thickness measurement of masticatory mucosa in vivo. Int Dent J. 1971;21:430–41.
7. Katz JL, Meunier A. Scanning acoustic microscopy of human and canina cortical bone microstructure at high frequencies. In: Lowet G, et al., editors. Bone research in biomechanics. Amsterdam: IOS Press; 1997. p. 123–33.
8. Spranger H. Ultrasonic diagnosis of marginal periodontal diseases. Int Dent J. 1971;21:442–55.
9. John C. Directing ultrasound at the cement-enamel (CEJ) of human teeth: I. Asymmetry of ultrasonic path length. Ultrasonics. 2005;43:467–79.
10. Fukukita H, Yano T, Fukumoto A, Sawada K, Fujimosa T, et al. Development and application of an ultrasonic imaging system for dental diagnosis. J Clin Ultrasound. 1985;13:597–600.
11. Bab IA, Feuerstein O, Gazit D. Ultrasonic detector of proximal caries. Caries Res. 1997;31:32.
12. Gazit D, Ziv V, Bab I, Feuerstein O, Findler M, et al. In vitro/in vivo assessment of approximal caries using ultrasonic surface waves. J Dent Res. 1998;77:766.
13. Ziv V, Gazit D, Beris D, Feuerstein O, Aharonov L, et al. Correlative ultrasonic histologic and roentgenographic assessment of approximal caries. Caries Res. 1998;32:294.
14. Baum G, Greenwood I, Slawski S, Smirnov R. Observation of internal structures of teeth by ultrasonography. Science. 1963;139:495–6.
15. Ng SY, Ferguson MWJ, Payne PA, Slater P. Ultrasonic studies of unblemished and artificially demineralized enamel in extracted human teeth: a new method for detecting early caries. J Dent. 1988;16:201–9.
16. Lees S, Barber FE, Lobene RR. Dental enamel: detection of surface changes by ultrasound. Science. 1970;169:1314–6.
17. Fontana M, Caliskan Yanıkoglu F, Ozturk F, Ando M, Hayran O, Gonzalez-Cabezas C, Haider A, Baldridge LA, Stookey GK. Comparison of QLF, ultrasound and confocal microscopy in the measurement of demineralization/remineralization of enamel lesions developed on natural smooth surfaces. In: Proceedings of the 4th annual Indiana conference on early detection of dental caries II, Indianapolis, Indiana, 19–22 May 1999.
18. Caliskan FY, Ozturk F, Hayran O, Analoui M, Stookey GK. Detection of natural white spot caries lesions by an ultrasonic system. Caries Res. 2000;34:225–32.
19. Ozturk F, Tagtekin D, Kucukkeles N, Sur H, Yanikoglu F. In vivo ultrasonic detection of early enamel lesions: a pilot study. In: 49th Congress of the European Organisation for Caries Research (ORCA) (Abst. No: 57), Naantali, Finland, 4–6 July 2002.
20. Caliskan Yanıkoglu F, Ozturk F, Hayran O, Analoui M, Stookey GK. Detection of natural white spot caries lesions by ultrasonic system. In: Stookey GK, editor. Proceedings of the 6th annual Indiana conference on early detection of dental caries III, Spring Dot, Ohio, 1999. p. 107–12.
21. Tagtekin DA, Ozturk F, Lagerweij M, Hayran O, Stookey GK, Yanikoglu FC. Thickness measurement of worn molar cusp by ultrasound. Caries Res. 2005;39:139–43.
22. Ozturk FB, Tagtekin DA, Hayran O, Stookey GK, Yanıkoglu FC. Accuracy of ultrasound measurement of progressive change in occlusal enamel thickness. Oral Surg Oral Med Oral Pathol Oral Radiol Endod. 2005;99:101–5.

23. Tagtekin DA, Ozyoney G, Baseren M, Ando M, Hayran O, Alpar R, Gokalp S, Yanikoglu FC, Stookey GK. Caries detection with DIAGNOdent and ultrasound. Oral Surg Oral Med Oral Pathol Oral Radiol Endod. 2008;106(5):729–35.
24. Bozkurt FO, Tagtekin D, Yanıkoglu F, Fontana M, Gonzalez-Cabezas C, Stookey GK. Capability of an ultrasonic system to detect very early caries lesions on human enamel. Marmara Dent J. 2013;1:16–9.
25. Korkut B, Yanikoglu F, Tagtekin D. *In vitro* assessment of dimensional alterations of worn human incisors. Paripex Ind J Res. 2015;4:218–22.
26. Avcı H, Yanıkoglu F, Tagtekin D. Ultrasonic system as a diagnostic method on flat surface caries with different depths. In: 64th Congress of the European Organisation for Caries Research (ORCA) (Abst. No: 2993), Oslo Norway, 5–8 July 2017.
27. Yanikoglu F, Durmusoglu O, Tagtekin D, Hayran O. Ultrasound may aware us about initial root caries lesion. Ann Clin Lab Res. 2017;5(4):210.
28. Turkmen E, Tagtekin D, Yanikoglu F. Remineralization potential of a new toothpaste containing ginger and honey on different depth of enamel lesions. In: 65th Congress of the European Organisation for Caries Research (ORCA) (Abst. No: 15), Copenhagen, Denmark, 4–7 July 2018.
29. Caliskan Yanıkoglu F, Arslantunalı D, Akant O, Stookey GK. Early detection of enamel caries and its fluoridation by an ultrasonic system: a pilot study. In: Stookey GK, editor. Proceedings of the 6th annual Indiana conference on early detection of dental caries III, Spring Dot, Ohio, 1999. p. 112–6.
30. Bilgin G, Yanikoglu F, Tagtekin D, Hayran O, Stookey GK, Schemeron BR. Remineralization potential of herbal medicaments and assessment by ultrasound. In: 59th Congress of the European Organisation for Caries Research (ORCA) (Abst. No: 122), Brasil, 2012.

22 Bioluminescence Technology to Aid Lesion Activity Assessment

Christopher Longbottom and Bruce Vernon

22.1 Introduction

The CALCIVIS Imaging System is a novel device designed to enhance the assessment and management of demineralization due to dental caries and erosion. By indicating the presence of calcium ions, the system allows the "live" visualization of active enamel demineralization. Previous research has shown that active caries lesions exhibit ongoing demineralization of the enamel structure, leading to a loss of calcium ions from the hydroxyapatite of dental enamel [1]; therefore, the CALCIVIS Imaging System is intended to act as a model for assessing demineralization of teeth.

In cases where enamel is undergoing active demineralization, elevated levels of "free" calcium ions are present in the fluid-filled pores of dental enamel [2]. The system is designed to detect such "free" calcium ions via a calcium-sensitive photoprotein, and in response to this interaction between the calcium ions and the protein solution, a bioluminescent signal is emitted (Fig. 22.1) [3]. The device camera detects this luminescence—as a result of which a demineralization map of the tooth can be generated and presented to the user.

$$3Ca^{2+} + \text{Protein} \xrightarrow{h\upsilon \;\; \text{Blue Light}} \text{Apo-protein} + \text{Cofactor} + CO_2$$

Fig. 22.1 CALCIVIS photoprotein mode of action

C. Longbottom (✉)
King's College London Dental Institute, London, UK
e-mail: Christopher.longbottom@kcl.ac.uk

B. Vernon
Calcivis Ltd., Edinburgh, UK

© Springer Nature Switzerland AG 2019
A. Ferreira Zandona, C. Longbottom (eds.), *Detection and Assessment of Dental Caries*, https://doi.org/10.1007/978-3-030-16967-1_22

22.2 Detection of Calcium Ions

The primary mode of action of the CALCIVIS system is the bioluminescent emission from the photoprotein following binding of free calcium ions.

22.2.1 Bioluminescence

Figure 22.2 shows the images captured using the CALCIVIS system following the application of photoprotein solution to stock solutions of aqueous calcium chloride.

Using specialist imaging software [4], the intensity of the luminescence from each digital image can be quantified and plotted against calcium concentration, as shown in Fig. 22.3.

From this plot, a clear relationship can be observed between luminescence intensity and calcium ion concentration over a specific range limited by the photoprotein concentration (100 μg/mL). From this data, the limit of detection (LOD) and other key parameters can be calculated.

22.2.2 Acid Erosion (Ex-Vivo Teeth)

Sample extracted teeth have been subjected to successive acid challenges, using 30% phosphoric acid, 10 μL application to the occlusal surface. Figure 22.4 shows an example of the images obtained from one tooth using the CALCIVIS system.

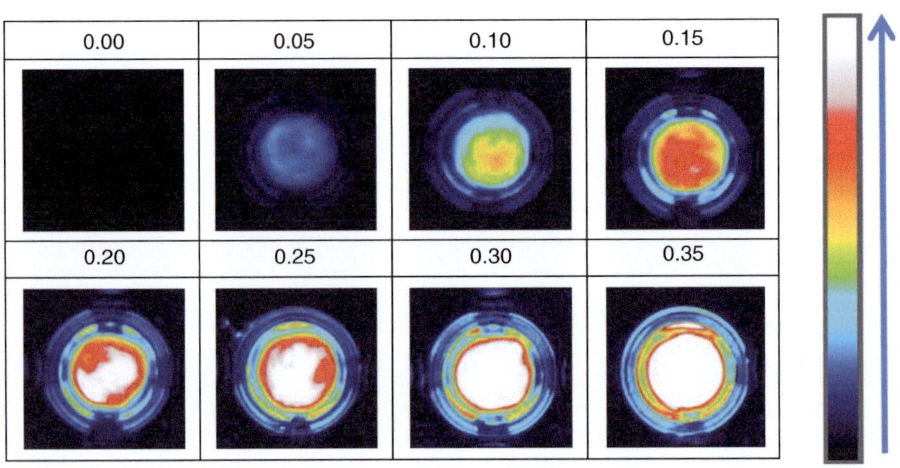

Fig. 22.2 Detection of calcium ions in solution (values given are equal to concentration of calcium chloride (mM)). A false-colored luminescence scale is provided for reference (Images owned and reproduced by kind permission of Calcivis Ltd., Edinburgh, UK)

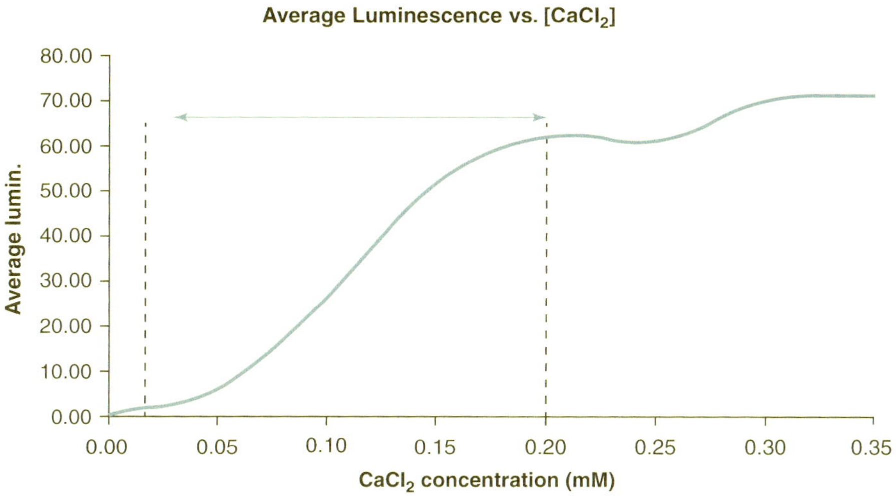

Fig. 22.3 Plot of average luminescence vs. calcium concentration (solution phase) (Image owned and reproduced by kind permission of Calcivis Ltd., Edinburgh, UK)

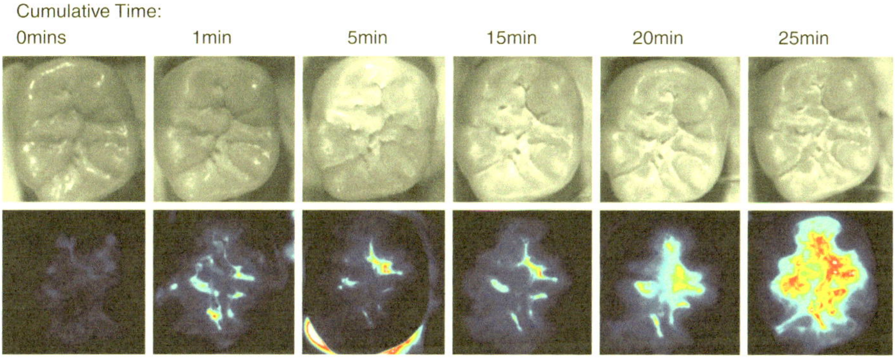

Fig. 22.4 Ex vivo teeth acid challenge results (Images owned and reproduced by kind permission of Calcivis Ltd., Edinburgh, UK)

The images captured show an increasing luminescent signal following successive acid challenge treatments, illustrating the relationship between acid demineralization and increased detection of free calcium ions.

22.2.3 Artificial Caries Lesion Demineralization

The CALCIVIS Imaging System has been used to evaluate the activity of in vitro caries lesions developed on sample enamel blocks (Fig. 22.5a) [5].

Figure 22.5b shows the results from using the CALCIVIS Imaging System on blocks with lesions at various stages of development.

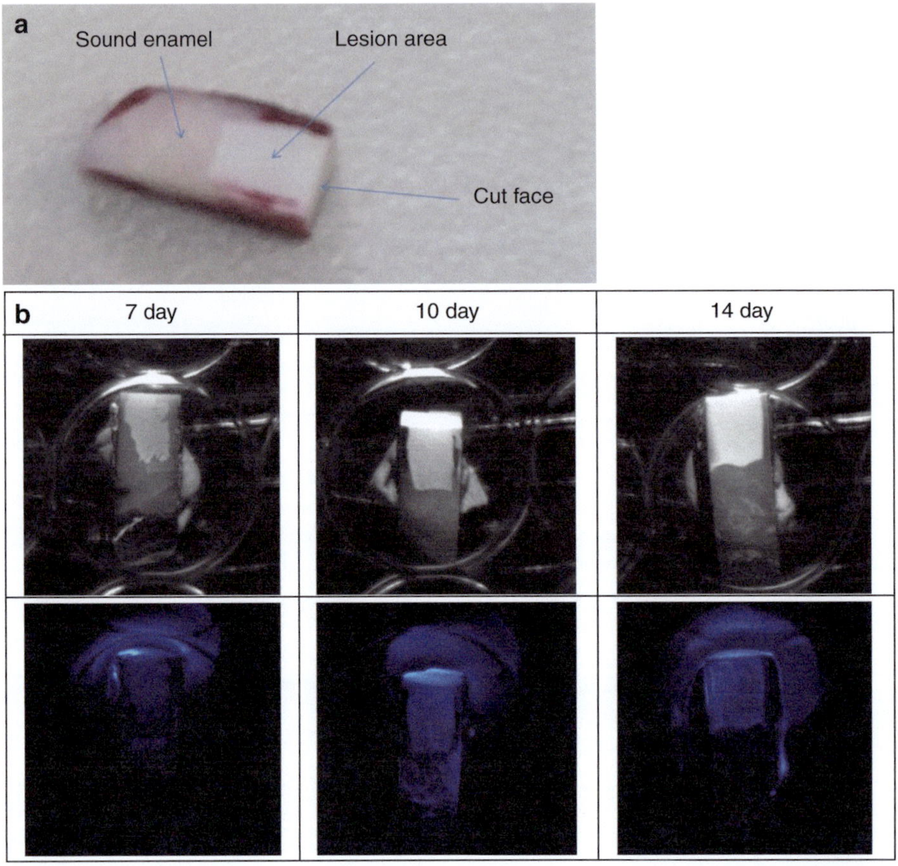

Fig. 22.5 (**a**) Enamel block. (Image owned and reproduced by kind permission of Calcivis Ltd., Edinburgh, UK). (**b**) CALCIVIS images of an enamel block as an in vitro caries lesion are generated (Images owned and reproduced by kind permission of Calcivis Ltd., Edinburgh, UK)

Blocks were prepared at a major oral care company's laboratories and imaged at CALCIVIS. The results show a significant increase in luminescence within the lesion area from the 10-day and 14-day samples compared to the 7-day sample, indicating progression of the lesion and increased demineralization of the enamel surface.

22.3 Caries Activity

The development of the natural caries lesion is a gradual and dynamic process where individual factors such as enamel structure, saliva composition, and oral hygiene may interfere in the lesion's development. Previous research has established a link between the development of active caries lesions and elevated calcium ion concentration within the fluid-filled pores of dental enamel [6]; therefore, the CALCIVIS System has the potential to be an effective tool for measuring a lesion's activity.

22.3.1 Active Lesions

Figure 22.6 shows sample images from ex vivo teeth with active lesions as identified by an experienced cariologist, according to ICDAS caries activity assessment guidelines.

The CALCIVIS System shows increased luminescence around the areas of the tooth displaying active caries lesions.

The images have been shown to be remarkably reproducible and persistent. Repeated imaging of the same tooth surface shows reproducible persistence of signal for up to five or six consecutive images, after which the signal starts to diminish due to depletion of the pool of available calcium ions available to the photoprotein.

22.3.2 Inactive Lesions

Figure 22.7 shows sample images from ex vivo teeth with inactive lesions as identified by an experienced cariologist.

The images above show no increased luminescence in the areas of interest, in these cases indicated by areas of dark staining. Even tactile examination of these teeth would present some difficulty in conclusively determining whether the lesions were still active or not. Using the CALCIVIS system, it is clear from the low level of luminescent response that no increased levels of calcium ions are present.

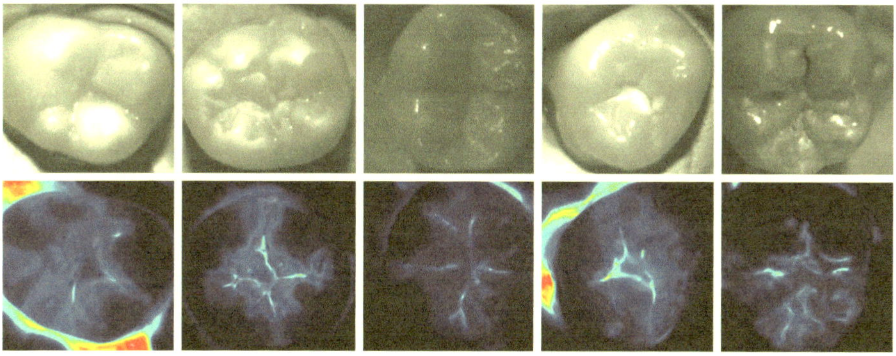

Fig. 22.6 Active caries lesions in five sample ex vivo molars imaged with the CALCIVIS Imaging System (Images owned and reproduced by kind permission of Calcivis Ltd., Edinburgh, UK)

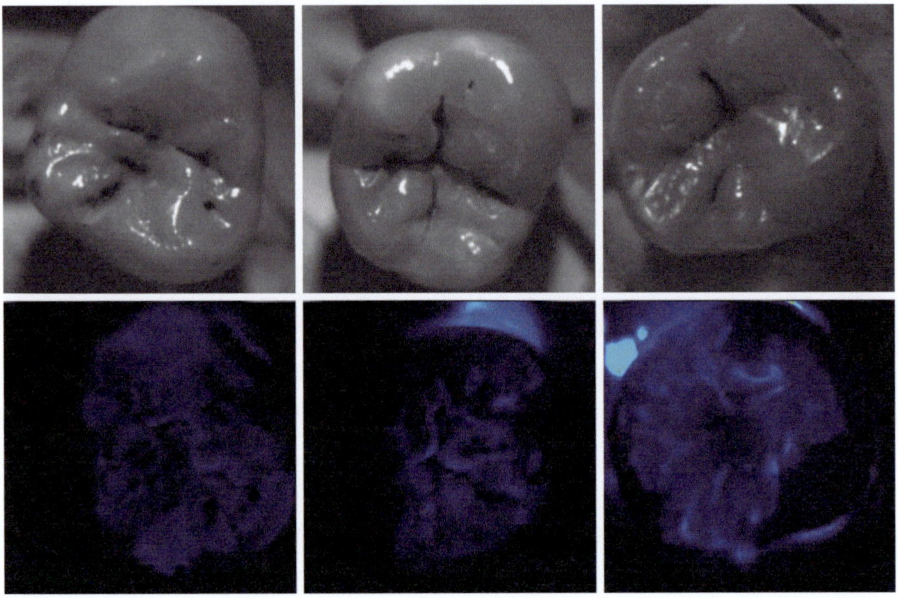

Fig. 22.7 Inactive caries lesions in three sample ex vivo molars imaged with the CALCIVIS Imaging System (Images owned and reproduced by kind permission of Calcivis Ltd., Edinburgh, UK)

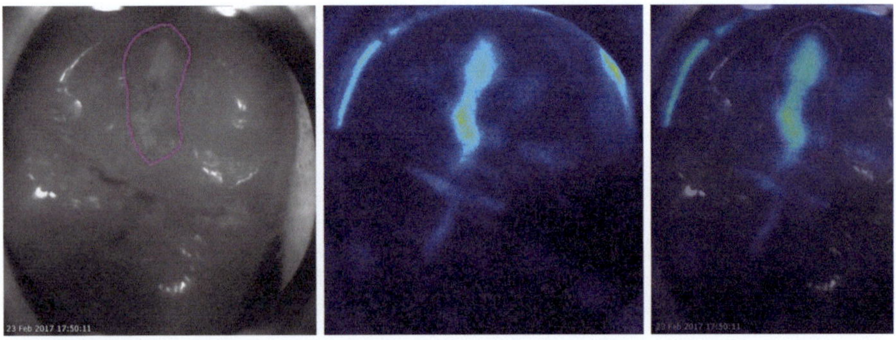

Fig. 22.8 Active caries lesions in a sample in vivo molar imaged with the CALCIVIS Imaging System (Images owned and reproduced by kind permission of Calcivis Ltd., Edinburgh, UK)

In vitro studies have shown that the calcium in saliva and the dental biofilm do not act as confounders in vivo provided the tooth being imaged is cleaned, isolated from saliva and gently air-dried prior to imaging with the CALCIVIS System.

22.3.2.1 In Vivo Images

Figure 22.8 shows an example of the types of images generated in vivo by the CALCIVIS Imaging system. From left to right, a lower molar has been imaged,

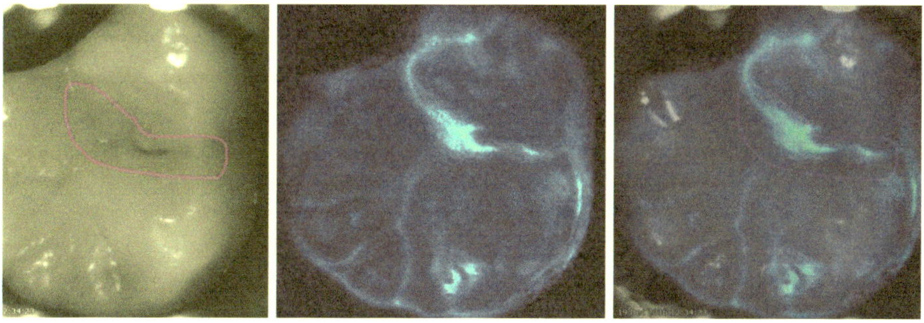

Fig. 22.9 Active caries lesion in a sample in vivo molar imaged with the CALCIVIS Imaging System (Images owned and reproduced by kind permission of Calcivis Ltd., Edinburgh, UK)

producing first a black and white image with an area (outlined in purple) indicated by a general practitioner as containing an *active* white spot lesion. The middle image shows the false-colored luminescence image, displaying specific areas of increased luminescence. The image on the right is the merged (overlapped) image of the first two images and shows that the area of the greatest increase in luminescence corresponds to the site of the active white spot lesion. Other areas of active demineralization are present within the fissure system of the tooth.

Figure 22.9 shows a further example of a set of CALCIVIS images generated when imaging a molar in vivo. As in Fig. 22.8, the highlighted suspected *active* lesion displays an increased luminescent signal, indicating active demineralization is present, with other aspects of the fissure system displaying increased luminescence compared to the adjacent sound enamel.

22.4 Concluding Remarks

The above evidence shows the system's capability to detect free calcium ions liberated from the crystalline enamel structure as a result of dental demineralization, for example, during caries formation and erosion. The bioluminescent emission from the photoprotein following binding of free calcium ions is proportional to the concentration of calcium ions present and can therefore be used to assess the extent of demineralization during erosive challenge and caries lesion formation.

In addition, time course studies in vitro have demonstrated the system's ability to monitor both demineralization and remineralization of the enamel surface.

A technique to identify ***active*** demineralizing lesions (compared to techniques and technologies to ***detect*** caries lesions which *may or may not be active*) is of critical importance in aiding clinicians in their diagnostic assessments and therapeutic/treatment decision-making within the arena of preventive dental healthcare. Ongoing further research into the novel CALCIVIS Imaging System will help determine the extent of its potential role in aiding dental practitioners, particularly in the field of preventive dentistry.

References

1. Fejerskov O, Kidd E. Dental caries: the disease and its clinical management. Hoboken: Wiley; 2008. p. 211.
2. Fabregas R, Rubinstein J. On the initial propagation of dental caries. J R Soc Interface. 2014;11:20140809.
3. Deng L, Markova SV, Vysotski ES, Liu ZJ, Lee J, Rose J, Wang BC. Crystal structure of a Ca2+-discharged photoprotein. J Biol Chem. 2004;279(32):33647–52.
4. ImageJ Software by National Institutes of Health, USA. https://imagej.nih.gov/ij/.
5. Lynch RJM, Mony U, ten Cate JM. Effect of lesion characteristics and mineralizing solution type on enamel remineralization in vitro. Caries Res. 2007;41:257–62.
6. Featherstone JD, Holmen L, Thylstrup A, Fredebo L, Shariati M. Chemical and histological changes during development of artificial caries. Caries Res. 1985;19(1):1–10.

Part V

Treatment Decision After Detection

Clinical Decision-Making in Caries Management: Role of Caries Detection and Diagnosis

23

Margherita Fontana and Marie-Charlotte D. N. J. M. Huysmans

23.1 The Role of Caries Detection and Diagnosis in the Process of Clinical Decision-Making

Dental caries is a multifactorial, dynamic disease process that results from a dysbiosis in the biofilm, driven by exposure to sugars and other carbohydrates, which over time leads to demineralization of dental hard tissues [1, 2]. As explained in earlier chapters, this disease process is characterized by the formation of caries lesions, located in different tissues (i.e., enamel vs. dentin) and surfaces (e.g., occlusal, proximal, and root), which allow for different clinical accesses. If the disease is allowed to continue unchecked, caries lesions of increased severity will develop. However, as the disease activity can vary over time, lesions can also go through stages of progression and arrest. The accurate detection and assessment of existing caries lesions, and their monitoring over time, is an essential step in the diagnostic process leading to a clinical decision about how to best manage, in a patient-centered manner, both the disease and the resulting caries lesions. In fact, it has been stated that as modern caries management stresses a conservative and preventive evidence-based philosophy, with patient-centered risk-based disease management, early detection of caries lesions and efforts to remineralize and/or arrest lesions are crucial in order to preserve tooth structure and maintain health [3, 4]. Furthermore, this caries management philosophy is the basis for current cariology education frameworks worldwide [5, 6].

M. Fontana (✉)
Department of Cariology, Restorative Sciences and Endodontics, University of Michigan School Dentistry, Ann Arbor, MI, USA
e-mail: mfontan@umich.edu

M.-C. D. N. J. M. Huysmans
Department of Dentistry, Radboud University Medical Center, Nijmegen, Netherlands
e-mail: marie-charlotte.huysmans@radboudumc.nl

© Springer Nature Switzerland AG 2019

A. Ferreira Zandona, C. Longbottom (eds.), *Detection and Assessment of Dental Caries*, https://doi.org/10.1007/978-3-030-16967-1_23

23.2 Clinical Decision-Making: Definition

Although there are numerous definitions in the healthcare literature of clinical decision-making, they all agree decision-making involves a process that results in choosing between options for clinical care. This process is not simple, but rather complex. It is based on information that needs to be first gathered (e.g., caries lesion characteristics from caries detection tools), then it needs to be analyzed to help identify potentially effective, evidence-based alternative solutions, and these then need to be weighted as to their risks and consequences for a particular individual, to then reach a judgment or decision (together with the patient) on how to manage the disease in a personalized manner [7]. Thus, clinical decision-making is a process that includes clinical reasoning or critical thinking [8–10]. Critical thinking involves scrutinizing, differentiating, and appraising information and evidence, as well as reflecting on information to make judgments that will help problem-solving and inform clinical decisions [11].

Factors affecting this process are described next.

23.2.1 General Factors Influencing Clinical Decision-Making

23.2.1.1 Evidence

The move in the last several decades toward evidence-based medicine and dentistry has prompted a paradigm shift in clinical practice that calls for making informed clinical decisions based on best available evidence. As the amount of evidence available grows, learning how to find and access it, as well as how to interpret its quality and relevance has become paramount to clinical care. Courses on how to find and interpret evidence are now part of the dental curricula of many dental schools around the world; yet the busy clinician, even if trained, lacks in many cases the time to search and interpret findings for the many topics he/she needs to master in everyday practice. Moreover, many of the questions or problems are faced by the dental profession at large and should be addressed on a larger scale. Thus, national and international authorities or professional groups (e.g., the Institutes of Medicine [IOM], the World Health Organization [WHO], the American Dental Association [ADA], the National Institute for Health and Care Excellence (NICE), and the Centers for Disease Control and Prevention [CDC]) have a very important role to play. These groups have the expertise and resources to develop recommendations or evidence-based practice guidelines and other guidance documents (e.g., expert consensus statements) that can help decision-making as they synthesize evidence so that it can be used for clinical care. In fact in the last decades, numerous guidelines or systems have been developed for caries management (e.g., [12–16])

The difference between evidence-based practice guidelines and expert consensus statements will be described next. In 2011, the Institute of Medicine (IOM) [17] defined clinical practice guidelines as "statements that include recommendations intended to optimize patient care that are informed by a systematic review of evidence and an assessment of the benefits and harms of alternative care options." Thus, when evidence is available, a rigorous process including a systematic review and a systematic grading of levels of evidence is preferred (e.g., GRADE, [18]). There are many existing systematic reviews around different topics related to cariology, and sites like the Cochrane Library, which houses systematic reviews on multiple oral health topics, are an important resource for clinical decision-making, by clinicians, guideline developers, healthcare providers, and patients [19]. Systematically developed evidence-based practice guidelines, using the AGREE II instrument [20], are more robust than any other alternative, and when available these guidelines should be incorporated into the decision-making process.

However, when available evidence is limited or scarce, professional societies or expert-based groups are used to develop expert consensus guidance (also called consensus reports, task force position papers, or position statements) to aid clinicians in decision-making [21]. These consensus reports summarize the opinions of an expert panel on a particular topic that is generally narrower and more focused than that of a clinical guideline (e.g., expert-based recommendations on managing caries lesions [22]). In many cases, consensus among the experts needs to be reached, and consensus development methods, such as the Delphi process, nominal group technique, or consensus development conference, are then used [23].

In the future, as the complexity of evidence grows, decision-making will increasingly require decision support and computational systems to help guide the decision-making process. Electronic health systems can also be made to "learn" from applying evidence to solve clinical problems to individual cases, thus further helping to adapt evidence-based decision trees to local populations.

23.2.1.2 Patient

Clinical decision-making involves more than evidence; clinicians should understand the evidence and individualize decision-making according to individual patients' needs and desires. Thus, dentists must reconcile best evidence with patient characteristics and preferences, which results in a process in which individuals are informed of the best available evidence and all relevant options, and share in the decision-making. It is important to remember that evidence-based clinical practice guidelines are generally based on the "average patient," and the strength of the evidence and resulting recommendations will help guide the clinician to how much or not it is suggested this be generalized or not to individual patients. For example, using the GRADE criteria, for "strong recommendations," most people would want the recommended course of action, and only a small proportion would not. Formal decision aids are not likely to be needed to help people make decisions consistent with their values and preferences. On the other hand, for "conditional recommendations," it is important to recognize that different choices will be appropriate for individual patients and that clinicians must help each patient arrive at a management decision consistent with his or her values and preferences. Decision aids may be useful in helping people do this [15].

This process of negotiation between clinicians and patients in developing a treatment plan is referred to as shared decision-making. Shared decision-making is the basis for obtaining informed consent [24] and allows for a patient-centered approach in decision-making.

23.2.1.3 Dentist

Among the many factors that are related to treatment decisions, the dentists' knowledge and clinical expertise play a very important role in being able to identify alternatives and implement them. Attending continuing education courses, study clubs, etc. are examples of important ways for the dental professional to remain a lifelong learner, adapting to the ever changing evidence landscape in cariology.

23.3 Specific Factors Guiding Clinical Decision-Making for Caries Lesion Management

Decision-making for management of individual caries lesions is based on the same general factors discussed previously. In addition, there are specific individual- and tooth-level factors that also guide this decision-making process and are described next.

23.3.1 Risk Assessment

Risk assessment is an essential component in the decision-making process for the correct prevention and management of dental caries. Dentistry has entered an era of personalized care (i.e., "personalized dentistry"), in which targeting care to individuals or groups based on their risk has been advocated as a means to make use of limited existing recourses and avoid under- or overtreatment, especially when the disease process is unequally distributed among the population (i.e., there are groups in which dental caries prevalence and incidence are significantly higher). The process of assigning a level of risk of caries involves determining the probability of incidence of caries, and as a result the probability that there will be a progression of caries lesions [25]. Usually, demographic, social, behavioral, and biological variables, along with the clinical/radiographic examination and supplementary tests, are used to develop a caries risk profile or category (e.g., low, moderate, or high caries risk [26]). For a clinician, the concepts of assessment of risk and prognosis are important parts of clinical decision-making. In fact, the dentist's overall subjective impression of the patient might have good predictive power for caries risk [27].

23.3.2 Lesion Characteristics

Of utmost importance is to clearly define lesion thresholds and clinical conditions that separate restorative from non-restorative caries interventions, as these have immediate treatment consequences. The ability to differentiate between the stages of lesion development or to establish the appropriate detection thresholds for these stages depends on the detection method and/or criteria being used as discussed in previous chapters. A recent expert-based consensus report suggested the following lesion characteristics to aid the decision on when to intervene restoratively [22]:

(a) Lesion cavitation
(b) Level of cleansability
(c) Lesion activity

Although cavitation is at the top of this list, as mentioned below, cavitation in itself is not a strict criterion, but largely used as a surrogate for lesion activity. Lesion activity may be considered the main criterion, but it carries the complication that there are no evidence-based, validated, reproducible, and accurate diagnostic systems for its measurement.

Thus, the following are general expert-based recommendations [22] based on caries lesion detection and diagnosis to help guide the decision-making process:

(a) Arrested caries lesions do not require caries interventions (restorative or non-restorative), except to address issues associated with esthetics, function, or risk for pulp death.

    These lesions can be present in patients that are at high, moderate, or low risk of future caries. If at risk, patients should receive preventive advice or interventions to reduce the risk of developing future caries lesions (e.g., sealants for occlusal surfaces [16]).

(b) Non-cavitated active lesions should be treated using evidence-based non-restorative methods.

    Evidence-based practice guidelines for non-restorative treatment options are available [15]. In addition, patients with these lesions will be considered at risk for future caries lesions and thus should receive preventive interventions.

(c) Certain occlusal lesions might appear clinically non-cavitated but radiographically extend significantly into dentin. These lesions can be treated non-restoratively (i.e., using fissure sealants), but the integrity of the sealant needs to be monitored as there is a possibility, until more evidence has emerged, that a "trampoline" effect may lead to failure of the sealant and a restoration will be required.

(d) Most cavitated lesions are non-cleansable, and thus active. These lesions cannot normally be managed by biofilm removal, remineralization, or fissure sealing alone, and thus in general will need to be restored.

    Patients with these lesions will be considered at risk in the near future for future caries lesions and thus should receive preventive advice or interventions.

23.4 Concluding Remarks

Accurate detection and monitoring of lesions, determination of lesion progression/activity and thus the presence of disease, and a patient's risk of future disease are cornerstones of modern patient-centered caries decision-making with the goal of preserving tooth structure and maintaining health. The strength of the evidence, patient characteristics, patient preference, and dentist's expertise need to be considered in the decision-making process.

References

1. Fontana M, Wolff M, Feathertone JBD. Introduction to ICNARA 3. Adv Dent Res. 2018;29(1):3.
2. Selwitz RH, Ismail AI, Pitts NB. Dental caries. Lancet. 2007;369(9555):51–9.
3. Fontana M, Gonzalez-Cabezas C, Fitzgerald M. Cariology for the 21st century—current caries management concepts for dental practice. J Mich Dent Assoc. 2013;95:32–40.
4. Slayton RL, Fontana M, Young D, Tinanoff N, Nový B, Lipman RD, Robinson L. Dental caries management in children and adults. Discussion paper. Washington, DC: National Academy of Medicine; 2016. https://nam.edu/wpcontent/uploads/2016/09/Dental-Caries-Management-in-Children-and-Adults.pdf.
5. Fontana M, Guzman-Armnstrong S, Schenkel AB, Allen KL, Featherstone J, Goolsby S, Kanjirath P, Kolker P, Martignon S, Pitts N, Schulte A, Slayton RL, Young D, Wolff M. Development of a core curriculum in cariology for US dental schools. J Dent Educ. 2016;80(6):705–20.
6. Schulte AG, Pitts NB, Huysmans MC, Splieth C, Buchalla W. European core curriculum in cariology for undergraduate dental students. Eur J Dent Educ. 2011;15(1):9–17.
7. Tiffen J, Corbridge SJ, Slimmer L. Enhancing clinical decision making: development of a contiguous definition and conceptual framework. J Prof Nurs. 2014;30(5):399–405.
8. Croskerry P. Achieving quality in clinical decision making: cognitive strategies and detection of bias. Acad Emerg Med. 2002;9:1184–204.
9. Matteson P, Hawkins J. Concept analysis of decision making. Nurs Forum. 1990;25:4–10.
10. Orme L, Maggs C. Decision-making in clinical practice: how do expert nurses, midwives and health visitors make decisions? Nurse Educ Today. 1993;13:270–6.
11. Fontana M, Gonzalez-Cabezas C, de Peralta T, Johnsen D. Dental education required for the changing healthcare environment. J Dent Educ. 2017;81:eS153–61.
12. Ismail AI, Tellez M, Pitts NB, Ekstrand KR, Ricketts D, Longbottom C, Eggertsson H, Deery C, Fisher J, Young DA, Featherstone JDB, Evans W, Zeller GG, Zero D, Martingon S, Fontana M, Zandona A. Caries management pathways preserve dental tissues and promote oral health. Community Dent Oral Epidemiol. 2013;41(1):e12–40.
13. Pitts NB, Ekstrand KR, ICDAS Foundation. International caries detection and assessment system (ICDAS) and its international caries classification and management system (ICCMS)—methods for staging of the caries process and enabling dentists to manage caries. Community Dent Oral Epidemiol. 2013;41(1):41–52.
14. SIGN138. Scottish Intercollegiate Guidelines Network (SIGN). Dental interventions to prevent caries in children. Edinburgh: SIGN; 2014.
15. Slayton R, Urquhart O, Araujo MB, Fontana M, Guzman-Armstrong S, Nascimento MM, Novy B, Tinanoff N, Weyant R, Wolff MS, Young DA, Zero D, Tampi MP, Pilcher L, Banfield L, Carrasco-Labra A. Evidence-based clinical practice guideline on nonrestorative treatments for caries lesions: a report from the American Dental Association. J Am Dent Assoc. 2018;149(10):837–49.
16. Wright JT, Tampi MP, Graham L, Estrich C, Crall J, Fontana M, Gillette J, Novy B, Dhar V, Donly K, Hewlett E, Quinonez R, Chaffin J, Crespin M, Iafolla T, Griffin S, Siegal M, Carrasco-Labra A. Evidence-based clinical practice guidelines for the use of pit-and-fissure sealants: a report of the American Dental Association and the American Academy of Pediatric Dentistry. J Am Dent Assoc. 2016;147(8):672–82.

17. IOM (Institute of Medicine). Clinical practice guidelines we can trust. Washington, DC: The National Academies Press; 2011.
18. Alonso-Coello P, Oxman AD, Moberg J, et al. GRADE evidence to decision (EtD) frameworks: a systematic and transparent approach to making well informed healthcare choices, part 2: clinical practice guidelines. BMJ. 2016;353:i2089.
19. Worthington H, Clarkson J, Weldon J. Priority oral health research identification for clinical decision-making. Evid Based Dent. 2015;16:69–71.
20. Brouwers MC, Kho ME, Browman GP, Burgers JS, Cluzeau F, Feder G, Fervers B, Graham ID, Grimshaw J, Hanna SE, Littlejohns P, Makarski J, Zitzelsberger L, for the AGREE Next Steps Consortium. AGREE II: advancing guideline development, reporting and evaluation in healthcare. CMAJ. 2010;182:E839–42.
21. Kwong JSW, Chen H, Sun X. Development of evidence-based recommendations: implications for preparing expert consensus statements. Chin Med J. 2016;129(24):2998–3000.
22. Schwendicke F, Frenchen J, Bjørndal L, Maltz M, Manton DJ, Ricketts D, Van Landuyt K, Banerjee A, Campus G, Doméjean S, Fontana M, Leal S, Lo E, Machiulskiene V, Schulte A, Splieth C, Zandona A, Innes N. Managing carious lesions: recommendations on carious tissue removal. Adv Dent Res. 2016;28:58–67.
23. Black N, Murphy M, Lamping D, McKee M, Sanderson C, Askham J, et al. Consensus development methods: a review of best practice in creating clinical guidelines. J Health Serv Res Policy. 1999;4:236–48.
24. Bauer J, Spackman S, Chiappelli F, Prolo P. Evidence-based decision making in dental practice. J Evid Based Dent Pract. 2005;5(3):125–30.
25. Fontana M, Zero D. Assessing patients' caries risk. J Am Dent Assoc. 2006;137(9):1231–40.
26. Twetman S, Fontana M. Patient caries risk assessment. Monogr Oral Sci. 2009;21:91–101.
27. Fontana M. The clinical, environmental and behavioral factors that foster early childhood caries. Pediatr Dent. 2015;37:217–25.

Integrating Caries Detection Devices into Clinical Practice

24

Stephen Abrams

24.1 Introduction

Dental caries is a disease that results in the destruction of tooth structure. The right tools to detect those changes will allow detection and monitoring of caries lesions.

All detection techniques take advantage of a specific part of the electromagnetic spectrum (including light, heat, or ultrasound) and its interaction with sound and carious tooth structure. These fundamental interactions are classified in Fig. 24.1, from work published by Hall and Girkin in 2004 [1]. X-rays (see Chaps. 11–13) involve both transmission and scattering. The scattering occurs when they encounter calcified tissue and restorations. Visual examination (see Chaps. 5–8) involves the reflection and scattering of light from the tooth surface where the severity of decay can be inferred from examining teeth in wet and dry fields. The newer technologies are combinations of these various phenomena including fluorescence, absorption with heat production, etc.

Fluorescence (see Chaps. 16 and 17) is simply the emission of light from an object that has absorbed light at a specific wavelength [2]. These devices produce glow from the tooth surface when an LED or laser light is shone on the tooth. The literature indicates that the glow or fluorescence may be from one or more of the following, whether or not caries is present [2–8], fluorophores within the DEJ; bacterial porphyrins (bacterial breakdown product) [5]; stain; calculus; or food debris.

The original version of this chapter was revised. A correction to this chapter can be found at https://doi.org/10.1007/978-3-030-16967-1_27

S. Abrams (✉)
Quantum Dental Technologies Inc., Toronto, ON, Canada
e-mail: stephen@thecanarysystem.com

© Springer Nature Switzerland AG 2019

A. Ferreira Zandona, C. Longbottom (eds.), *Detection and Assessment of Dental Caries*, https://doi.org/10.1007/978-3-030-16967-1_24

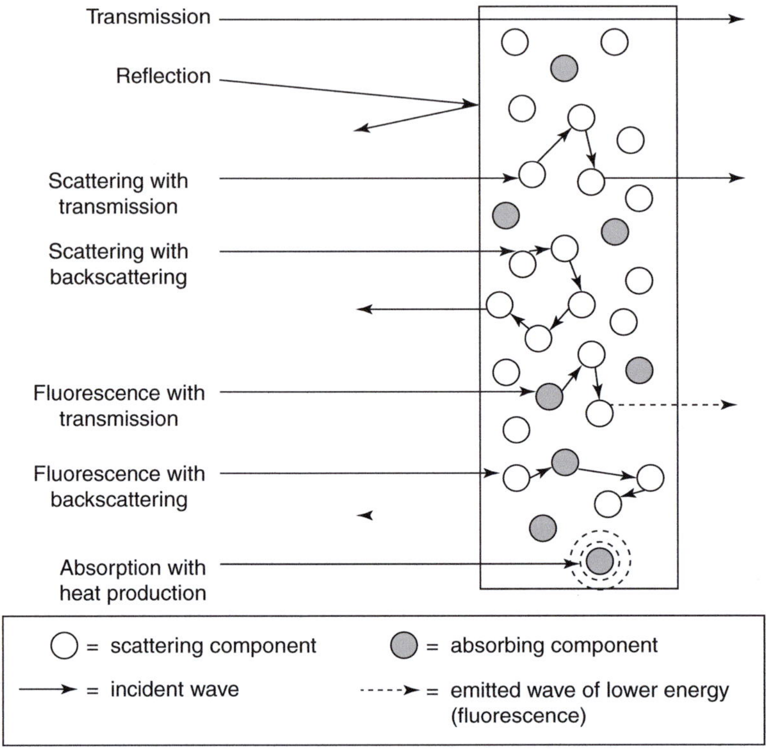

Fig. 24.1 Interaction of energy including light and heat with a material such as a tooth surface. Image is courtesy of Hall A, Girkin, J.M. A review of potential new diagnostic modalities for caries lesions. Journal of Dental Research 2004;83(Spec No C):C89–94

Many methods do not provide information regarding the crystal structure of the tooth. There are a number of other factors that influence the sensitivity of these detection systems such as the wavelength of light (portion of the electromagnetic spectrum), the resolution and sensitivity of the detection system, and the distance of the detector from the tooth surface. Longer wavelengths penetrate deeper into tooth structure but may miss small areas of decay. One needs to consider all these factors when considering the various caries detection systems on the market.

The final consideration is the area of the tooth being examined and the presence of existing restorations, sealants, or orthodontic brackets. Early interproximal lesions and caries around restorations present major challenges for some diagnostic systems. At times, the restoration may also interfere or reflect a particular wavelength of light from the restoration. This may interfere with the ability of the device to accurately examine the interface between the tooth and the restoration [9–15]. Detecting and monitoring caries under sealants also may have some challenges as the sealant may impede or block the particular wavelength of electromagnetic energy from penetrating the sealant [16–20]. Detecting early caries around orthodontic brackets may also present a challenge from some caries detection systems as the bracket may impede the signal [21, 22]. All these clinical situations should be assessed when deciding how to use and integrate a caries detection system into clinical practice.

24.2 Detection Tools and Patient Engagement

Some of the methods discussed in this book allow for patient engagement. Methods with imaging capability and quantification can more easily be explained to patients, helping both the operator and the patient to understand what is being measured. Radiographs (Chaps. 11–13) are familiar to patients and changes can be easily indicated, but usually no quantification is provided. At times, patients may not be able to see the small black or grey areas associated with early interproximal lesions. Near-infrared transillumination (Chap. 15) has the imaging capability but no quantification. The system based on photothermal radiometry and modulated luminescence, The Canary System (Chap. 18) has a voice which provides a number after each 5 s scan as well as imaging ability. Systems based on fluorescence (QLF) (Chap. 16) have the imaging capability and quantification ability, while others have the quantification ability but no imaging.

Integrating this data into existing electronic records is something that the clinician must consider. Most systems are standalone. Systems that rely on the cloud must meet HIPPA and PIPEDA privacy requirements that allows dental offices to view and manage their patient data. An example is the Canary Cloud, an online environment, where the Canary Scan data can be viewed for each patient by tooth number and surface over a given time period. Customized reports for the dental team, patient and third party carriers can be beneficial to vizuallized data and monitor changes.

24.2.1 How to Integrate These Systems into Clinical Practice

These diagnostic aids can be integrated in at least three ways [23]:

1. As part of the new patient exam or emergency examination to determine if the tooth is fractured or has caries which is causing pain on temperature changes or when chewing
2. As part of the preventive re-care examination
3. As part of a prevention program to detect, monitor, and document demineralization and remineralization [24, 25]

The systems can be used as a diagnostic tool during a new patient exam. Depending on the system selected it can be used to scan a number of suspected areas including around the margins of restorations, occlusal pits and fissures, smooth surfaces, and interproximal areas. It is very important to note that many systems cannot be used across all surfaces, in both coronal and root caries or around restorations. Some systems like The Canary allow the information to be stored on the cloud and the patient is given a report or can access their information online following the appointment. Others will require notes in the patient chart or importing images. In most practices, new patient exam is completed before a dental hygiene appointment. As stated in Chap. 2, teeth need to be clean before an accurate examination can be performed. For patients with significant biofilm buildup, a professional brushing or dental prophylaxis would be indicated prior to an exam with most of the methods described, with few exceptions (like radiographs or The Canary System).

During the re-call appointment, the devices can be used to scan a few selected teeth. If caries are found that require restoration, one then arranges for further treatment. If there are white spots, brown spots, and other areas of demineralization, the chosen method can be performed on only a few areas. The patient can then return for either a more complete examination or begin a customized remineralization program using the initial assessments as bench marks to measure and monitor the outcomes of the remineralization therapy. Since many of the devices do not have quantification abilities, it is important to write copious notes of findings. For systems which have a quantification, the initial numbers can be used to monitor the lesions.

If a practice were going to have the patient involved in a remineralization program, it could begin the program right at the re-call visit by applying an in-office therapy and dispensing home-based products. If there are large areas of demineralization, they could arrange to have the patient back for a 30 min visit where they could scan a number of teeth and then apply the remineralization therapy [26].

Integrating new technology and new diagnostic devices into a clinical practice may take some additional time. There needs to be time set aside to train staff both on the use and interpretation of the findings from the device. There also needs to be time set aside to take the various measurements and record the findings in a clinical chart. Finally there is also need to introduce this technology to patients with a very short and simple explanation and also an interpretation of the findings from the examination. The American and Canadian Dental Associations have now introduced billing codes which allow providers to bill for a caries examination that does not use radiographs.

24.2.2 American Dental Association Billing Code D0600

In April 2016, The American Dental Association (ADA) Code Maintenance Committee approved the addition of a procedure code for caries detection (D0600) with the following nomenclature:

> ***"Non-ionizing diagnostic procedure capable of quantifying, monitoring, and recording changes in structure of enamel, dentin and cementum."***

24.2.3 Canadian Dental Association Billing Code 04220–04229

In January 2018, The Canadian Dental Association added a new group of codes 04220–04229 to its uniform list of codes and services. The codes are based upon 15 min units of time and have the following nomenclature:

> ***"Non-ionizing scanning procedure to detect caries and capable of quantifying, monitoring and recording changes in enamel, dentin, and cementum, which includes diagnosis and interpretation of findings."***

Before using the ADA or Canadian Dental Association code for caries examination, the dentist should validate with the manufacturer of the particular device that they meet all the criteria for these codes.

24.3 Concluding Remarks

Detection of dental caries, a common procedure in clinical practice, needs new technologies to help detect lesions throughout the entire caries process and monitor the changes in lesion volume and size over time. Detecting these changes involves exposing the tooth to various portions of the electromagnetic spectrum and understanding the interaction of a particular portion of the spectrum with the tooth structure. Diagnosis of caries involves using the results obtained from these systems and integrating this with our knowledge of the dental history and associated risk factors of our patients. Dental caries is a very common oral disease and the placement of restorations does not treat the disease only the outcome from the disease process. New caries detection devices can help the dental team to detect, measure, and monitor lesions over time as they respond to various interventions within the oral environment. When the lesions are large, these devices will allow the dental team to determine what is the appropriate restorative therapy.

Conflicts of Interest and Sources of Funding Statement S. Abrams is President and Co-Founder and shareholder of Quantum Dental Technologies, the manufacturer of The Canary System, and did not receive any compensation for this publication.

References

1. Hall A, Girkin JM. A review of potential new diagnostic modalities for caries lesions. J Dent Res. 2004;83(Spec No C):C89–94.
2. Rechmann P, Rechmann BM, Featherstone JD. Caries detection using light-based diagnostic tools. Compend Contin Educ Dent. 2012;33(88):582–93.
3. Lussi A, Imwinkelried S, Pitts N, Longbottom C, Reich E. Performance and reproducibility of a laser fluorescence system for detection of occlusal caries in vitro. Caries Res. 1999;33(4):261–6.

4. Lussi A, Hibst R, Paulus R. DIAGNOdent: an optical method for caries detection. J Dent Res. 2004;83(Spec No C):C80–3.
5. Verdonschot EH, van der Veen MH. Lasers in dentistry 2. Diagnosis of dental caries with lasers. Ned Tijdschr Tandheelkd. 2002;109(4):122–6.
6. König K, Flemming G, Hibst R. Laser-induced autofluorescence spectroscopy of dental caries. Cell Mol Biol (Noisy-le-Grand). 1998;44(8):1293–300.
7. Alwas-Danowska HM, Plasschaert AJ, Suliborski S, Verdonschot EH. Reliability and validity issues of laser fluorescence measurements in occlusal caries diagnosis. J Dent. 2002;30(4):129–34.
8. Ástvaldsdóttir Á, Tranæus S, Karlsson L, Peter Holbrook W. DIAGNOdent measurements of cultures of selected oral bacteria and demineralized enamel. Acta Odontol Scand. 2010;68(3):148–53.
9. Rodrigues JA, Neuhaus KW, Hug I, et al. In vitro detection of secondary caries associated with composite restorations on approximal surfaces using laser fluorescence. Oper Dent. 2010;35(5):564–71.
10. Neuhaus KW, Rodrigues JA, Seemann R, Lussi A. Detection of proximal secondary caries at cervical class II-amalgam restoration margins in vitro. J Dent. 2012;40(6):493–9.
11. Sichani AV, Javadinejad S, Ghafari R. Diagnostic value of DIAGNOdent in detecting caries under composite restorations of primary molars. Dent Res J (Isfahan). 2016;13(4):327–32.
12. Simon JC, Lucas S, Lee R, et al. Near-infrared imaging of secondary caries lesions around composite restorations at wavelengths from 1300–1700-nm. Dent Mater. 2016;32(4):587–95.
13. Abrams TE, Abrams SH, Sivagurunathan KS, Silvertown JD, Hellen WMP, Elman GI, Amaechi BT. In vitro detection of caries around amalgam restorations using four different modalities. Open Dent J. 2017;11:609–20.
14. Spagnulo G. Detecting caries around amalgam restorations with the canary system. Ont Dent. 2016;93(4):24–5.
15. Abrams T, Abrams S, Sivagurunathan K, et al. Detection of caries around resin-modified glass ionomer and compomer restorations using four different modalities in vitro. Dent J (Basel). 2018;6(3).
16. Rodrigues JA, Diniz MB, Hug I, Cordeiro RC, Lussi A. Relationship between DIAGNOdent values and sealant penetration depth on occlusal fissures. Clin Oral Investig. 2010;14(6):707–11.
17. Sonmez IS, Oba AA, Erkmen M, Ekici S. Effects of different fissure sealant applications on laser fluorescence measurements. Int J Paediatr Dent. 2011;21(1):29–34.
18. Markowitz K, Rosenfeld D, Peikes D, Guzy G, Rosivack G. Effect of pit and fissure sealants on caries detection by a fluorescent camera system. J Dent. 2013;41(7):590–9.
19. Silvertown JD, Wong BP, Abrams SH, et al. Comparison of the canary system and DIAGNOdent for the in vitro detection of caries under opaque dental sealants. J Investig Clin Dent. 2017;8(4).
20. Mansour S, Ajdaharian J, Nabelsi T, Chan G, Wilder-Smith P. Comparison of caries diagnostic modalities: a clinical study in 40 subjects. Lasers Surg Med. 2016;48(10):924–8.
21. Dorfman JM. Cement composition effects on enamel demineralization adjacent to orthodontic brackets: an in vitro study using the canary system [Dissertation/thesis]. ProQuest Dissertations & Theses Global. (1951782587): Temple University; 2017.
22. Almosa NA, Lundgren T, Aldrees AM, Birkhed D, Kjellberg H. Diagnosing the severity of buccal caries lesions in governmental and private orthodontic patients at debonding, using the ICDAS-II and the DIAGNOdent Pen. Angle Orthod. 2014;84(3):430–6.
23. Glor K. Measuring caries quantitatively: a product review and case report. Dentistry IQ. 2017;
24. Abrams SH. Integrating 21st century caries detection into your clinical practice. Oral Hygiene. 2012:21–25.
25. Maragliano-Muniz P. Review: the canary system by Quantum Dental Technologies. Dentistry IQ. 2015.
26. Abrams SH. Remineralization of carious lesions—it really does work. Oral Health. 2012;102(12):38–44.

Part VI

Conclusion

Concluding Remarks

25

Christopher Longbottom and Andrea Ferreira Zandona

Since the late 1960s, with the increasing exposure of populations to fluorides, especially to fluoride toothpastes, not only has the prevalence, incidence, and distribution of dental caries lesions changed, but the very presentation of these lesions has altered the classical detection methods of visual and radiographic examinations/assessments.

Fluorides have impacted the recognized oscillating demineralizing–remineralizing flux of the caries process—influencing the general speed of progression of lesions, as well as the resistance of the enamel "surface layer". These changes affect the surface integrity of the enamel, the breakdown at micro and macro cavitation levels. The detection of dental caries lesions at the earliest stage is not a simple task and requires careful and systematic visual techniques to identify the subtle changes in the various characteristics of tooth tissues brought about by the pathological processes involved. Each tooth site being examined should be clean, dry (dried), and well illuminated for optimum visual assessment. Even then, meticulous visual examination is not sufficient to totally accurately detect all lesions and assess the stage of each lesion at different sites. There are well-recognized patterns of susceptibility of tooth sites to caries attack in both the permanent and primary dentitions. Knowledge of these site-risk patterns will aid the clinician in the optimization of the visual assessment method of caries lesion detection. These factors helped to stimulate a search for methods of improving the detection of lesions at the earliest stages, in order to facilitate the more effective use of secondary preventive measures

C. Longbottom
King's College London Dental Institute, London, UK
e-mail: Christopher.longbottom@kcl.ac.uk

A. Ferreira Zandona (✉)
Department of Comprehensive Care, Tufts University School of Dental Medicine, Boston, MA, USA
e-mail: azandona@email.unc.edu

© Springer Nature Switzerland AG 2019

A. Ferreira Zandona, C. Longbottom (eds.), *Detection and Assessment of Dental Caries*, https://doi.org/10.1007/978-3-030-16967-1_25

designed to arrest and possibly reverse the progression of lesions prior to their cavitation.

Numerous technologies, including optical, radiographic, electrical, and ultrasound-based methods, have been and continue to be developed with the objective of detecting lesions at various stages of the caries process. The visual assessment method remains the universal fundamental method of assessment and can be supplemented relatively simply and inexpensively to improve the validity of lesion detection. Additional, more sophisticated technologies, with their inherent expense, are available for increasing the yield of detection information for the different tooth sites, e.g., approximal sites, root caries, and CARS lesions, and these have been covered in preceding chapters.

However, detection of lesions is an initial stage in the diagnostic process—characterization of lesions in order to aid in the assessment of the ***activity status*** of lesions is a crucial stage in the diagnostic process which seeks to identify the most appropriate treatment option for a detected lesion. This characterization can involve directly assessing the physical, chemical, optical (including visual and radiographic), or electrical properties of the surface of lesions and/or comparing time-domain measurements/assessments of lesion depth and/or volume. Accurate time-domain comparative measurements require meticulous repositioning methods which can be challenging in a general practice environment.

The fundamental process involved in the progression of a caries lesion is the loss of the constituent chemicals of the mineral from the enamel (or dentin)—this produces the *effects of* increasing the porosity within the enamel (or dentin) and increasing the ionic concentration of the constituent elements of hydroxyapatite within the expanded fluid-filled enamel (or dentin) nano- and micropores, in addition to disturbing the original structural integrity of the micromorphology of the tooth surface. Thus, the successful development and commercialization of technologies which can be used to assess these effects will ultimately provide clinicians with tools to help identify which particular detected lesions are actively progressing, requiring some form of specific preventive intervention to arrest and/or reverse this progression, and which lesions require only monitoring at specified appropriate intervals. Such technologies are being developed and are at different stages of development and commercialization. Once these tools reach general practitioners, their application should transform the diagnosis of caries lesions and the therapies and treatments applied to such lesions.

Caries lesion detection is the first step in a three-stage process, which involves lesion characterization and subsequent assimilation of the lesion information, together with patient data, to lead the clinician to a diagnosis relating to the activity (or otherwise) of any detected lesion(s) and his/her subsequent treatment decision with regard to each lesion.

The parallel development of advances in remineralization technologies should integrate with the diagnostic developments to transform how dentistry is practiced.

Part VII

Appendices

26 Definitions

Marie-Charlotte D. N. J. M. Huysmans

In the past decades, there has been a gradual change in the way caries diagnosis has been viewed and the chosen emphasis on certain aspects of the disease and the diagnostic process. Caries has been recognized as a condition or disease already for centuries, and by the end of the nineteenth century, the role of bacterial acid production from sugary foods had taken hold. GV Black, who has often been portrayed as only considering operative treatment of dental caries, already mentioned preventing and arresting the early disease by tooth brushing [1]. However, in everyday dental practice, in a world where caries was ubiquitous and usually rapidly progressive, the emphasis lay on detecting the advanced lesions and treating them operatively.

More recently, in most developed countries, caries progression has been significantly reduced by the use of fluoride in tooth paste and sometimes in water, and more attention is given to the early stages of lesion progression, to prevention and management, and to the aspect of disease activity. Not only has this led to the development of many new diagnostic techniques, aimed at early detection and assessment, as this book clearly shows, it has also subtly changed the language we use in describing the disease and its key features. Because these changes are so slow and subtle, there is a real danger of miscommunication and it was deemed useful to clarify the definition of some terms used in this book.

26.1 Dental Caries

Dental caries is the localized destruction of susceptible dental hard tissue by acidic by-products from bacterial fermentation of dietary carbohydrates [2].

This the most concise definition found in recent years. Some definitions have tended to emphasize the occurrences in the dental biofilm; however, this might

M.-C. D. N. J. M. Huysmans (✉)
Department of Dentistry, Radboud University Medical Center, Nijmegen, Netherlands
e-mail: Marie-Charlotte.Huysmans@radboudumc.nl

© Springer Nature Switzerland AG 2019

A. Ferreira Zandona, C. Longbottom (eds.), *Detection and Assessment of Dental Caries*, https://doi.org/10.1007/978-3-030-16967-1_26

suggest that even in the absence of a tooth, the disease may be present. The proteolytic component of the disease, when caries occurs in dentin, is only very rarely mentioned in definitions, which focus on the demineralization component.

26.2 Caries Lesion

A caries lesion is the localized destruction of tooth tissue, which is the clinical manifestation or sign of the disease caries [3].

There is little discussion on the definition of a caries lesion. The term "carious lesion" is also used.

26.3 Caries Process

The caries process is the progressive involvement of dental tissue by the disease, for instance the progression of a lesion from the tooth surface towards the pulp.

For a while, around the turn of the century, there was a trend to define the caries process as the disbalance in the dental biofilm driving the disease ("These metabolic events are the carious process," [4]*). Often, the term was also used to the lesion progression through tooth tissue. More recently, the "disbalance" approach has been abandoned again* [5].

26.4 Caries Lesion Detection

Lesion detection is the process of recognizing changes in the tooth tissue, which are consistent with being caused by the disease caries.

The first step in caries lesion detection is differentiating the observed signs from other conditions (differential diagnosis). As there are few conditions with similar signs, little attention is usually given to this stage of the diagnostic process. There is no consensus of the level of damage required for a lesion to be considered a lesion. Traditionally, in epidemiology only "advanced" lesions with obvious cavitation or dentinal involvement were detected and scored. Over time, earlier lesions were detected with visual methods, and in future highly sensitive additional detection methods may be able to detect even earlier changes. It may be questioned in how far such "sub-clinical" lesion detection is relevant in individual patient care.

26.5 Caries Lesion Assessment

Caries lesions assessment involves assessment of the characteristics of a caries lesion once it has been detected.

Caries lesion assessment may involve characteristics such a color, surface gloss and integrity, and extension, but also physical aspects such as electrical conductance, fluorescence, and attenuation of X-rays. It may be used to draw conclusions about lesion stage (depth) and activity, and for monitoring progression.

26.6 Caries Diagnosis

The human professional summation of all relevant information regarding history, signs and symptoms, test results, and probable causes to arrive at an identification of the **past or present** occurrence of the disease caries.

In a previous definition [3], *the summation was restricted to signs and symptoms, which appears to ignore other sources of information increasingly used in clinical practice, such as patient background information, presence of risk factors, and results of diagnostic tests* [6]. *Including both past and present disease is logical when one realizes that caries lesion formation is reversible only to a relatively small degree and most disease experience remains visible in arrested lesions ("scars") and fillings or missing teeth. However, this also implies that past and present disease must be explicitly separated in order for diagnosis to sensibly inform treatment decisions.*

26.7 Caries Activity

When there is **present** occurrence of the disease caries, this may be called caries activity.

Caries activity is usually a general term, describing the condition of a single patient, but it is sometimes used as a specific term, describing a localized condition (e.g., caries activity in partially erupted third molars). It implies the progression of existing caries lesions and the development of new lesions.

26.8 Active Caries Lesion

An active caries lesion is a caries lesion currently (recently) progressing.

In a previous definition [3], *it was pointed out that the word activity might also imply regression. However, as was pointed out by the authors, this is not a clinically helpful interpretation, and only progression should be linked with activity.*

References

1. Black GV. A work on operative dentistry. Vol. 1. The pathology of the hard tissues of the teeth. 4th ed. Chicago: Medicodental Publishing Company; 1920.
2. Selwitz RH, Ismail AI, Pitts NB. Dental caries. Lancet. 2007;369:51–9.
3. Longbottom CL, Huysmans MC, Pitts NB, Fontana M. Glossary of key terms. Monogr Oral Sci. 2009;21:209–16.
4. Fejerskov O, Kidd E. Dental caries. 2nd ed. Hoboken: Wiley Blackwell; 2008.
5. Fejerskov O, Nyvad B, Kidd E. Dental caries. 3rd ed. Hoboken: Wiley Blackwell; 2015.
6. Schulte AG, Pitts NB, Huysmans MCDNJM, et al. European core curriculum in cariology for undergraduate dental students. Eur J Dent Educ. 2011;15:9–17.

Correction to: Integrating Caries Detection Devices into Clinical Practice

Stephen Abrams

Correction to:
Chapter 24 in: A. Ferreira Zandona, C. Longbottom (eds.), ***Detection and Assessment of Dental Caries,*** **https://doi.org/10.1007/978-3-030-16967-1_24**

Dr. Stephen Abrams name had been misspelt in the original version of the book in chapter 24. The author's name has now been corrected.

The updated online version of this chapter can be found at
https://doi.org/10.1007/978-3-030-16967-1_24

© Springer Nature Switzerland AG 2019

A. Ferreira Zandona, C. Longbottom (eds.), *Detection and Assessment of Dental Caries*, https://doi.org/10.1007/978-3-030-16967-1_27

MIX
Papier aus verantwortungsvollen Quellen
Paper from responsible sources
FSC® C105338

If you have any concerns about our products,
you can contact us on
ProductSafety@springernature.com

In case Publisher is established outside the EU,
the EU authorized representative is:
Springer Nature Customer Service Center GmbH
Europaplatz 3, 69115 Heidelberg, Germany

Printed by Libri Plureos GmbH
in Hamburg, Germany